CRICE 18

D1568022

Design
of
Microcomputer-Based
Medical Instrumentation

Based onWILLIS J. TOMPKINS AND JOHN G. WEBSTER, EDS.

Department of Electrical and Computer Engineering
University of Wisconsin—Madison

PRENTICE-HALL, INC., Englewood Cliffs, New Jersey 07632

Library of Congress Cataloging in Publication Data

Main entry under title:

Design of microcomputer-based medical instrumentation.

Includes bibliographies and index.
1. Medical electronics. 2. Microcomputers.
3. Medical instruments and apparatus—Design and
construction. I. Tompkins, Willis J. II. Webster,
John G. [DNLM: 1. Computers. 2. Biomedical
engineering—Instrumentation. 3. Equipment and
supplies. W26 D457]
R856.D47 1981   681'.761   80-16513
ISBN 0-13-201244-8

Editorial/production supervision and interior design
    by Barbara A. Cassel
Manufacturing buyer: Anthony Caruso

© 1981 by Prentice-Hall, Inc., Englewood Cliffs, N.J.   07632

All rights reserved. No part of this book
may be reproduced in any form or
by any means without permission in writing
from the publisher.

Printed in the United States of America
10 9 8 7 6 5 4 3 2

PRENTICE-HALL INTERNATIONAL, INC., *London*
PRENTICE-HALL OF AUSTRALIA PTY. LIMITED, *Sydney*
PRENTICE-HALL OF CANADA, LTD., *Toronto*
PRENTICE-HALL OF INDIA PRIVATE LIMITED, *New Delhi*
PRENTICE-HALL OF JAPAN, INC., *Tokyo*
PRENTICE-HALL OF SOUTHEAST ASIA PTE. LTD., *Singapore*
WHITEHALL BOOKS LIMITED, *Wellington, New Zealand*

List of Contributors

John P. Abenstein
Hossein Baharestani
Kevin R. Colwell
Dhruba P. Das
Gregory S. Furno
Peter D. Gadsby
Yongmin Kim
Steven L. Paugh
Alan V. Sahakian
Gary V. Sprenger
Nitish V. Thakor
Handayani Tjandrasa
James D. Woodburn
Michael J. Yanikowski

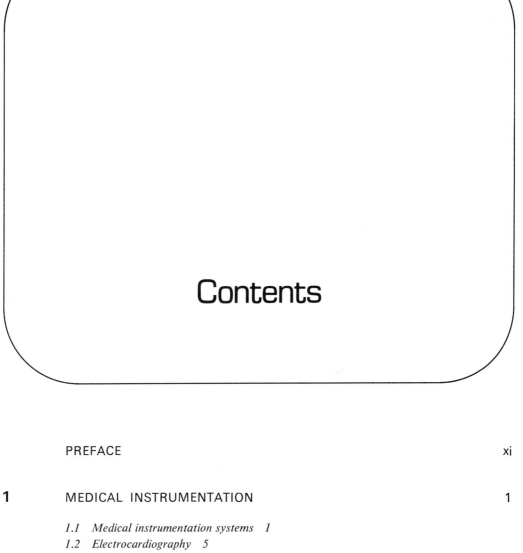

Contents

6   A DETAILED DESIGN EXAMPLE—
        AMBULATORY ECG MONITORING   390

APPENDICES   465

INDEX   481

Preface

This book will help you design medical instruments using microcomputers. It helps you assess each medical instrument and decide whether or not it is a likely candidate for a microcomputer. It helps you select the proper microcomputer for the job and the necessary size of memory and peripherals. It explains the costs and time required to implement both hardware and software. It points out both the costs and advantages of using various software development packages. Finally, it guides you step by step through the detailed design of a complex medical instrument involving analog circuits and microcomputer hardware and software.

Chapter 1 provides you with the characteristics of all medical instrument signals. For the electrocardiogram it shows you correct use of analog elements, such as electrodes and amplifiers, and digital elements, such as cardiotachometers and nonfade displays. It informs you of pulmonary instrumentation, including likely candidates for microcomputers, such as apnea monitors and ventilators. It provides a wealth of material on anesthesia machines, surgical monitoring, EEG monitoring, blood pressure, and clinical chemistry. Microcomputers are used in all these areas.

Once you have the analog signal, you must convert it into digital form. Chapter 2 shows you how to translate the analog signal to the proper range for an analog-to-digital converter. It explains the various number systems used by converters and how the different types work. It shows you the advantages and disadvantages of all types and how to interface them with a microcomputer. It explains how digital-to-analog converters work and optimal filters for smoothing their output transitions. It details the many errors that may appear so that you can evaluate manufacturers' specifications.

Chapter 3 shows you how to design filters. In addition to describing various analog filter types, it provides design equations and tables for the design of a second-order active filter. The section on digital filters is made to order for microcomputer users. You give it your filter requirements and it takes you step by step through both recursive and nonrecursive filter designs. The chapter also shows you the algorithms to use and applications for differentiation, integration, and the fast Fourier transform.

Chapter 4 shows you both the hardware and software required to implement a microcomputer system. It explains microcomputer architecture and tristate logic. You will learn how to use interrupts and stacks. It shows you how to select memory types and input/output hardware, such as modems, keyboards, and displays. It provides software instruction, so you can use branching, addressing, and look-up tables. It helps you decide which software development tools are right for you, such as editors, assemblers, compilers, simulators, and emulators. It details the low-power COSMAC because it is the only 8-bit microcomputer capable of long-term battery operation in portable instruments. It also details the Z80, because it is the most powerful single-chip 8-bit microcomputer and can perform very intelligent, sophisticated signal processing. A working knowledge of these microcomputers will let you generalize readily to other microcomputers.

Chapter 5 provides you with multiple ideas for using microcomputers in medical instrumentation. It details about 100 examples where commercial manufacturers have incorporated microcomputers to boost sales or researchers have demonstrated feasibility. It shows you how microcomputers are used in intensive-care monitoring, pulmonary instruments, anesthesia machines, clinical chemistry laboratories, sensory testing, prosthetics, and a host of other areas. In addition to suggesting many potential applications, it provides a wealth of detail to guide you in your specific design.

Chapter 6 is the kind of nuts-and-bolts information that few books provide. We take a problem statement and follow it step by step through all the phases of the project. You learn the reasons for trade-offs between analog and digital circuitry and how to design both the analog circuits and microcomputer hardware. It shows you the algorithm development, flowcharts, and software implementation. You learn how to perform system tests and evaluate complete systems.

We assume that you know electronics, including operational amplifier design, digital logic design, and assembly language programming. In addition to electrical engineering students, the book should have wide appeal to practicing design engineers in the medical equipment industry and users of medical equipment in hospitals and medical research centers.

We would welcome your suggestions for corrections and improvement of subsequent printings and editions.

WILLIS J. TOMPKINS / JOHN G. WEBSTER
*Department of Electrical
and Computer Engineering
University of Wisconsin
Madison, Wisconsin 53706*

Design
of
Microcomputer-Based
Medical Instrumentation

1

Medical
Instrumentation

This chapter presents an overview of the field of medical instrumentation. We describe the way medical instrumentation operates without using microcomputers. Even when medical instrumentation uses microcomputers, it still requires much of the hardware described in this chapter. Thus, when in Chapter 5 we describe applications of microcomputers in medical instrumentation, we will build upon the information contained in this chapter. However, rather than attempt to cover all medical instrumentation, we emphasize only those measurements that have already demonstrated applications for microcomputers.

1.1 MEDICAL INSTRUMENTATION SYSTEMS*

Imagine what would happen if we were to go into any hospital today and ask a physician working there to refrain from using any medical instrumentation for 24 hours. He or she would be very upset because a physician's diagnostic and thera-

*Section 1.1 written by Gregory S. Furno.

1

peutic skills depend heavily on the numbers obtained by use of medical instrumentation. Before we describe these instrumentation systems and their design, let us look at the practice of medicine and see just how medicine has become dependent upon instrumentation.

Medical procedures

We can define medicine as a multistep procedure performed on an individual by a physician, group of physicians, or an institution, and repeated until the symptoms disappear. These steps are:

1. Collection of data.
2. Analysis of data.
3. Decision making.
4. Treatment instituted from the decision.
5. Repeat.

Medical instruments play a role in several of these steps. They regularly collect signals, analyze signals, display information, and control treatment.

In the data-collection step, the physician gathers all the facts he or she can about the patient. Some items are easily obtained, such as the patient's appearance and skin color, the sound of a cough, or the location of wounds. But for many other types of data, the physician's senses are not sensitive enough, or precise enough, to collect all the data. For instance, he or she cannot detect some types of broken bones or high blood pressure. The physician may note that a patient is breathing heavily but will need to know more about what is happening within the patient than his or her senses can discern.

Medical instrumentation assists the physician by extending the senses, and in some cases providing new senses that he or she can use to collect data. Simple instruments such as the stethoscope, or complex radiographic imaging devices such as the CAT (computerized axial tomography) scanner, extend the physician's senses (sound and sight, in this case). Instruments that detect biopotentials (potentials on and in the body) and sensors that respond to acidity (pH), the partial pressure of CO_2 (PCO_2), and the partial pressure of O_2 (PO_2) give the physician additional senses and supply him or her with a more complete picture of the patient's condition. Figure 1.1 lists typical values of physiological signals.

Medical instrumentation also helps the physician to analyze the data. For example, in Chapter 6 we describe a device that can analyze a person's heartbeat continually and determine when life-threatening abnormalities occur. The advent of the microcomputer has greatly increased the ability of medical instruments to analyze data. These microcomputer-based instruments can perform sophisticated mathematical operations on the data they collect. In addition, with medical instruments collecting and processing ever-increasing amounts of data, it becomes important that this information be presented to medical personnel in a clear and

Primary signal ranges and characteristics

Cardiovascular System

Blood pressure, direct method

Frequency range: dc to 200 Hz; dc to 60 Hz usually adequate. Pressure range, arterial: 40 to 300 mm Hg; venous: 0 to 15 mm Hg.

Blood pressure, indirect method, intermittent systolic and diastolic

Auscultatory criterion (Korotkoff sounds): 30 to 150 Hz usually adequate. Palpatory criterion: 0.1 to 60 Hz. Both require additional signal showing occluding pressure.

Pulse waves, indirect method, peripheral artery

Frequency range: 0.1 to 60 Hz usually adequate. Pulse trace similar to blood pressure, direct, but without baseline zero.

Plethysmogram (volume measurements)

Frequency range: dc to 30 Hz.

Heart rate

Average rate, human: 45 to 200 beats/min; lab animal: 50 to 600 beats/min.

Oximetry

Frequency range: 0 to 60 Hz; 0 to 5 Hz usually adequate.

Cardiac output

Frequency range: 0 to 60 Hz; 0 to 5 Hz usually adequate.

Electrocardiogram

Frequency range: 0.05 to 100 Hz. Signal range: 10 μV (fetal) to 5 mV (adult).

Respiratory system

Flow rate (pneumotachogram)

Frequency components to 40 Hz. Normal flow range: 250 to 500 ml/s; maximum 8 liters/s.

Breathing rate calculated from record (with approximate relative respiratory volume)

Average rate: human, 12 to 40 breaths/min; lab animal, 8 to 60 breaths/min.

Tidal volume (measured per breath or integrated to provide volume/min)

Typical volume, adult human: 600 ml/breath; 6 to 8 liters/min.

CO_2, N_2O or halothane concentration in respired air

Normal range, CO_2: 0 to 10%; end-tidal CO_2, human: 4 to 6%. N_2O: 0 to 100%. Halothane: 0 to 3%.

Dissolved gases and pH

Partial pressure of dissolved O_2, in vivo or in vitro

Frequency range: dc to 1 Hz usually adequate. Normal measurement range: 0 to 800 mm Hg PO_2. Hyperbaric PO_2 range: 800 to 3000 mm Hg.

pH, in vitro

Signal range: 0 to ± 700 mV covers pH range.

Partial pressure of dissolved CO_2, in vitro

Normal signal range: 0 to ± 150 mV covers range from 1 to 1000 mm Hg PCO_2.

FIGURE 1.1   Biophysical signals and ranges. (From Strong, P. 1970. Biophysical measurements. Beaverton, OR: Tektronix.)

Bioelectric potentials

Electroencephalogram	Frequency range: dc to 100 Hz; major diagnostic components lie in range 0.5 to 60 Hz. Normal signal range: 15 to 100 μV.
Electromyogram (primary signal)	Frequency range: 10 to 200 Hz. Pulse duration: 0.6 to 20 ms.
Electromyogram (averaged)	An average of the primary signal, after full-wave rectification.
Electroretinogram	Frequency range: dc to 20 Hz adequate. Normal signal strength: $\frac{1}{2}$ μV to 1 mV.
Electrocardiogram	(See listing under cardiovascular system.)
Electronystagmogram	Direct: frequency range, 0 to 20 Hz. Typical signal strength, 100 μV/10° eye movement. Derivative or velocity: frequency range, 0 to 20 Hz. Signal derived from direct reading.

Physical quantities

Body temperature	20 to 45°C.

FIGURE 1.1   (continued)

direct manner so that they may more effectively carry out their decision-making responsibilities.

In the treatment of patients, many mechanical and electrical devices perform treatments that would be difficult or impossible to do by the unaided physician. Direct control of treatment by machine is not widespread, as most treatment cannot yet be effectively carried out by machine. However, simple tasks, such as drug administration, can be handled.

Generalized medical instrumentation system

Figure 1.2 shows the block diagram of a generalized medical instrument. The stimulator block contains a stimulus source. If the instrument is going to examine a particular response, then repeated stimuli can initiate responses so that they can be studied. The next block contains the sensors. Here specialized transducers convert the various signals of Fig. 1.1 into electrical signals. These signals travel to the processor block, where operations such as amplification, filtering, interference rejection, and computer analysis are carried out. Information then flows to the display, recorder, and distribution blocks, where the information is displayed to others in the immediate vicinity of the device, recorded on paper or other media for permanent storage, and distributed to other, more distant areas. Finally, the processed data flows to a controller block to control patient treatment or patient stimulus.

In the chapters that follow, we fill in the details of this diagram by describing some of the present techniques and future directions of implementation.

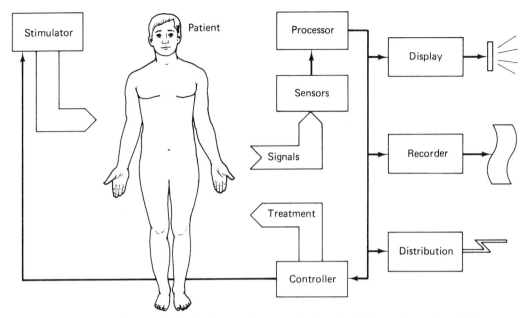

FIGURE 1.2 Block diagram of a generalized medical instrument or system. Note how the controller block completes a feedback loop.

1.2 ELECTROCARDIOGRAPHY*

The leading cause of death in the United States is heart disease. Physicians and researchers spend considerable effort in treating and trying to further understand this disease. One of their main tools is the electrocardiograph (ECG) machine. What makes this machine so valuable is that it can examine many conditions of the heart noninvasively—without exposing the heart. For example, the ECG machine displays data for determining heart rate—its speed in beats per minute—and any rhythm irregularities. It is useful for locating within the heart many defects in the heart's electrical conduction system. These can lead to inefficient pumping action and, in some cases, a complete failure in pumping. The ECG machine is also useful for detecting defects or damage in the heart muscle itself, which may have come about by an earlier disease process or temporary failure. We consider how the ECG machine accomplishes these functions by describing how the various blocks of Fig. 1.2 are filled to form the ECG machine.

The ECG machine obtains an electrical signal that is related to cardiac electrical activity. Electric currents accompany heart-muscle contraction and produce a time-varying electric field, which results in potentials on the skin. Electrodes on the skin pick up these potentials for input to the ECG machine.

---

*Section 1.2 written by Gregory S. Furno.

Electrodes

In order to detect body potentials, electrodes must convert the ionic currents in the body into electron current in the wire. Electrodes perform this conversion, and two electrodes are required to make a measurement. Electrodes may be classified as either polarizable or nonpolarizable. Common electrodes have characteristics that lie between these extremes. Polarizable electrodes behave as capacitors. A constant current flowing through them causes a continually increasing voltage (offset potential) across them. Nonpolarizable electrodes behave as resistors. A constant current flowing through them causes a constant offset potential across them.

Figure 1.3 shows two of the most common electrode types, one of which consists of a german silver metal plate and the other a snap fastener plated with silver and coated with a film of silver chloride. The metal plate closely approximates a polarizable electrode, while the silver–silver chloride (Ag–AgCl) electrode closely

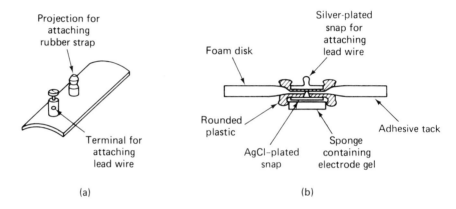

(a)   (b)

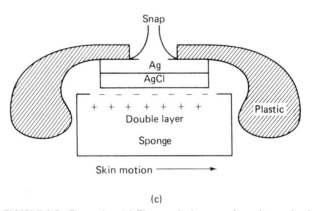

(c)

FIGURE 1.3 Electrodes. (a) The metal-plate type for wrists and ankles is attached with rubber straps. (b) The foam-disk type sticks on the chest. (c) Recessing the electrode double layer away from motion prevents changes in offset potential.

approximates a nonpolarizable electrode. Figure 1.3(c) shows a double layer of electric charge that exists between the metal and the electrolyte. The AgCl layer permits easy flow of current so that the offset potential is constant. Recessing this double layer prevents skin motion from disturbing it and changing the offset potential. On the other hand, skin motion can disturb the double layer of electric charge of metal plate electrodes, and the resultant large offset potential changes can mask the signal of interest. By stabilizing the double layer of electric charge, recessed Ag–AgCl electrodes provide more artifact-free signals than other electrodes.

Lead systems

Frontal plane leads. The heart generates an electric field which can be represented mathematically by a vector having a magnitude and a direction. Cardiologists (physicians who specialize in studying the heart and related systems) have standardized ways of looking at this electric field. Their approach is based upon the work of Dutch physiologist Willem Einthoven, who first developed the vector concept shown in Fig. 1.4(a). By measuring the potential differences between the arms and between each arm and the left leg (i.e., along each side of Einthoven's triangle), we can reconstruct the magnitude and direction of the cardiac vector. Measurements of potentials along the sides of Einthoven's triangle are known as standard frontal plane (bipolar limb lead) measurements and are commonly referred to as leads I, II, and III. Another set of measurements, known as augmented unipolar limb leads, measures the potential at one corner of Einthoven's triangle with respect to the average of the other two, as shown in Fig. 1.4(b).

Unipolar chest leads. The leads we have described so far have only examined the cardiac vector in the frontal plane—the plane that is parallel to the earth when lying down. Six more measurements, called the V-lead measurements, examine the cardiac vector in the transverse plane—the plane that is parallel to the earth when standing up. Figure 1.4(c) shows the electrode positions for the V leads. A Wilson central terminal is formed by averaging the RA, LA, and LL leads together. A trained cardiologist normally takes a standard 12-lead ECG, consisting of the six V leads, the three augmented unipolar limb leads (aVR, aVF, aVL), and the three bipolar limb leads (I, II, III), carefully scrutinizing them for any abnormalities.

The electrocardiogram. Figure 1.5 shows a typical ECG signal. The heart's electrical conduction system initiates an electrical impulse in the SA (sinoatrial) node located in the atria (top of the heart). A wave of excitation spreads over the atria, producing the P wave and causing the atria to contract. The excitation is then delayed in the AV (atrioventricular) node, resulting in the P-R interval. Then the wave of excitation spreads over the ventricles, causing them to contract and produce the QRS complex. Recovery of ventricular depolarization produces the T wave.

When the SA node triggers all these events, we state that sinus rhythm exists.

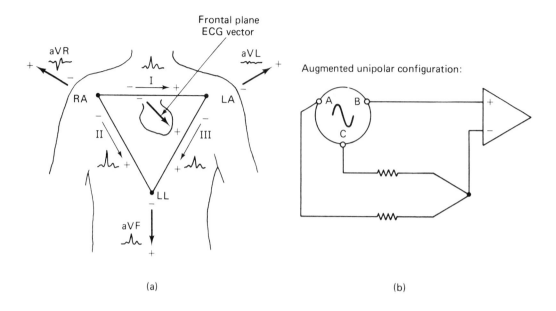

Augmented unipolar configuration:

(a)

(b)

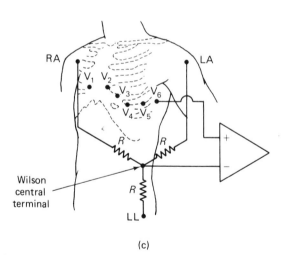

Wilson central terminal

(c)

FIGURE 1.4 The standard 12-lead electrocardiogram. (a) The Einthoven triangle and associated lead measurements. Electrodes placed on the LL (left leg), LA (left arm), and RA (right arm) are considered to pick up signals at the corners of the Einthoven triangle. (b) An equivalent circuit of augmented unipolar limb leads. Potential input to amplifier equals $B - (A + C)/2 = (2B - A - C)/2$. (c) V lead positions. Each of the six V leads is measured with respect to the Wilson central terminal. [Frames (a) and (b) from Strong, P. 1970. Biophysical measurements. Beaverton, OR : Tektronix. Frame (c) from Ganong, W. F. 1979. Review of medical physiology, 9th ed. Los Altos, CA : Lange. Used with permission.]

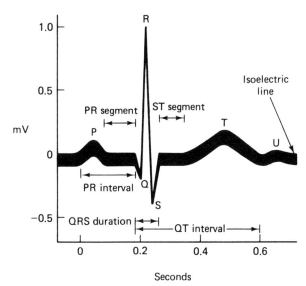

FIGURE 1.5 Typical lead II ECG wave. (From Ganong, W. F. 1979. Review of medical physiology, 9th ed. Los Altos, CA: Lange. Used with permission.)

Abnormal rhythms are called arrhythmias and their detection is important for diagnosis and treatment. Sinus bradycardia is an abnormally slow rhythm, while sinus tachycardia is an abnormally fast rhythm.

Disease may cause failures in the cardiac conduction system. First-degree heart block exists when the P-R interval is lengthened because of delay in the AV node. Second-degree (partial) heart block exists when some impulses do not conduct to the ventricles and the ventricles beat at their own slower rhythm (intermittent dissociation). Third-degree (complete) heart block exists when no impulses conduct to the ventricles. Heart block may be treated by pacemakers, as described in Section 5.13.

Even when the conduction system is intact, the heart may generate aberrant beats. The atria may contract early—an atrial premature beat (APB), or the ventricles may contract early—a premature ventricular contraction (PVC). In an intensive-care ward, a cardiac monitor may monitor one lead (usually lead II) and count the number of PVCs per minute to provide information required for drug therapy.

Vectorcardiogram. Another method of analyzing the electrical activity of the heart involves obtaining three ECGs along axes at right angles to each other and displaying any two of them as a time-varying vector display on an oscilloscope. This display is called a vectorcardiogram (VCG). Figure 1.6(a) shows a spatial VCG and its projections in the standard planes. Figure 1.6(b) shows a common VCG electrode arrangement known as the Frank lead system. The resistor weighting network compensates for electrical inhomogeneities of the human torso. A few

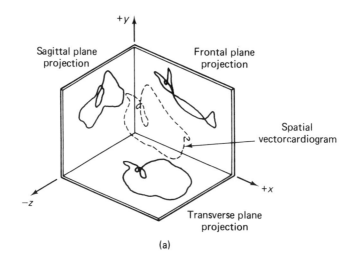

(a)

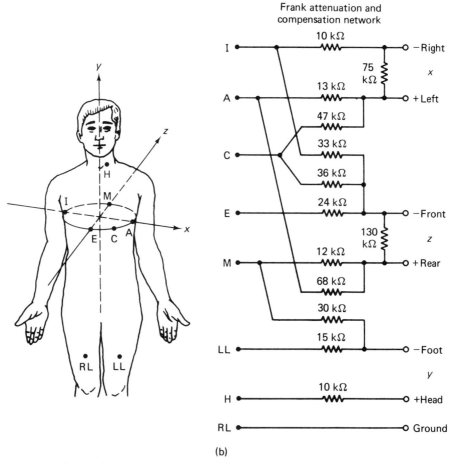

(b)

FIGURE 1.6 The vectorcardiogram. (a) The three-dimensional path traced by the tip of the cardiac vector is projected onto three two-dimensional planes. (b) In the Frank lead system, signals are passed through unity-gain buffers to prevent loading by the resistor weighting network. (From Strong, P. 1970. Biophysical measurements. Beaverton, OR : Tektronix.)

cardiologists now use the VCG in preference to the 12-lead ECG in their examination of the heart's electrical activity.

Basic signal processing

We next discuss the processing block in Fig. 1.2. One of the simplest forms of processing is amplification of the ECG signal from its low values on the body's surface to levels large enough for use by output devices and the rest of the instrument's circuitry.

Figure 1.7 shows the block diagram of a typical ECG machine. The electrodes are applied to the patient. Protection circuits block the high voltages induced by electrosurgical and defibrillation units. The lead selector switching system selects one of the 12 standard leads to be amplified.

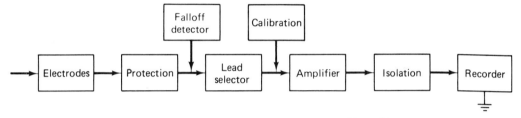

FIGURE 1.7 Block diagram of an ECG machine.

Amplifier.   The differential amplifier amplifies the ECG and rejects electrical interference. This stage may also contain a variable gain control. The amplifier also performs the important processing task of bandpass filtering. Occasionally, electrodes have a dc offset potential that reaches a level of 300 mV. This potential can drive the amplifier circuits into saturation. By filtering out frequencies below about 0.05 Hz, this dc offset potential is eliminated, thus allowing high gain of the ac ECG. Also, by filtering out frequencies above about 100 Hz, the amplifier bandwidth is limited just enough to adequately pass the ECG. This procedure results in the optimal signal-to-noise ratio, because artifact (undesired signal) such as electrical voltages generated by muscle activity (which fall in a range from 30 to 2000 Hz) is greatly reduced. If the low corner frequency is too high, or if the high corner frequency is too low, frequency distortion occurs. Figure 1.8 shows some of the effects of frequency distortion.

Figure 1.9 shows a simple ECG amplifier. The first two operational amplifiers on the left form a high-input-impedance differential amplifier. The 100-kΩ potentiometer compensates for resistor imbalances. Switch S_1 discharges the 1-μF capacitor in the high-pass filter network in case of overload. The 10-nF capacitor forms a low-pass filter in conjunction with the 150-kΩ resistor, thus limiting the high-frequency response.

Amplifiers for use with patients require the isolation circuits shown in Fig. 1.7. These circuits isolate the patient and amplifier from recorder ground and prevent currents larger than 10 μA from flowing through the patient.

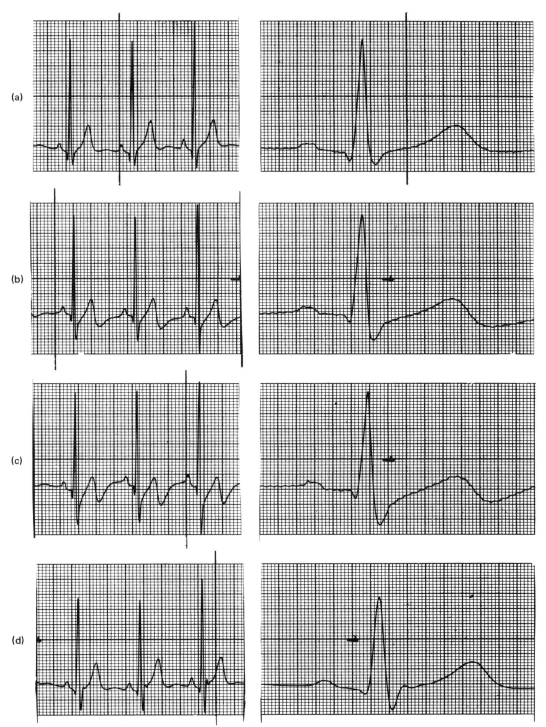

FIGURE 1.8 Effects of frequency distortion on the ECG. Left traces are at a chart speed of 25 mm/s. Right traces are at 125 mm/s. (a) Diagnostic bandwidth of 0.05 to 100 Hz. (b) Monitoring bandwidth of 0.5 to 50 Hz. This signal has both high- and low-frequency distortion. (c) Bandwidth of 1 to 100 Hz shows the effect of low-frequency distortion alone. (d) Bandwidth of 0.05 to 25 Hz shows effect of high-frequency distortion alone.

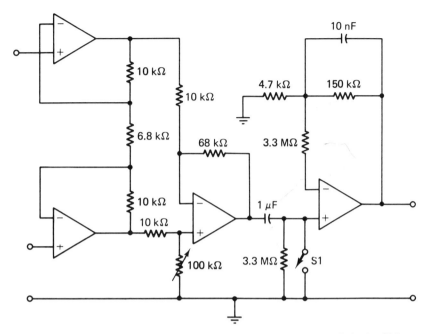

FIGURE 1.9 This ECG amplifier has a gain in the dc-coupled stages limited to 26.8 to prevent electrode offset voltages from saturating the op amps. The ac-coupled stage limits the frequency response and provides a gain of 33.

Interference. An important task of processing is the reduction of interference. One major source of interference is the electrical power system. Power lines in the walls, floor, and ceiling, as well as cords connecting various pieces of equipment in the room, all radiate electric and magnetic fields. Electric fields are present when voltage is on the lines, even though no current is flowing through the lines. Capacitance between the power lines and the equipment couples current into the patient, wires, and machine. Rejection of this electric field interference depends mostly upon the ability of the differential amplifier in the ECG machine to reject common-mode voltages—voltages that appear at both inputs to the amplifier at the same time. Only those voltages not in common—the differential voltages—are amplified. Figures 1.10 and 1.11 show how electric field interference can be reduced by using amplifiers having both high input impedance and good common-mode rejection, and by minimizing the input electrode impedances, and the differences between them. Interference can also be reduced by shielding the leads and grounding the shields at the electrocardiograph.

Another source of interference from power lines is magnetic induction. Current in magnetic fields induces voltage into the loop formed by the patient leads. The induced voltage is proportional to the field strength and the coil area. Reducing this interference requires that the field strength be reduced by moving the equipment and leads (difficult to do in practice) or that the coil area be reduced by twisting the lead wires together all along their length. Figure 1.12(a) shows 60-Hz interference.

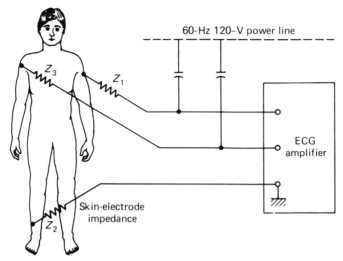

FIGURE 1.10 The power line capacitively couples 60-Hz current into the patient leads. This current flows through the skin-electrode impedances on the way to ground. The resulting voltage drops cause 60-Hz interference.

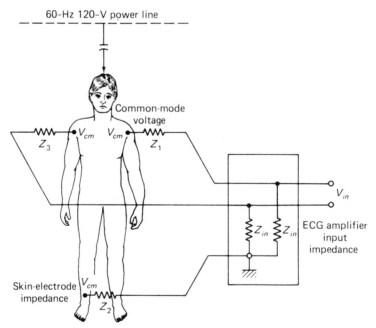

FIGURE 1.11 The power line capacitively couples 60-Hz current into the body. This current flows through the skin-electrode impedance on the way to ground. The resulting common-mode voltage on the body converts to differential voltage when the patient-lead skin-electrode impedances are unequal.

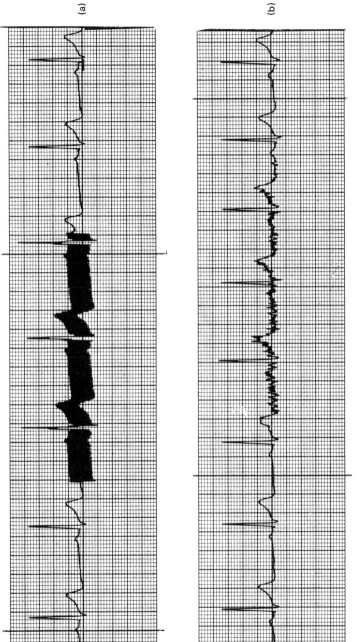

(a)

(b)

FIGURE 1.12 Effects of noise on the ECG. (a) 60-Hz power-line interference. (b) Electro-myographic artifact.

Electromagnetic interference radiating from nearby high-power radio, television, radar, electrosurgical, or diathermy equipment may appear on the ECG record because the nonlinear semiconductor junctions (and occasionally the electrode–electrolyte interface) rectify and demodulate the RF power. Frequently, this interference can be eliminated by shunting the amplifier input terminals with small capacitances which act as short circuits to the RF power and as open circuits to the ECG signals.

Artifact. Electromyographic signals (potentials developed by contracting muscles) can also cause artifact in the ECG recording [see Fig. 1.12(b)]. This muscle artifact can be reduced by either minimizing muscle contractions or by attaching the ECG electrodes farther up the limbs. Another source of artifact is the motion of electrodes with respect to the skin. This occurs because movement disturbs the double layer of electric charge, thus shifting the electrode offset potential. Use of nonpolarizable electrodes such as the Ag–AgCl electrodes and construction of recessed electrodes to physically stabilize the electrode–electrolyte interface minimizes this artifact. Ac coupling of the amplifier circuits also helps to reduce the resulting drift by filtering out the relatively slowly changing offset potential. Movement of the skin causes a similar movement artifact because the potential difference between the inside and outside of the skin varies with skin movement. This artifact can be minimized by mild skin abrasion.

Overload. If a large transient voltage change occurs at the amplifier input, due either to motion artifact or a defibrillator spike, the capacitors in the high-pass filter circuit charge up, causing the amplifiers to temporarily overload and saturate. Figure 1.13 shows that this causes lost data during a critical procedure. ECG machines now have manual or automatic reset circuits that quickly discharge the capacitors in the filter circuit and return the trace.

Advanced signal processing

We first discuss some techniques of heart-rate detection. When the physician or nurse determines a heart rate, they usually count the number of heartbeats in a fixed unit of time and convert this to beats per minute. For a physician, the easiest way to obtain the number of heartbeats is to count the pressure pulses at the radial artery at the wrist. For an ECG machine, the easiest way to obtain the number of heartbeats is to count some identifying feature of the ECG. The most distinguishing feature of the ECG is the sharp spike known as the QRS complex. Spectrum analysis of the ECG signal reveals that most of the frequencies contained in the QRS complex lie near 16 Hz. Therefore, we can use a bandpass filter to emphasize the QRS complexes. It rejects the P and T waves, the high-frequency interference, and low-frequency artifacts and baseline drift.

Averaging cardiotachometer. Figure 1.14 shows a block diagram of an averaging cardiotachometer. The averaging cardiotachometer determines average heart rate

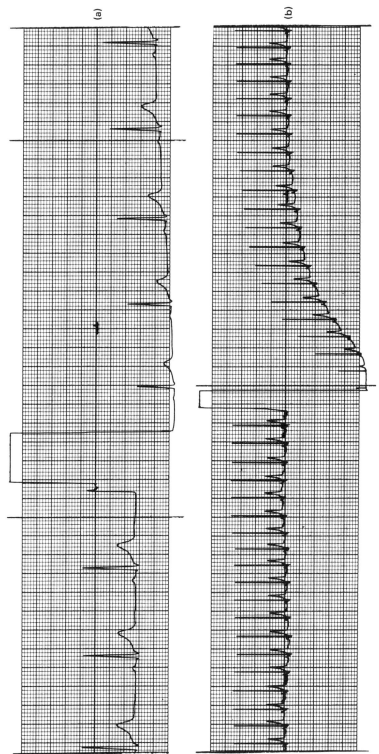

FIGURE 1.13 Effect of a voltage transient on an ECG recorded on an electrocardiograph in which the transient causes the amplifier to saturate. A finite period of time is required for the charge to bleed off enough to bring the ECG back into the amplifier's active region of operation. (a) Initiation and recovery of a transient at a chart speed of 25 mm/s. (b) Similar transient at a chart speed of 125 mm/s shows first-order recovery of the system.

by counting the number of QRS complexes over a known period of time. The threshold circuit triggers the pulse generator when the filter output exceeds a preset threshold level. The pulse generator produces a pulse of constant width, which is longer than the QRS complex to allow only one pulse per complex. The resulting string of pulses is fed to a low-pass filter which determines their average amplitude. The time constant of the filter should be several beats long, typically 5 to 15 s in duration, to reduce output ripple. The output is then fed to an indicator, usually a meter, which is calibrated in beats per minute. Most cardiotachometers have alarm circuits which warn the personnel when heart rates have gone above or below preset levels.

Beat-to-beat cardiotachometer. In Fig. 1.15, a beat-to-beat cardiotachometer finds the time between each beat and inverts it, presenting it as an instantaneous heart rate. Changes in the time interval appear as changes in instantaneous heart rate. The bandpass filter and threshold circuit operate as in Fig. 1.14. The threshold circuit triggers the first monostable, and the falling edge of this pulse triggers the second monostable. These two pulses control the circuitry in such a way that register 2 contains the number of 1-kHz clock pulses that have occurred between QRS complexes. Thus register 2 contains the number of clock pulses, or time per beat, which is inversely proportional to the number of beats per unit time, which is the heart rate. The current output of the variable resistance digital-to-analog converter is $i = V/R$, which is inversely proportional to R. Thus i is proportional to the heart rate and can be sent to a meter for display. Alarms may be activated by this circuit with either an analog comparator, which looks at the converted output, or with a digital comparator, which compares the digital output of register 2 with a preset digital level. Beat-to-beat cardiotachometers respond much more rapidly to changes in heart rates than do averaging cardiotachometers. This is because they compute a new value for every beat. For simple trend monitoring, however, an averaging cardiotachometer would be adequate.

Electrode falloff detector. Another useful processing technique is a method for detecting poor electrode connections. Figure 1.16 shows the block diagram for such an electrode falloff detector. The 50-kHz current source passes several milliamperes through the electrodes, and if the connection is poor or nonexistent, the voltage across the generator rises. The current is not dangerous because at 50 kHz the sensitivity of the body's excitable tissue is low. Any 50-kHz voltage rise due to increasing electrode resistance triggers the threshold detector and sets off an alarm.

Fetal ECG. A special processing technique is used to obtain the fetal ECG. Figure 1.17 shows the problem. The maternal ECG is superimposed upon the fetal ECG and it is difficult to separate them. The system diagrammed in Fig. 1.18 first detects the maternal ECG and then uses it to blank out the maternal ECG from the combination of maternal and fetal ECGs. Special circuits can then compensate for any fetal beats that may have been blanked out with the maternal signal and reconstruct the fetal heart rate.

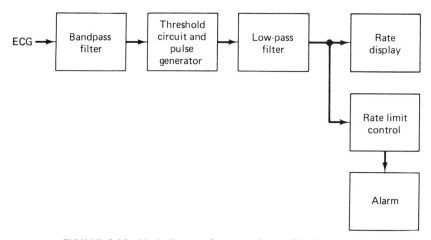

FIGURE 1.14 Block diagram of an averaging cardiotachometer.

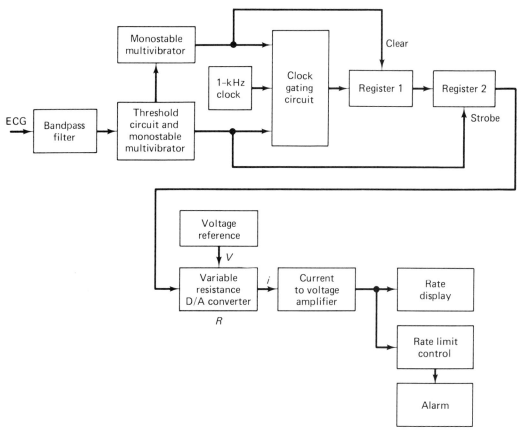

FIGURE 1.15 Block diagram of a beat-to-beat instantaneous cardiotachometer.

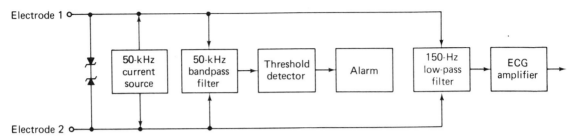

FIGURE 1.16 Block diagram of a system for use with cardiac monitors to detect either increased electrode impedance or electrode falloff.

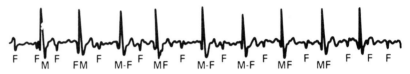

Abdominal leads

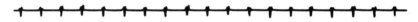

Fetal ECG (direct)

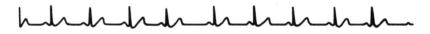

Maternal ECG

FIGURE 1.17 Typical fetal ECG as obtained from the maternal abdomen. F represents fetal QRS complexes and M represents maternal QRS complexes. The maternal ECG and the fetal ECG (recorded directly from the fetus) are included for comparison. (From Roux, J. F., Neuman, M. R., and Goodlin, R. C. 1975. Monitoring of intrapartum phenomena. Crit. Rev. Bioeng. 2:119–158. © The Chemical Rubber Co. Used by permission of C.R.C. Press, Inc.)

Memory loops. A final processing technique utilizes memory loops to continuously record about 15 s of ECG waveform so that should an alarm occur, it automatically switches on a chart recorder and gets a record of the events leading up to that particular pattern. Memory loops are usually implemented either as a continuous tape loop 15 s long or as a digital shift register where the analog signal has been changed to digital form and then clocked in and shifted around in a 15-s loop. Reconversion to analog form allows the delayed signal to be recorded. While tape systems have the advantage of simplicity of design, they have been largely replaced by digital systems, which do not have the maintenance problems associated with tape.

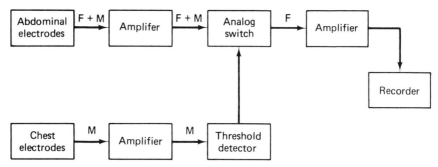

FIGURE 1.18 Block diagram of a scheme for isolating the fetal ECG from the abdominal signal that contains both fetal and maternal ECGs. (From Roux, J. F., Neuman, M. R., and Goodlin, R. C. 1975. Monitoring of intrapartum phenomena. Crit. Rev. Bioeng. 2:119–158. © The Chemical Rubber Co. Used by permission of C.R.C. Press, Inc.)

Display and recording. The display and recorder blocks of Fig. 1.2 allow the ECG machine to communicate with the doctors and nurses who use it. One of the most common recording devices is the pen recorder. This device uses a moving pen to deposit ink on a graduated chart passing under it. Some recorders have a heated stylus contacting heat-sensitive paper, leaving a trace. Other recorders have introduced pressurized-ink systems to avoid the problems of clogged pens, which made previous ink recorders undesirable. Pen recorders offer a permanent record of the ECG but require paper and ink supplies.

Another common display device is the CRT or cathode-ray-tube display. In this display, the ECG waveform can be traced out on a screen that has a long-persistence phosphor which presents recent information brightly, and past information dimly. This screen takes a relatively long time to fade (most traces fade before the next one comes along). In this fading or "bouncing ball" display, it is difficult to examine complete physiological waveforms.

Nonfade displays use electronic memory (Section 4.3), together with other digital and analog circuitry, to hold and display complete waveforms. Commonly, the nonfade display mimics the familiar pen recorder, with the waveform parading from right to left on the display screen. The most recent value of the measured signal thus appears at the right edge of the screen as the oldest is pushed off the left. To make the display seem continuous, even though the phosphor image fades, the screen is refreshed (reswept) frequently (typically 256 or 512 times each second). The electrical signal to be displayed is sampled at this same rate, and each sample is converted to a digital value by an A/D converter (Section 2.3). Thus every sweep of the display screen is accompanied by the arrival of a new value to be stored in the memory (updating it) and the exit of the oldest value. Typically, the entire display consists of 1024 values from one side of the screen to the other.

A recirculating shift register is the most common memory device used in the nonfade display. Using the shift register, a typical screen-sweep and memory-update cycle would be as follows. With the shift register initially circulated to the most recent value, a sweep (right to left) of the screen begins. Every 1024th of the way across the screen the shift register is advanced to the next older value and this value is used to drive the CRT vertical deflection plates. When the 1024th value (the oldest) has been displayed at the left side of the screen, the beam of the CRT is blanked (gated off) and retraced (returned to the right edge of the screen). While the CRT is being retraced, the incoming value from the A/D converter is written into the shift register at the present location (where the oldest value was), and the display sequence begins again, starting with this (the most recent) value at the right side of the screen.

Since each time the screen is swept, every stored value of the waveform becomes one cycle older (one more position farther from the most recent value in the register), the waveform appears to move slowly across the screen. With a 10-cm-wide screen, a 1024-value shift register, and sample rates of 256 and 512 values/s, the apparent display speeds are 25 mm/s and 50 mm/s, respectively.

It is also possible to "freeze" the display at any time by not performing the update during the retrace period, but rather advancing the shift register one position (to the value with which the sweep began). In this way each sweep is identical to the previous, and the display waveform can be viewed indefinitely.

Other display devices emit audible tones or "beeps," either as an indication of the presence of heartbeats or as alarms. Audible devices must be chosen with care so that patients do not become concerned and personnel are not confused by the different sounds.

Indicator lights provide a convenient means for displaying status information, especially if they are clearly marked and uncluttered.

Distribution. Distribution of ECG data can take place over telephone lines, radio airways, and specially dedicated data lines. For a complete discussion of telephone transmission, see Section 5.2.

Transmission of data by wireless link is called radiotelemetry and can link a patient with a majority of the signal-processing components. A miniature radio transmitter relays patient data to a receiver over the area of a hospital ward, thus giving the patient full mobility.

Specially dedicated digital data lines can connect, for example, separate bedside monitors with a central monitor or nurses' station in an intensive-care unit. The data lines can be serial, where data flows sequentially over one pair of lines, or the lines can be parallel, where many data bits can flow at once over several parallel paths. The approach taken depends upon the amount of data to be transferred and how quickly it must be moved.

1.3 PULMONARY INSTRUMENTATION*

This section describes the instruments that measure pulmonary flow, volume, gas concentration, and respiratory rate. It also describes ventilators, which are used for respiratory therapy.

---

*Section 1.3 written by Dhruba P. Das.

Physiological considerations

Figure 1.19 shows the gross anatomy of the human respiratory system. This system supplies body cells with O_2 and removes CO_2. The inspired air passes through the nasal passages, pharynx, trachea, and bronchi to the alveoli, where gas exchange takes place to the pulmonary blood circulation by simple diffusion processes.

A first-order model of the normal respiratory system during quiet breathing is adequate for most pulmonary function tests. The inhaled air passes through the pneumatic resistance of the airways to fill the compliant lung and thoracic wall.

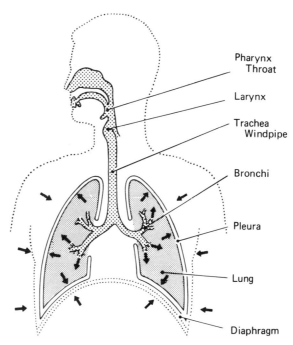

Pharynx
Throat

Larynx

Trachea
Windpipe

Bronchi

Pleura

Lung

Diaphragm

FIGURE 1.19 Anatomy of the respiratory system. (From Jacobson, B., and Webster, J. G. Medicine and clinical engineering. © 1977, p. 56. Reprinted by permission of Prentice-Hall, Inc.)

Pressure measurement

Dynamic pressure can be conveniently measured with a diaphragm-type pressure transducer. Figure 1.20 shows the diaphragm, which must be large and thin to measure pressures of a few centimeters of water. One side of the transducer is exposed to the respiratory gas and the other side is usually at atmospheric pressure, except when pressure difference between two sites is to be measured. The diaphragm movement is usually sensed by strain gages or a differential transformer. The high-frequency limit for such a system is typically about 40 Hz (Cotes, 1975).

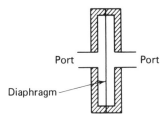

FIGURE 1.20   Diaphragm-type pressure transducer.

Flowmeters

A respiratory gas flowmeter must be able to measure bidirectional flow rate and must have a low back pressure so that it does not influence the breathing pattern. It must be able to withstand the high pressure applied to the airway during assisted ventilation. The calibration must not change with changes in gas composition and temperature. The dead space must be small so that the patient does not rebreathe his or her expired air. Most commonly used respiratory gas flowmeters can be classified into the following three categories.

Thermal dissipation devices.   A heated wire or a heated thermistor is placed in the airstream. Increased air velocity results in convective cooling that lowers the sensor temperature. The resistance change due to this cooling is related to the air flow. Since the cooling effect is the same irrespective of air direction, this device can only measure unidirectional flow.

Differential pressure devices.   When flow passes through a flow resistance, there is a pressure drop. Flowmeters based on this relationship are flow-resistance, venturi, and pitot-tube flowmeters. Flow-resistance flowmeters are more linear and accurate than the others and are the most extensively used. To ensure laminar flow, the resistance elements consist of a wire mesh or a bundle of capillary tubes or channels placed axially (Fleisch head) in the flow path as shown in Fig. 1.21. The Fleisch pneumotachometer is the most accurate clinical flowmeter (Blumenfeld et al., 1975). The pressure tap in both types of flow-resistive elements can be obtained from single holes through the wall on each side of the screen or bundle. For flow-resistance pneumotachometers the flow $Q = \Delta P/R$, where ΔP is the pressure drop across the resistance and we assume that the flow resistance R is constant. However, this resistance may increase significantly, owing to the accumulation of condensed expired water vapor. To overcome this problem it is a common practice to heat the pneumotachometer element. However, this heating also affects the gas temperature and therefore the transducer calibration. Pneumotachometers also rely on a consistent, if not uniform flow pattern in the near region on each side of the resistance element. The placement of the pressure ports and the configuration of the tubing are critical in determining the pressure drop/flow relationship and are important when we use alternating and/or high-frequency flow patterns.

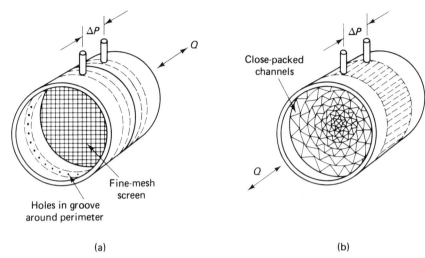

(a)   (b)

FIGURE 1.21   Pneumotachometer flow-resistance elements. (a) Screen. (b) Capillary tubes or channels. (From *Medical Instrumentation: Application and Design* by John G. Webster et al. Copyright © 1968 by Houghton Mifflin Company. Reprinted by permission of the publisher.)

Ultrasonic flowmeters.   Acoustic waves traveling with the air velocity arrive at a receiving piezoelectric transducer sooner than those traveling against the air velocity. Ultrasonic flowmeters built using this transit-time principle alternately transmit upstream and downstream between two transducers. The transducers may be mounted axially (Blumenfeld et al., 1975) or at an angle to the flow (Statham Instruments SP5004). Problems with baseline drift have limited the application of these devices.

Volume measurements

The changes in lung volumes during various phases of breathing and the absolute volume of the lung shown in Fig. 1.22 are widely used indices for determining the mechanical status of the ventilatory system. The lungs have a total capacity (TLC) of about 5 to 6 liters. After quiet expiration, the lung volume is the functional residual capacity (FRC). After forced expiration the lung volume is the residual volume (RV). The amount of air that enters the lungs or moves out of the lungs at rest in each respiratory cycle is called tidal volume (TV) and is about 0.5 liter. Other volumes shown are the inspiratory capacity (IC), the expiratory reserve volume (ERV), and the vital capacity (VC).

The most widely used method for measuring slow volume changes of the lung is by physical integration of the volume-flow rate and the device used is called a spirometer (static spirometry). Figure 1.23 shows that the bell is like a bucket upside down in water which is statically counterbalanced by a weight. The soda-lime cannister and the one-way rubber valves prevent CO_2 buildup during rebreath-

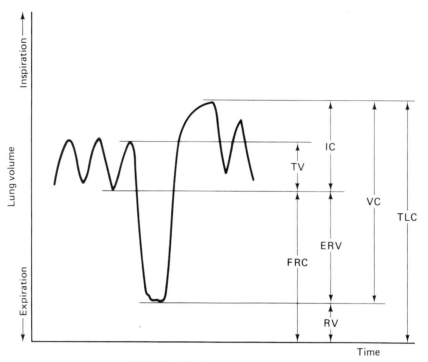

FIGURE 1.22 Static lung volumes.

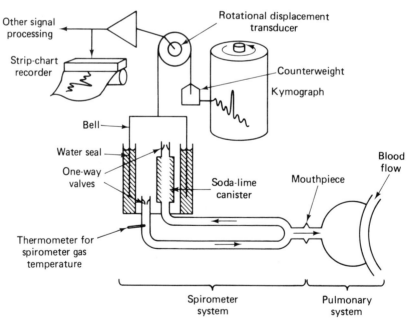

FIGURE 1.23 Water-sealed spirometer set up to measure slow lung-volume changes. (From *Medical Instrumentation: Application and Design* by John G. Webster et al. Copyright © 1968 by Houghton Mifflin Company. Reprinted by permission of the publisher.)

ing. As the volume changes due to respiration, the volume inside the sealed chamber changes. The bell displacement is linearly proportional to these volume changes. The volume changes are most frequently recorded directly on the kymograph. However, for further signal processing and display, often a single-turn rotational displacement potentiometer is coupled to the pulley. The electrical output can be recorded on a strip-chart (pen) recorder.

Pneumographs

Instruments that simply detect respiratory activity are known as pneumographs, and the resulting recordings are known as pneumograms. Various pneumograph techniques use such parameters as change in the size of thoracic wall, temperature of inspired and expired gas, thoracic impedance, and EMG from intercostal muscles.

The thermistor pneumograph requires placement of a thermistor inside the nostrils, which irritates the subject. Strain gage and resistance pneumographs detect changes in the length of a band that encircles the chest. However, body movements cause dimensional changes unrelated to lung volume changes and cause artifacts. The impedance pneumograph is the most extensively used, not only because artifacts are lower but also because the electrodes that are used to monitor breathing may also be used to simultaneously record the electrocardiogram.

Impedance pneumograph. Although the impedance method is not suitable for accurate measurement of lung volume changes, it is useful for relative changes.

During inspiration, the lung tissue fills with air and becomes more resistive. Also, the chest wall becomes thinner and its circumference increases. Both effects increase the impedance. The transducers are simple, appropriately placed electrodes.

If we passed low-frequency current through the thorax, the patient might perceive it as a shock. Moderate currents (0.3 mA) above 20 kHz are not perceived or dangerous, so currents with frequencies of 50 to 100 kHz are normally used. The demodulator can be a simple diode detector, but a carrier system that uses a phase-sensitive demodulator is a better choice because of its ability to reject noise and 60-Hz interference. The output of the demodulator yields both the undesired baseline impedance Z and the much smaller desired change ΔZ. Capacitive coupling with a time constant long enough to pass respiratory frequencies (0.1 to 2 Hz) is used to extract ΔZ.

Monitoring apnea. Apnea means respiratory arrest. An apneic episode is a cessation of airflow at the nose and mouth enduring for at least 10 s (Guilleminault et al., 1976). Apnea frequently occurs in prematurely born infants (Stein and Shannon, 1975) and is prominent in the age group 9 to 16 weeks (Steinschneider, 1976). Recent studies suggest that apnea is associated with the sudden infant death syndrome (SIDS). Any method that can reliably detect respiratory activity may be used for monitoring apnea. The impedance pneumograph is widely used because of its reliability and relative versatility. However, false signals may occur because of electrode or chest-wall movement.

Figure 1.24 shows a block diagram of an apnea monitor for a laboratory animal. Each breath resets the integrator. If no breath occurs for a duration set by the variable direct voltage, the alarm sounds.

Figure 1.25 shows the block diagram of a circuit that can be used to monitor

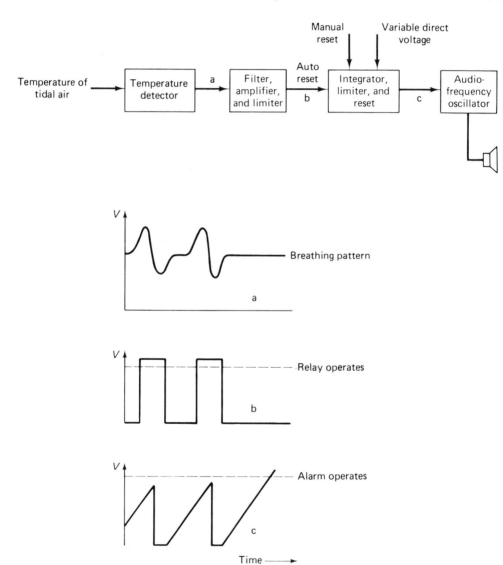

FIGURE 1.24 Apnea monitor for a laboratory animal. A thermistor is placed in a tracheal cannula and connected in a resistance bridge.

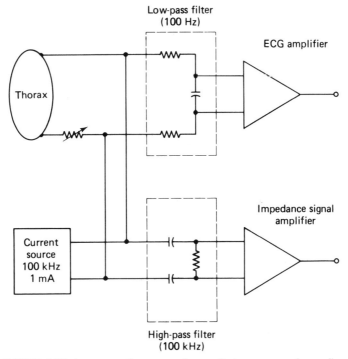

FIGURE 1.25 Instrumentation system for monitoring apnea and recording ECG simultaneously.

apnea and the ECG simultaneously using the same pair of electrodes. The filters separate the ECG and the impedance signals.

Figure 1.26 shows recordings obtained from an impedance pneumograph. The small-amplitude waveforms during apneic episodes are due to the heart pulsations; thus heart rate can be determined from the respiratory signal during the episode.

Sleep-associated apnea results in a rapid drop of heart rate, so a cardiac monitor is also useful in detecting sleep apnea.

Measurements of concentrations of respiratory gases

Measuring techniques for respiratory gases can be classified into chemical and physical methods. Chemical methods are highly accurate, so they are often used for calibrating new devices. Physical methods are faster and easier to use and have largely replaced chemical methods.

Discrete gas or blood samples are analyzed in the blood-gas laboratory. Continuous analysis requires close proximity of the instrument and the patient. Since the sensor portion of most instruments is large, it cannot be placed directly at the site of the gas to be analyzed. Therefore, the gas must be transported from the

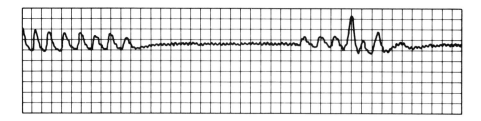

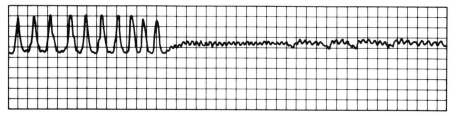

FIGURE 1.26 Top : Recording of two apneic episodes (left, 17 s ; right, 8 s) in an
infant. Heart rate, 135 beats/min. Bottom : Recording of an apneic episode in the
same infant. Apnea lasted 29 s and heart rate fell from 135 to 80 beats/min. (From
Stein, I. M., et al. The pediatric pneumogram : a new method for detecting and quantitating apnea in infants. Pediatrics 55 : 599–603. © American Academy of Pediatrics,
1975. Used with permission.)

respiratory system via a catheter or tube to the sensor site in the instrument, which
introduces problems such as time delay and condensation of water vapor inside
the catheter (Primiano, 1978).

Mass spectroscopy.   Figure 1.27 shows the essential parts of a mass spectrometer.
It separates the various components of a gas mixture into a spectrum of individual
components using the differences in mass-to-charge ratios. The outputs are proportional to the quantities of each component. The components must be separated
by at least one mass unit. The instrument has difficulty separating CO and N_2 or
N_2O and CO_2 since they have about the same molecular weight. A typical response
time is about 0.1 s. A portion of the gas drawn by the sampling inlet pump diffuses
into the ionization chamber, where it is ionized by collisions with the electron
stream effusing from a heated cathode to an anode. Then the positive ions are
focused into a beam and accelerated into a dispersing magnetic or electric field,
which separates the beam into component beams. The quantity of each component
is measured either by focusing each component beam on a single collector at a
different point in time or by using multiple collectors. The different ion currents are
proportional to the partial pressures, and the results can be expressed in molar
fractions by incorporating a summing circuit.

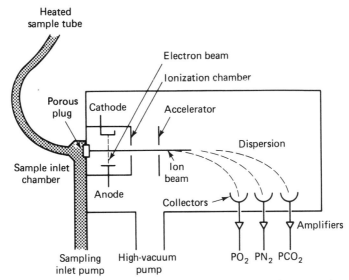

FIGURE 1.27 The medical mass spectrometer separates respiratory gas into its components and measures the partial pressure of each component.

Gas chromatography. A mixture of the component gas of interest and a carrier gas pass through a heated column at a constant volume flow. Figure 1.28 shows that those gases that are least soluble in the column material travel through the column fastest; hence the gases are separated. Since thermal conductivity changes with the composition of the mixture, each gas may be detected with a sensor that measures thermal conductivity.

The system can analyze only discrete samples and requires several minutes for one analysis. Thus this method cannot be used for continuous or on-line measurements. However, it requires a small sample (< 1 ml), gives a very accurate analysis, and is much less expensive than the mass spectrometer.

Absorption spectroscopy. The principle of this method is that various chemical species, whether in gaseous form or in liquid form, absorb power from certain regions of the electromagnetic spectrum. The power transmitted through the substance is given by Beer's law (see Section 1.7) and is related to the molar fraction of the substance. Figure 1.29 is a schematic of the instrument. The two infrared beams are modulated by the chopper at the rate of 60 Hz and pass through both the reference cell and the test cell. The test cell is filled with the test gas. The reference cell has a gas mixture which does not include the test gas. Both cells are irradiated by the infrared beams. Depending upon the absorption in the cells, the detector chambers heat differentially and the expanding gas bends the diaphragm toward the side of lower pressure, changing the capacitance of the capacitor microphone. The output after the linearizer is proportional to the concentration of the test gas.

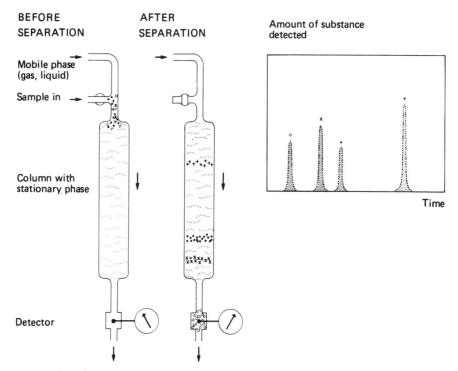

FIGURE 1.28 Principle of gas chromatography. The components in the sample separate as a result of their different migration velocities when the mobile phase passes over the stationary phase. (From Jacobson, B., and Webster, J. G. Medicine and clinical engineering. © 1977, p. 311. Reprinted by permission of Prentice-Hall, Inc.)

Emission spectroscopy.   Figure 1.30 shows a schematic of the emission spectrometer. A sample of a gas mixture is drawn into the ionization chamber through the needle valve. The gas is ionized and emits light of intensities proportional to the concentrations. The band of light emitted lies between 310 and 480 nm for respiratory gases. Reflecting surfaces direct the light through a set of filters that absorb the unwanted spectra of the light. The filtered beam falls on a phototube and the resulting current is nonlinearly related to the concentration of the gas of interest. After passing through a linearizer circuit an output proportional to the gas concentration is obtained.

This method is usually used for N_2. A commercially available device may have a transport and rise-time delay of the order of 40 ms to a step change in N_2 concentration. The steady-state error of the device in the range 0 to 8% is as low as 0.5% rms (Primiano, 1978).

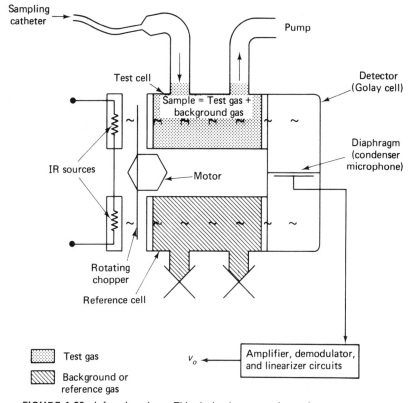

Sampling catheter

Pump

Test cell

Detector (Golay cell)

Sample = Test gas + background gas

Diaphragm (condenser microphone)

IR sources

Motor

Rotating chopper

Reference cell

Test gas

Background or reference gas

v_o

Amplifier, demodulator, and linearizer circuits

FIGURE 1.29 Infrared analyzer. This device is commonly used to measure gas-phase concentrations of gases such as CO_2, CO, N_2O, and halothane. (From *Medical Instrumentation: Application and Design* by John G. Webster et al. Copyright © 1968 by Houghton Mifflin Company. Reprinted by permission of the publisher.)

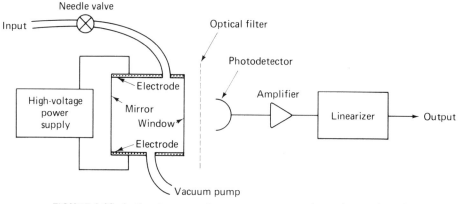

Needle valve

Input

Optical filter

Photodetector

High-voltage power supply

Electrode

Mirror

Window

Electrode

Amplifier

Linearizer

Output

Vacuum pump

FIGURE 1.30 In the nitrogen analyzer, a vacuum pump draws the gas through a chamber. A high voltage ionizes the gas. An optical filter selects the ultraviolet given off by nitrogen and passes it to the photodetector.

Therapeutic devices

Respiratory therapy depends to a large extent on automatic ventilators for the lungs. These devices are typically used for either short-term assist or prolonged artificial ventilation. They can be broadly classified into two groups: the controller and the assister. A controller completely determines the respiratory ventilation for the patient as programmed. In the case of the assister the patient has control over the device to augment his or her own ventilation. Figure 1.31 shows a positive-pressure ventilator. Air is forced into the lungs by increasing the pressure in the trachea and then the lungs recoil as the positive pressure is removed. Ventilators can be time-cycled, volume-cycled, or pressure-cycled (Hill and Dolan, 1976). There are available more than 80 different commercial ventilators (Mushin et al., 1969).

Engelman and Cook (1977) have described a digital electronic control system with a 1 % accuracy for rate, ratio, and sigh functions, and with a 5 % accuracy for volume controls (normal and sigh). It provides independence of rate, ratio, and

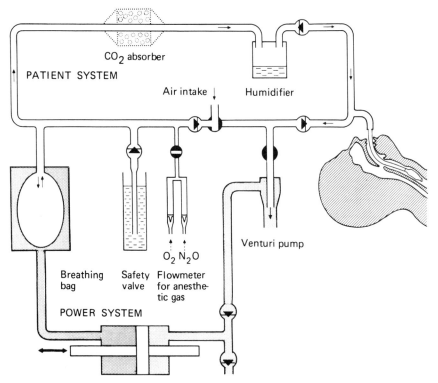

FIGURE 1.31 Simplified diagram showing the principle of the Engström ventilator. The patient system and the power system are separated by the breathing bag. (From Jacobson, B., and Webster, J. G. Medicine and clinical engineering. © 1977, p. 547. Reprinted by permission of Prentice-Hall, Inc.)

tidal volume controls. Figure 1.32 shows how the respiratory rate is adjusted by varying T, the total period. The ratio is adjusted by selecting a different inspiration time, which is adjusted independent of the rate. The tidal volume adjustment is also independent of the other controls.

The system consists of the four major blocks shown in Fig. 1.33. The rate block contains the master oscillator and rate scalars, and operator-controlled switch S_1 sets the rate. The ratio block has an input from operator switch S_2 to set the inspiration time. The sigh block provides operator control of sigh rate, sigh/hour, sigh/interval, and sigh volume through switches S_4 through S_7.

The ratio and sigh-block outputs control the duration of first 256 pulses from the rate block to set inspiration time, while the next 256 pulses set expiration time (when the ratio is 1 : 1). Then a reset pulse starts a new respiratory cycle.

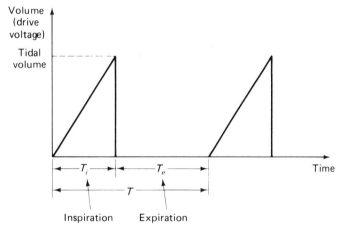

FIGURE 1.32 Timing diagram of a digital electronic control system for a ventilator. (From Engelman, F. A., Jr., and Cook, A. M. 1977. Digital electronic control of automatic ventilators. IEEE Trans. Biomed. Eng. BME-24 : 188–190.)

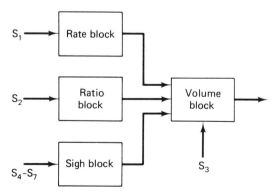

FIGURE 1.33 Block diagram of a digital electronic control system for a ventilator.

The volume block contains a digital-to-analog converter, and the output is a voltage that varies during T_i. The maximum amplitude (the tidal volume) can be adjusted with S_3. During T_e this voltage is reduced to 0 V. The control voltage goes to a linear driven piston, whose position is proportional to the voltage applied. In this way the system provides a volume-versus-time drive signal.

The use of a fixed clock and variable-rate scalars eliminates problems connected with variable RC oscillators, such as nonlinearities and drift. This feature provides extremely stable and accurate control of respiratory rate. Note also that the rate and ratio controls are independent.

1.4 ANESTHESIA MACHINES
AND SURGICAL MONITORING*

Administration of inhalation anesthetics is accomplished using an anesthesia machine. Features common to all anesthesia machines are vaporizers for liquid anesthetics, gas flowmeters to monitor oxygen and nitrous oxide, carbon dioxide absorbers, and gas reservoir bags.

As well as ensuring that the patient is adequately anesthetized, the anesthetist must monitor the physiological state of the patient during surgical procedures. Commonly monitored variables are the electrocardiogram (Section 1.2), heart or pulse rate (Section 1.2), blood pressure (Section 1.6), cardiac output (Section 3.3), respiratory volumes and rates (Section 1.3), and temperature.

Vaporizers

Most general anesthetics are volatile liquids at room temperature and pressure. The task of the vaporizer is to convert a liquid to its gaseous form and to control the amount of vapor delivered to the patient. To understand how vaporizers work, we must first consider the physical properties governing the vaporization of liquids—vapor pressure, temperature, and heat of vaporization. We will then discuss two common types of vaporizers.

Figure 1.34(a) shows a volatile liquid inside a vessel closed to the atmosphere. If we keep the temperature of the closed system constant, a number of molecules of the liquid have enough energy to escape and move into the air above. The molecules in the gas phase are collectively called a vapor. Collision of these molecules with the walls of the container results in a net outward pressure on the walls. Collision of these molecules with the liquid results in their movement back into the liquid. A state of equilibrium is reached when the number of molecules escaping the liquid phase to the gas phase and the number of molecules recaptured by the liquid phase become equal (no net movement into or out of the liquid phase). The partial pressure exerted on the walls of the container by the vapor at equilibrium is defined as the vapor pressure of the liquid at that temperature.

---

*Section 1.4 written by Gary V. Sprenger.

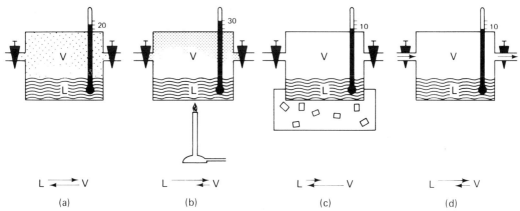

FIGURE 1.34 Vaporization of liquids. (a) The liquid and vapor are in equilibrium. (b) The application of heat causes the equilibrium to shift so that more molecules enter the vapor phase, as illustrated by the increased density of dots above the liquid. (c) Lowering the temperature causes a shift toward the liquid phase and a decrease in vapor pressure. (d) Effect of carrier gas flow. Passing a carrier gas over the liquid shifts the equilibrium toward the vapor phase because vapor is carried away from the system. The temperature falls as heat is lost during vaporization. (From Dorsch, J. A., and Dorsch, S. E. Understanding anesthesia equipment: construction, care, and complications. © 1975. Williams & Wilkins Co., Baltimore. Used with permission.)

If we now heat the container as shown in Fig. 1.34(b) we supply more energy to the molecules of the liquid and the equilibrium shifts to the right, where the net number of vapor molecules increases. Conversely, if we cool the liquid (remove energy) the equilibrium shifts to the left, where the net number of vapor molecules decreases. Hence the measure of the energy of the liquid—its temperature—plays an important role in vaporization. Furthermore, vapor pressure assumes no significance unless the temperature is specified. The temperature at which a liquid's vapor pressure becomes equal to atmospheric pressure is defined as the boiling point of the liquid. Oxygen, carbon dioxide, and nitrous oxide are gases at room temperature and pressure.

Knowing the vapor pressure and temperature of an anesthetic agent and the ambient atmospheric pressure, we can express the amount of anesthetic vapor in terms of its partial pressure or that part of the total pressure contributed by the vapor. That is, the total pressure of a mixture of gases is equal to the sum of the partial pressures of its constituents. The concentration of a vapor may also be expressed in terms of its volume percentage in the total gas mixture:

$$\frac{\text{partial pressure of the vapor}}{\text{total pressure}} \times 100 = \text{volume } \%$$

The amount of heat necessary to vaporize 1 g of a particular volatile liquid is defined as its heat of vaporization.

The heat to vaporize an anesthetic agent comes from the liquid itself. Consequently, as the agent vaporizes, the temperature of the liquid falls. In actual practice, heat from the surroundings is supplied to the liquid and an equilibrium is established where no further change in liquid temperature occurs. Heat-transfer factors thus become important in the selection of materials for use in a vaporizer and affect its efficiency directly.

The vaporization of an anesthetic agent would be of little use if the vapor could not be transported to the patient in doses large enough to produce the desired effect. Two basic schemes are currently used to accomplish this task. Both systems use oxygen as the "carrier" gas.

Figure 1.34(d) shows the "flow-over" approach. As the anesthetic agent vaporizes it is carried away by the oxygen flowing above it. The temperature of the liquid falls in proportion to the amount of vapor produced and the vapor pressure of the liquid also falls. Therefore, proportionately less liquid vaporizes at the lower temperature. Unless heat is supplied to the liquid continually, less vapor is produced and supplied to the patient. The magnitude of this problem is also directly related to carrier gas flow rate and the gas–liquid interface area. Hence the management of actual anesthetic concentrations is difficult at best.

A somewhat different approach to the problem is the "bubble-through" method. Here the carrier gas is passed directly through the liquid as small bubbles. Considerable improvement in vaporizer efficiency is possible if the total surface area of the bubbles is large with respect to total carrier gas flow. Temperature changes with vaporization still present a problem, however. The inescapable conclusion is that temperature stability of vaporizers is mandatory. This is sometimes accomplished by specifying intermittent carrier gas flow, which allows the temperature to stabilize during the intervals of no carrier gas flow.

Measurement of gas flow—the rotameter

The most common flowmeter in use for gases associated with anesthesia is the rotameter. Simple in design, the rotameter consists of a hollow tapered tube containing a float. As gas flows through the rotameter, the buoyant forces caused by pressure and drag on the float oppose the force of gravity and cause it to rise to a section of the tapered tube that has a larger cross section. Then the forces are equal. The float is then used as a pointer to read the flow rate from the side of the tube. Figure 1.35 illustrates these relationships for a typical rotameter. A needle valve is used to set the desired flow rate. Although reliable in operation, the rotameter is useful only for the particular gas for which it is designed and calibrated. Viscosity and density of gases directly affect the buoyant forces applied to the float. Since no two gases have the same viscosity–density characteristics, the rotameter can only be used with one gas. Temperature stability is also mandatory because changes in temperature affect viscosity and density of gases.

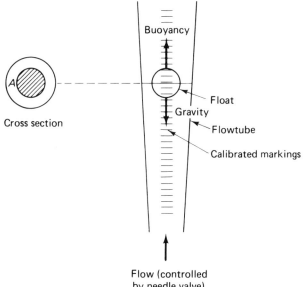

FIGURE 1.35 Rotameter. Flow through the rotameter is proportional to the gas velocity and the annulus area (*A*). When the upward buoyant forces are equal to the downward force due to gravity, the float is at equilibrium and the flow is read from the calibrated markings on the flowtube. These forces depend upon the geometry of the flowmeter and the physical properties of the gas and the float.

Carbon dioxide absorbers

Soda lime is the carbon dioxide absorbent that is most widely used. It relies on the dissolution of the carbon dioxide into a thin film of water within the absorber and subsequent reactions that result in the conversion of the carbon dioxide to a solid. The reactions are highly exothermic and great amounts of heat are generated.

Gas reservoir bag

The primary purpose of the gas reservoir bag is to allow for volume changes occurring within the breathing circuit. It may also be used to assist ventilation in the deeply anesthetized patient. Ventilators (Section 1.3) adapted for use in anesthesia are also available.

Breathing systems

Up to now we have investigated the various parts of the anesthesia machine that control the gas mixture supplied to the patient. Two systems used to deliver the gas mixture to the patient are the rebreathing and partial rebreathing systems.

Rebreathing system. The rebreathing system is totally closed. Theoretically, the closed nature of the device conserves anesthetic gases as well as preventing their leakage to the ambient atmosphere. It also buffers sudden changes in anesthetic concentration that might be harmful to the patient because the anesthetic is diluted by the exhaled air before being rebreathed.

The circle ventilation approach shown in Fig. 1.36 is a unidirectional flow device. Exhaled air is passed through a carbon dioxide absorber and mixed with fresh oxygen and anesthetic. The mixture is then inhaled by the patient after passage

REBREATHING SYSTEM

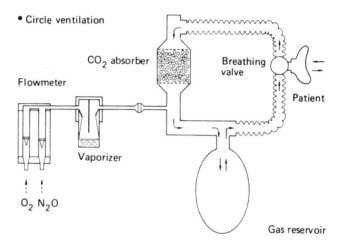

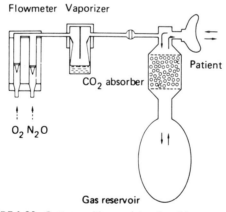

FIGURE 1.36 Systems with complete rebreathing are entirely closed. Exhaled CO_2 is absorbed and consumed oxygen is replaced. (From Jacobson, B., and Webster, J. G. Medicine and clinical engineering. © 1977, p. 515. Reprinted by permission of Prentice-Hall, Inc.).

through the gas reservoir bag. While dead space within the system is small, the resistance to ventilation is substantial.

Unlike circle ventilation the to-and-fro approach shown in Fig. 1.36 is typified by a small resistance to ventilation. Exhaled gas passes through the carbon dioxide absorber to the reservoir bag. The flow direction reverses upon inhalation and results in the gas passing through the absorber twice. This flow pattern necessitates replacement of the absorber cartridge more frequently because of increasing system dead space as more carbon dioxide is absorbed.

Partial rebreathing system.   Unlike the rebreathing system, part of the exhaled gas is vented to the atmosphere with each breath. The volume lost with each breath is replaced with a fresh gas mixture of oxygen and anesthetic. Figure 1.37 shows circle and to-and-fro types of partial rebreathing systems. Since anesthetic is released to the ambient atmosphere, we must consider the effects of the anesthetics on attending personnel.

Patient monitoring during anesthesia or surgery

The choice of appropriate methods for monitoring during anesthesia or surgery depends upon a complex set of circumstances involving the patient, the anesthesiologist, and the available equipment. These factors include the patient's condition with regard to pathological states, the anesthetic agent(s), the operative procedure, the available equipment, and the expertise and experience of the anesthesiologist.

Cardiovascular system monitoring.   The integrity of the cardiovascular system is often estimated by monitoring the ECG (Section 1.2), arterial and venous blood pressure (Section 1.6), and cardiac output.

The thermodilution method of estimating cardiac output utilizes a Swan–Ganz catheter. Its tip is inserted into an arm vein and advanced through the right heart into the pulmonary artery. A bolus of cold physiological saline is injected into the right atrium via the catheter. After mixing in the right heart the cooled blood passes by a thermistor contained in the tip of the catheter. Figure 1.38 shows the catheter placement, output curve, and calculation formula. Section 3.3 contains a detailed discussion of another method of cardiac output estimation—the dye-dilution method.

Temperature monitoring.   Temperature monitoring may be indicated in cardiovascular surgery and is mandatory in pediatric and hypothermia procedures. Skull temperature may be obtained by placement of a thermal probe into the nasopharynx near the base of the skull. Core temperature may be obtained from a probe inserted into the esophagus.

PARTIAL REBREATHING

• Circle ventilation

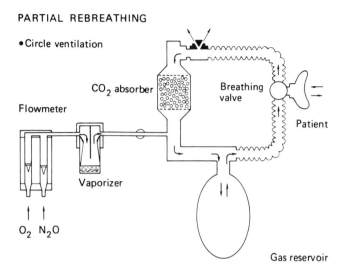

• To-and-fro ventilation

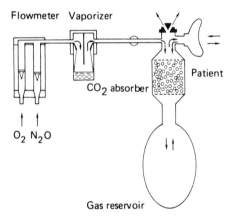

FIGURE 1.37 In systems with partial rebreathing, a fresh volume of gaseous mixture is constantly added. (From Jacobson, B., and Webster, J. G. Medicine and clinical engineering. © 1977, p. 516. Reprinted by permission of Prentice-Hall, Inc.)

1.5 EEG MONITORING*

The electroencephalogram (EEG) is a recording of the electrical activity of the brain as measured at the scalp with electrodes. Unlike the ECG, EEG recordings cannot be directly associated with a single electrical phenomenon within the brain, because the recordings represent the summation of the electrical activity of a large

*Section 1.5 written by Gregory S. Furno.

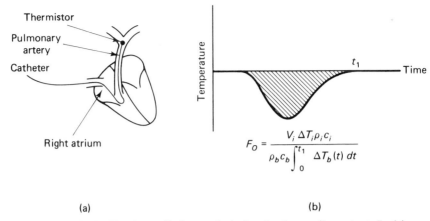

Thermistor
Pulmonary artery
Catheter
Right atrium

Temperature

Time

$$F_O = \frac{V_i\,\Delta T_i \rho_i c_i}{\rho_b c_b \displaystyle\int_0^{t_1} \Delta T_b(t)\,dt}$$

(a)   (b)

FIGURE 1.38 The thermodilution method of estimating cardiac output, F_o. (a) Catheter placement. (b) Output curve. V_i is the volume of injected saline. ΔT_i is the instantaneous temperature difference of the blood-injectate mixture at the thermistor relative to average blood temperature. ρ is specific gravity. c is heat capacity. The subscripts i and b indicate injectate and blood, respectively.

number of individual neurons. Arising from slow potential changes in the cortex (outer layer) of the brain, the EEG is useful for diagnosis of epilepsy, tumor, and brain death.

Characteristics of the EEG

The frequency content of the EEG varies with state of alertness and mental activity. To assist in EEG analysis, the normal EEG frequency range of 0.5 to 30 Hz has been subdivided into five bands, as follows:

Delta	δ	0.5–4 Hz
Theta	θ	4–8 Hz
Alpha	α	8–13 Hz
Beta	β	13–22 Hz
Gamma	γ	22–30 Hz

In addition to these frequency bands, certain characteristic waveforms are observed. During sleep, if the subject is dreaming, the EEG exhibits rapid, low-voltage waves that resemble those obtained in alert subjects. This is called rapid-eye-movement (REM) sleep. During nondreaming periods, the EEG exhibits bursts of alpha-like activity, called sleep spindles.

The pathological EEG during grand mal epilepsy exhibits high-magnitude synchronous waves of about 10 Hz. Petit mal epilepsy exhibits a spike-and-dome (spike-and-slow-wave) pattern that repeats at about 3 Hz.

Sensing

Figure 1.39 shows the locations of electrodes. They are placed at 10% or 20% intervals of the way around the head or over the top of the head. The scalp is cleaned, and a cone-shaped Ag–AgCl electrode is glued to the scalp with quick-drying collodion adhesive. The electrode is filled with a conductive gel and the scalp abraded until the impedance measures less than 5 kΩ. This preparation keeps interference and artifacts to a minimum.

Figure 1.39 shows three common recording modes. Of the three, the bipolar mode has the sharpest localization.

Processing

Most of the information in Section 1.2 on ECG processing applies as well to the EEG. For the EEG, the smaller signal levels require higher amplifier gains. Most EEG recordings are multichannel, with from 6 to 32 channels, but the most common numbers for routine work are 8 and 16. EEG amplifier frequency response extends from 0.1 Hz to 100 Hz. The techniques for artifact and interference reduction described in Section 1.2 also apply here.

Advanced processing

Evoked cortical potentials, like EEG potentials, arise from within the brain, but the evoked potentials result from applying a stimulus to the body's sensory system and are localized to a particular area of the brain. Typical stimuli are a light flash or a sharp sound. Unfortunately, other EEG activity usually masks the brain's response to a single stimulus. However, the use of repetitive stimuli and the technique of signal averaging discussed in Section 5.1 can yield an evoked response.

Another advanced EEG processing technique involves computing the frequency spectrum of EEG signals at discrete-time intervals and plotting the results in a frequency–time–amplitude plot known as the compressed spectral array (CSA). See Section 3.4 for a more complete description of this technique. At present the CSA is finding application in diagnosis and in monitoring depth of anesthesia during surgery.

1.6 BLOOD PRESSURE*

Blood-pressure measurements in the heart chambers and in the vascular system help the physician assess the function of the cardiovascular system as a whole. Figure 1.40 shows the pressures that occur during the cardiac cycle. Three type of measurements can be performed: direct (invasive), indirect (noninvasive), and relative (uncalibrated indirect).

---

*Section 1.6 written by Gregory S. Furno.

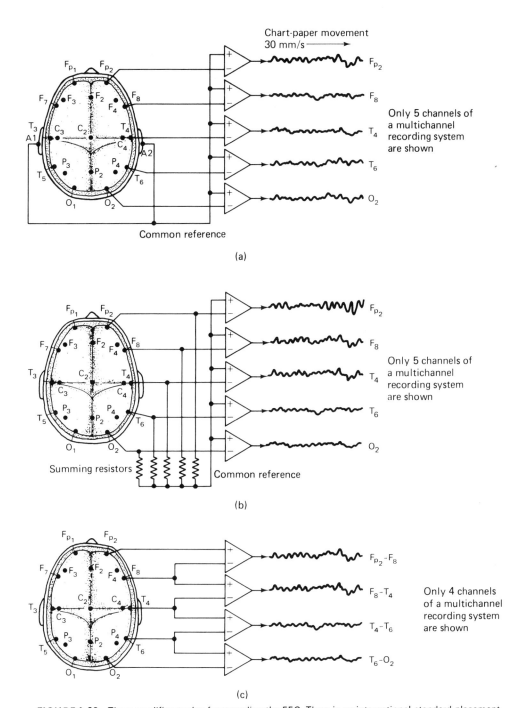

FIGURE 1.39 Three amplifier modes for recording the EEG. There is an international standard placement for the electrodes. The letters indicate brain lobes or areas: F is frontal, C is central, P is parietal, O is occipital, and T is temporal. (a) Unipolar EEG recording configuration. (b) Average EEG recording configuration. (c) Bipolar EEG recording configuration. (From Strong, P. 1970. Biophysical measurements. Beaverton, OR: Tektronix.)

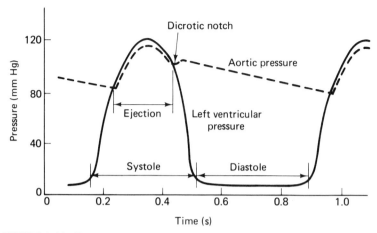

FIGURE 1.40 The cardiac cycle. When the left ventricular pressure exceeds the aortic pressure, the aortic valve opens and blood is ejected into the aorta.

Direct blood-pressure measurement

Figure 1.41 shows the most common method for measuring the pulsatile blood pressure within the vessels. The liquid-filled catheter transmits the pressure from the sensing port at its tip to the diaphragm within the transducer. Because the catheter invades the vessels, it is necessary to flush the tip every few minutes to prevent blood clotting. The catheter also limits the frequency response of the system to about 20 Hz (depending upon the catheter and transducer dimensions and the presence of air bubbles).

Catheter-tip pressure transducers incorporate a miniature diaphragm at the tip and obtain very high frequency response. However, they are expensive and prone to breakage.

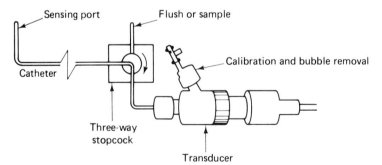

FIGURE 1.41 Extravascular pressure-transducer system. A catheter couples heparinized saline through a three-way stopcock to the extravascular-transducer element. The three-way stopcock is used to flush the catheter and take blood samples. (From *Medical Instrumentation: Analysis and Design* by John G. Webster et al. Copyright © by Houghton Mifflin Company. Reprinted by permission of the publisher.)

Strain gages commonly measure transducer diaphragm motion, but other principles such as linear variable differential transformer and variable capacitance have been used.

Replacement of the transducer by a saline-filled manometer yields a low-cost, low-frequency-response measurement of central venous pressure.

Indirect blood-pressure measurement

Indirect pressure measurements are commonly made with a sphygmomanometer. Figure 1.42 shows the features of this method. The sphygmomanometer cuff is pressurized, thus cutting off or occluding arterial flow. The pressure is then slowly bled off, and below systolic pressure as blood begins to squirt through the partially occluded arteries, the turbulence generates Korotkoff sounds, which can be heard with a stethoscope. When the cuff pressure falls below the diastolic pressure, no sounds are heard because the blood flow is then laminar. This so-called auscultatory method is also suitable for automation. The usual procedure is to have a cuff pump rapidly inflate the cuff to a pressure about 30 mm Hg above the suspected systolic pressure. Cuff pressure is then slowly reduced until the first Korotkoff

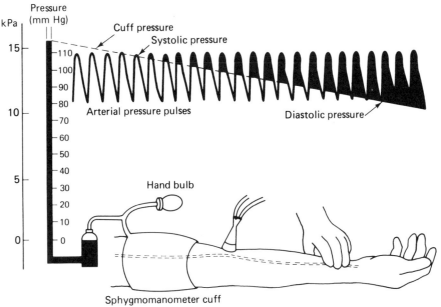

FIGURE 1.42 Typical indirect blood-pressure measurement system. Sphygmomanometer cuff is inflated by a hand bulb to pressures above the systolic level. Pressure is then slowly released and blood flow under the cuff is monitored by a microphone or stethoscope placed over a downstream artery. The first Korotkoff sound detected indicates systolic pressure, while the transition from muffling to silence brackets diastolic pressure. (From Rushmer, R. F. 1970. Cardiovascular dynamics, 3rd ed. Philadelphia: Saunders. Used with permission.)

sound is detected by a microphone placed beneath the cuff. The machine stores the value of the cuff pressure in a memory. Cuff pressure then continues its decline until the muffling and silent period of the Korotkoff sounds is detected, at which time the machine stores the value of the cuff pressure in a different memory location. The instrument then displays the systolic and diastolic pressures for a few minutes while it recycles. Variations of this method involve changes in the Korotkoff detection method. For example, some systems detect the pulsations in cuff pressure with pressure sensors during the Korotkoff sound period, rather than using a microphone. Other detectors use ultrasound to detect the arterial wall motion.

Relative blood-pressure measurement

When an external object partially collapses a pressurized flexible-walled vessel, the circumferential stresses in the vessel wall are removed, and the internal and external pressures are equal. This is the basic principle of tonometry. Figure 1.43 shows how

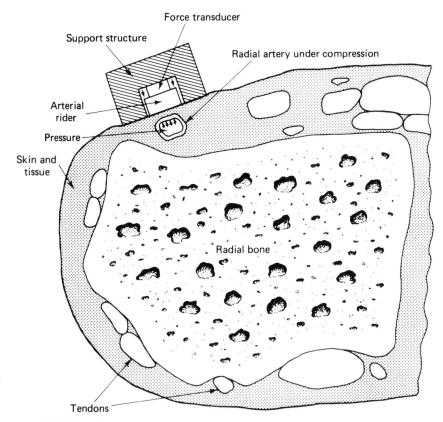

FIGURE 1.43 Arterial tonometer and partial cross section of the right wrist. The support structure holds the force transducer and flattens the surrounding tissue to minimize tissue forces on the radial artery.

the tonometer applies pressure to the radial artery in the wrist. The arterial pressure is proportional to the force on an arterial rider divided by its area. Present tonometer designs can only measure relative pressures, and must be calibrated by direct or indirect means. This is because the arterial rider also compresses intervening tissue. Thus the force on the transducer is greater than the force on the artery. Therefore, the pressure indicated by the device would be greater than that actually present within the artery were the readings not scaled down. Also, for 30% of the people tested with the tonometer, the tonometer failed to work satisfactorily. This may be due to small tendons that overlay the artery or to excessive intervening tissue.

1.7 CLINICAL CHEMISTRY*

Many clinical laboratory determinations are based upon measurements of radiant power emitted, transmitted, absorbed, or reflected under controlled conditions. Collection of specimens for analysis is an integral part of these quantitative procedures (Tietz, 1976).

In this section we cover determinations of serum protein, serum cholesterol, uric acid, bicarbonate, pH, blood PCO_2 and blood PO_2. We describe the main principles involved in clinical laboratory determinations.

Spectrophotometer

The spectrophotometer is used to measure the concentration of a given substance in solution. When blood is used as a sample, it is centrifuged to remove the cells and measurements are made on the resulting plasma. Colorless compounds are converted to colored reaction products by reaction with a suitable compound, called a reagent. Measurements are usually made in the visible wavelength spectrum from 380 to 780 nm. The advantage of spectrophotometry is that discrete portions of the spectrum can be isolated and used for measurements. A solution containing two unknown substances can be analyzed to determine the concentration of each substance if they each absorb maximally at different wavelengths.

Beer's law. The spectrophotometer uses Beer's law to measure concentrations. Consider an incident light beam with intensity I_0 passing through a cuvette containing a solution of a compound that absorbs light maximally at a given wavelength (λ). The intensity of the light transmitted through the solution I_S is less than the incident light I_0. The transmittance of light is defined as I_S/I_0. Some incident light is reflected by the surface of the cell or absorbed by the solvent. This factor is removed when a reference cell is used which contains only the compound solvent. The transmittance through this reference cell is I_R/I_0, where I_R is the intensity of the transmitted light beam through the reference cell. The transmittance for the com-

---

*Section 1.7 written by Peter D. Gadsby.

pound in solution is defined as I_S/I_R. We place the reference cuvette in the spectro-photometer and adjust the instrument to read 100% transmittance. We read the sample in percent transmittance. Since the transmittance varies inversely and logarithmically with sample concentration, it is more convenient to convert percent transmittance into a linear relationship called absorbance (A).

$$A = -\log \frac{I_S}{I_R} = -\log T = 2 - \log \%T$$

The absorbance of a solution also varies with the cuvette width that the incident light has to pass through. This is taken into account by Beer's law:

$$I_S = I_0 \exp(-\alpha c x)$$

where α = absorptivity, which is constant for a species and wavelength
       c = concentration, moles/liter
       x = path length, cm, through which the incident light beam passes

Instruments. An instrument that uses a filter to select the desired wavelength is called a filter photometer or colorimeter. The diffraction grating shown in Fig. 1.44 selects a narrower bandwidth and the instrument is then called a spectrophoto-meter. The light source is usually a tungsten lamp. The intensity of the output of the lamp varies with the wavelength. Hence the light-intensity control is used to give the phototube the proper level of illumination.

     The term "monochromer" refers to all the components from the entrance slit to the exit slit. The purpose of the monochromer is to supply the sample with light that is close to one wavelength. The diffraction grating separates the polychro-

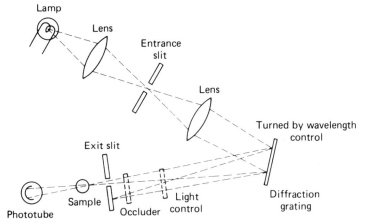

FIGURE 1.44 The spectrophotometer uses slits plus a diffraction grating or prism to select the desired wavelength.

matic white light into its component wavelengths. The desired wavelength is then focused on the exit slit. Monochromatic light is important because Beer's law does not hold for polychromatic light. The phototube then converts the transmitted light to an electrical signal. A Pyrex cuvette normally contains the sample.

The dual-beam spectrophotometer (Tietz, 1976) is used to overcome problems associated with the tungsten bulb. These problems include metallic vapor condensation, oil, dust, and heat, which alter the characteristics of the optical system. The single lamp output is split into two beams. One passes through the sample and the other through a reference cuvette. Finally, the ratio of the two outputs is used to compute transmittance. Ultraviolet and infrared spectrophotometry use different light sources for their measurements.

Fluorimetry

In a photofluorometer, ultraviolet light passes through a filter to screen out light of longer wavelengths. Part of the light is absorbed by the substance in solution. The emitted light, which is of longer wavelength, passes through a second filter at right angles to the ultraviolet beam and is measured photometrically.

Fluorometric methods have been developed for hundreds of compounds of potential clinical interest, including drugs and drug metabolites.

Turbidimetry

Turbidimetry and nephelometry are both used to measure particle concentrations within a solution. Turbidimetry measures the amount of light blocked by particulate matter in the sample as light passes through the cuvette. Nephelometry measures the light scattered by the particles at right angles to the beam incident on the cuvette.

Autoanalyzer

The name Autoanalyzer is a registered trademark of the Technicon Instruments Corporation. Those instruments that were initially designed to process many tests at the same time are designated sequential multiple analyzers (SMA) with a numerical qualification to indicate the number of tests that may be made simultaneously, and the number of samples per hour (e.g., SMA 12/60). Figure 1.45 shows a block diagram of an Autoanalyzer.

The four important design principles of the Autoanalyzer are (Tietz, 1976):

1. Spaghetti tubing of different diameters and a peristaltic pump provide several constant flow rates of samples and reagents through the tubes.
2. Air bubbles are introduced to separate the sample and reagent streams into segments.

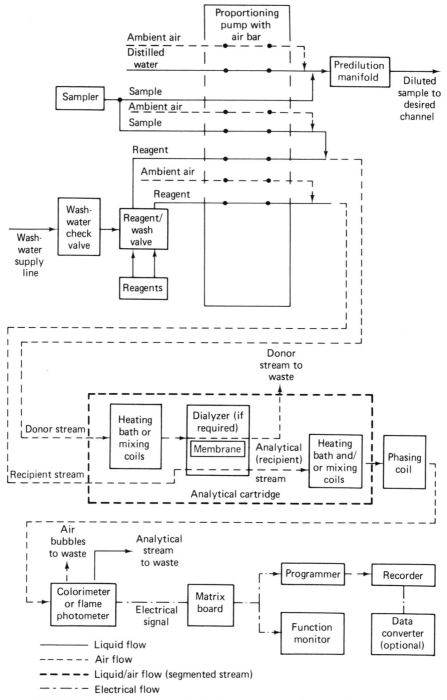

FIGURE 1.45 Block diagram of the Technicon SMA 12/60 Autoanalyzer. (Technicon and SMA are trademarks of Technicon Instruments Corporation, Tarrytown, N.Y. 10591)

3. Dialysis is carried out through a semipermeable membrane to separate proteins from analytes. This procedure helps to eliminate interference of protein with chemical reactions.

4. The key to the analyzer design is a modular construction which permits easy replacement of a faulty module or substitution of one module for another for different procedures.

Samples are placed into cups in the sampler unit. Aliquots (fixed-volume samples) are removed through the sample pickup tube of the manifold. Reagents and samples are mixed in fixed volume proportions and the fluid stream is segmented by air bubbles. The product formed after mixing of the dialyzed sample with the reagent, and after heating where necessary, is followed by measurement with the appropriate device, usually a spectrophotometer. As long as all samples and standards are handled exactly the same, it is not necessary to wait for the reaction to be complete before measurement. Results are displayed as a series of peaks on a strip-chart recorder.

Centrifugal analyzer

The high sensitivity of the centrifugal analyzer permits the use of capillary blood for routine tests on adults and children. Also, all time-related reactions such as enzyme kinetics can be monitored continuously (Tietz, 1976).

Figure 1.46 shows that the photometric measurements take place within a rotating centrifuge head. The rotor consists of an outer ring containing a number of cuvettes formed by a compression of an inert spacer between two plates of optically transparent material. Three concentric rows of cavities make up the transfer disk. Sample and reagent from the inner two cavities flow into the outer cuvette during centrifugation. Each set of three cavities and corresponding cuvette make up a reaction unit. A photometric system is arranged perpendicular to the rotor and cuvette. During centrifugation, the transmittance of each reaction mixture is measured against a reference blank in the first cuvette. The rotor makes a complete revolution every 50 to 100 ms. Generally, readings from eight consecutive revolutions are averaged. This instrument functions as a multichannel double-beam spectrophotometer. An internal computation system performs data acquisition, averaging, manipulation, and display.

Potentiometry and amperometry

Potentiometry refers to the measurement of an electrical potential difference between two electrodes in an electrochemical cell. This technique is employed to measure pH and PCO_2. Amperometry, on the other hand, is based on the measurement of a current flowing through an electrochemical cell when a constant electrical potential is applied to the electrodes. This technique is used to measure PO_2.

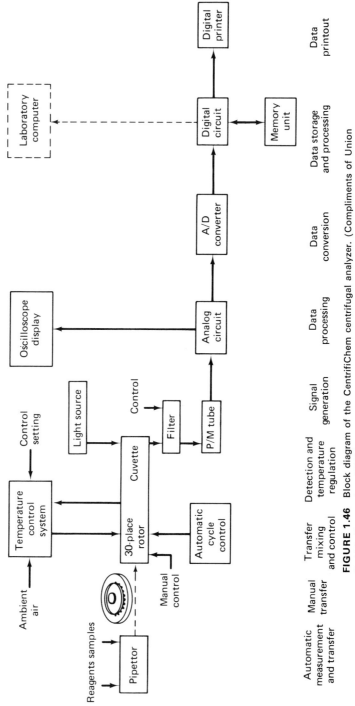

FIGURE 1.46 Block diagram of the CentrifiChem centrifugal analyzer. (Compliments of Union Carbide Corporation, 1979.)

Frequently, electrodes for pH, PCO_2, and PO_2 are packaged together in a single instrument, called a blood-gas analyzer.

pH measurement. When the body cannot blow off its CO_2, the carbonic acid, H_2CO_3 builds up in the blood and dissociates into hydrogen ions, H^+ and bicarbonate ions, HCO_3^-. To assess the patient's status, the increase in hydrogen ion concentration in moles/liter $[H^+]$ is measured as the pH, where

$$pH = -\log[H^+]$$

Figure 1.47(a) shows that the pH electrode uses a special glass membrane that behaves as if it were permeable only to H^+. The difference in $[H^+]$ on each side of the membrane produces a potential of about 60 mV/pH unit.

A calomel reference electrode is required to complete the circuit. The saturated Hg_2Cl_2 and KCl maintain a stable reference cell potential in spite of pH variations.

PCO_2 measurement. The PCO_2 electrode is a special application of the pH glass electrode. Figure 1.47(b) shows a silicone-rubber membrane, which is permeable to gas but not to solutions. The CO_2 gas diffuses from the test solution through the membrane and rapidly equilibrates with the bicarbonate solution, thus altering the pH. The relationship between PCO_2 and pH is given by the Henderson–Hasselbalch equation:

$$pH = -s \times \log PCO_2 - \log \alpha + pK' + \log[HCO_3^-]$$

where s = relative sensitivity of the electrode
$\quad\quad \alpha$ = solubility coefficient of CO_2
$\quad\quad K'$ = first dissociation constant of carbonic acid
$[HCO_3^-]$ = concentration of HCO_3^-

PO_2 measurement. Figure 1.47(c) shows the Clark PO_2 electrode. The cathode potential is adjusted to -0.67 V. In the absence of oxygen in the test solution the current is almost zero. When O_2 is present in the test solution, it diffuses through the membrane. The O_2 is reduced, consuming electrons, which are supplied by the cathode. The resulting current is amplified and displayed. The current is proportional to the PO_2 in the test solution.

The membrane prohibits movement of proteins and other oxidants which would poison the cathode and also restricts the diffusion zone to the membrane, thereby preventing variations in the diffusion coefficient of O_2.

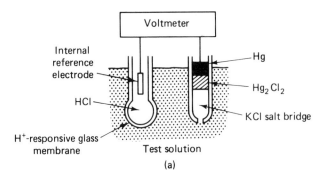

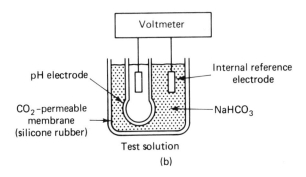

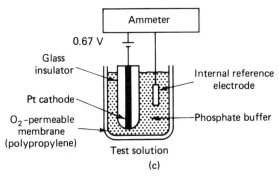

FIGURE 1.47 Electrodes. (a) pH differences across a glass membrane yield a voltage related to pH. (b) The PCO_2 electrode uses a gas-permeable membrane to cover a normal pH electrode. (c) The PO_2 electrode uses a platinum cathode to reduce oxygen and produce current flow.

REFERENCES

BENDER, G. T. 1972. Chemical instrumentation: a laboratory manual based on clinical chemistry. Philadelphia: Saunders.

BLUMENFELD, W., TUNNEY, S. Z., AND DENMAN, R. J. 1975. A coaxial ultrasonic pneumotachometer. Med. Biol. Eng. 13: 855–860.

CASTELLAN, G. W. 1971. Physical chemistry. Reading, MA.: Addison-Wesley.

COTES, J. E. 1975. Lung function. Oxford: Blackwell.

DORNETTE, W. H. L. (ED.). 1973. Monitoring in anesthesia. Clinical Anesthesia Series 9/2, 3. Philadelphia: Davis.

DORSCH, J. A., AND DORSCH, S. E. 1975. Understanding anesthesia equipment: construction, care, and complications. Baltimore: Williams & Wilkins.

ENGELMAN, F. A., JR., AND COOK, A. M. 1977. Digital electronic control of automatic ventilators. IEEE Trans. Biomed. Eng. BME-24: 188–190.

GANONG, W. F. 1979. Review of medical physiology, 9th ed. Los Altos, CA: Lange.

GUILLEMINAULT, C., EDRIDGE, F. L., SIMMONS, F. B., AND DEMENT, W. C. 1976. Sleep apnea in eight children. Pediatrics 58: 23–29.

HICKS, R., SCHENKEN, J. R., AND STEINRAUF, M. A. 1974. Laboratory instrumentation. New York: Harper & Row.

HILL, D. W., AND DOLAN, A. M. 1976. Intensive care instrumentation. New York: Grune & Stratton.

JACOBSON, B., AND WEBSTER, J. G. 1977. Medicine and clinical engineering. Englewood Cliffs, NJ: Prentice-Hall.

MASTERTON, W. L., AND SLOWINSKI, E. J. Chemical principles. Philadelphia: Saunders.

MUSHIN, W. W., BAKER, L. R., THOMPSON, P. R., AND MAPELSON, W. W. 1969. Automatic ventilation of the lungs, 2nd ed. Oxford: Blackwell.

NEUMAN, M. R. 1978. In J. G. Webster (ed.), Medical instrumentation: application and design. Boston: Houghton Mifflin.

PEURA, R. A. 1978. In J. G. Webster (ed.), Medical instrumentation: application and design. Boston: Houghton Mifflin.

PRIMIANO, F. P., JR. 1978. In J. G. Webster (ed)., Medical instrumentation: application and design. Boston: Houghton Mifflin.

ROTH, M. 1970. Methods in clinical chemistry. Baltimore: University Park Press.

ROUX, J. F., NEUMAN, M. R., AND GOODLIN, R. C. 1975. Monitoring of intrapartum phenomena. Crit. Rev. Bioeng. 2: 119–158.

RUSHMER, R. F. 1970. Cardiovascular dynamics, 3rd ed. Philadelphia: Saunders.

SHAW, A., GREGORY, N. L., DAVIS, P. D., AND PATEL, K. 1976. Flow-volume integrator for respiratory studies. Med. Biol. Eng. 14: 695–696.

STEIN, I. M., AND SHANNON, D. C. 1975. The pediatric pneumogram: a new method for detecting and quantitating apnea in infants. Pediatrics 55: 599–603.

STEINSCHNEIDER, A. 1976. A reexamination of "the apnea monitor business." Pediatrics 58: 1–5.

STRONG, P. 1970. Biophysical measurements. Beaverton, OR: Tektronix.

TECHNICON INSTRUMENTS. 1974. Product labeling for the SMA 12/60 multichannel bio-chemical analyzer, Vols 1–3. Tarrytown, NY.

TIETZ, N. W. 1976. Fundamentals of clinical chemistry. Philadelphia: Saunders.

UNION CARBIDE. 1979. Centrifichem instruction manual. Rye, NY.

WARD, C. S. 1975. Anesthetic equipment: physical principles and maintenance. London: Baillière, Tindall.

WEBSTER, J. G. (ED.). 1978. Medical instrumentation: application and design. Boston: Houghton Mifflin.

WYATT, G. M. 1974. Problems in the performance of anesthesia and respiratory equip-ment. International Anesthesiology Clinics 12(3). Boston: Little, Brown.

PROBLEMS

1.1 Refer to the multistep definition of medicine given at the beginning of Section 1.1. Describe the advantages and disadvantages of its closed-loop nature over a hypo-thetical open-ended system that does not have an ability to repeat the procedure.

1.2 The output signal from a transducer is in the form of a voltage. List the character-istics of this signal that you would need to know in order to design an amplifier. List the specifications for the amplifier itself.

1.3 Relabel the blocks in Fig. 1.2 so that it illustrates the multistep definition of medicine given at the beginning of Section 1.1.

1.4 Would a metal-plate electrode cause more motion artifact than a recessed electrode? Why?

1.5 Why is it possible to connect ECG electrodes to the wrists and ankles and record waveforms identical to those recorded with the electrodes placed on the shoulders and thighs?

1.6 Where on the body should electrodes be placed in order to record the R wave of maximum amplitude?

1.7 Figure P1.1 is a rudimentary input-protection circuit for a simple amplifier. If the 5-V Zener diodes are rated at 1-W dissipation, what value of R is necessary to safely limit the diode current should the input voltage rise to 6500 V (e.g., from a defibrillation pulse)?

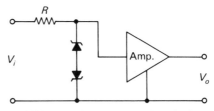

FIGURE P1.1 Input protection circuit.

1.8 Modern ECG amplifiers are designed to have an input current of 5 μA or less, even if the input load is connected to the 120-V line. This might occur for instance, if a patient touched a faulty piece of equipment. If we decide to put a resistor in series with the input load to limit the current, how big would it have to be? Is this a practical value? Why?

1.9 In Fig. 1.11 suppose that current flowing from the power line through the body created a common-mode voltage V_{cm} of 200 mV everywhere on the body. Now, if $Z_1 = Z_3 = 10\ \text{k}\Omega$, and $Z_{\text{in}} = 1\ \text{M}\Omega$, what would be the output voltage of an amplifier having perfect common-mode rejection [i.e., $v_o =$ amp gain $\times\ v_{\text{in}}$]? If Z_3 became 11 kΩ for some reason, what would be the new output voltage? Why does this happen?

1.10 Draw a block diagram of a filter for reducing 60-Hz interference after it has been amplified by the first stages of an ECG amplifier.

1.11 For the circuit of Fig. 1.9, we switch from a set of electrodes that has an offset voltage of 0 mV to another set that has an offset voltage of +300 mV. How long will it take for the circuit to recover after the transient has passed if the reset switch is *not* used? How long if it is used?

1.12 Compare the output of the averaging cardiotachometer in Fig. 1.14 to the output of the beat-to-beat cardiotachometer of Fig. 1.15 when the patient goes into cardiac arrest (i.e., the heart stops).

1.13 Consider the scheme presented in Fig. P1.2 for isolating the fetal ECG. Can such a scheme work? If not, why not?

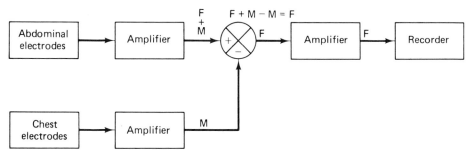

FIGURE P1.2 Alternative method for isolating the fetal ECG.

1.14 Redesign the ECG amplifier of Fig. 1.9 to work as an EEG amplifier. It should produce an output voltage of 1 V with an input voltage of 100 μV. The frequency range should extend from 0.1 to 100 Hz.

1.15 Would it be possible to devise an electrode arrangement to produce a vector EEG similar to the VCG of Section 1.2? Why or why not?

1.16 List the properties of the pressure transducer system of Fig. 1.41 that affect its dynamic response to pulsatile blood pressure.

1.17 If the blood pressure of an obese person were measured with a sphygmomanometer, would the indicated pressure tend to be higher than the actual pressure, lower, or the same? Why?

1.18 From the explanation given in the text about temperature/vapor pressure relationships of volatile anesthetic liquids, construct a curve showing these relationships.

Indicate with arrows the way you would expect the curve to move during vaporization without temperature compensation.

1.19 What is a possible disadvantage to partial rebreathing systems? How might it affect operating room personnel?

1.20 In Fig. 1.35 we show the three major forces on the rotameter float. The amount of drag is affected by the surface area of the float directly while the buoyant force is a function of the surface area presented to the gas flow. Redesign the float to minimize drag yet leave the buoyant forces unchanged.

1.21 What are the main differences between a photometer and a spectrophotometer? What factors should be considered in selecting one over the other for use in a clinical laboratory?

1.22 Draw a diagram of a double-beam spectrophotometer and explain how it differs from a spectrophotometer. Why is it important to use a blank channel?

1.23 Draw a diagram of fluorometer measurement system and describe the basics for measurement, the functional components, and the strengths and weaknesses of the measurement system.

1.24 Draw the sensors used in the *in vivo* blood-gas monitor and describe how they work.

1.25 On introduction of samples into an automatic clinical chemistry analyzer, air bubbles are interspersed between the different solutions. Why are these air bubbles introduced? Design a measurement system to detect them.

2

Analog-to Digital and Digital-to Analog Conversion

This chapter presents the intersection between the analog and digital worlds. Chapter 1 discussed analog techniques for obtaining the desired medical information. Chapters 3 to 6 emphasize digital techniques. Analog-to-digital and digital-to-analog conversion link together the analog and the digital worlds.

The primary purpose of this chapter is to help the designer use conversion techniques to sample data from analog transducers and convert them to a usable digital form for the microprocessor and to convert the processed digital data back to analog voltages. Following a review of basic conversion principles, we cover hardware aspects of digital-to-analog (D/A) converters, analog-to-digital (A/D) converters, and other devices that make up an analog-digital system.

---

*Chapter 2 written by Michael J. Yanikowski.

2.1 CONVERSION BASICS

The transducer in an instrument converts a physical value such as temperature, pressure, or flow into an electrical voltage or current. The electrical variable can be in the form of a slowly varying quantity, such as the voltage from a thermocouple or a potentiometer, or a rapidly varying waveform such as the output of a strain gage.

The analog–digital system

Figure 2.1 shows an example of an analog–digital conversion system. The parameters of temperature, pressure, and flow are converted by transducers to voltages proportional to signal amplitudes. These voltages are then amplified, filtered, and normalized to values that fall within the operating range of the analog multiplexer, the sample and hold, and the A/D converter. The analog multiplexer time multiplexes its set of input signals and presents each in turn to the sample-and-hold circuit. The sample and hold stores the input voltage level of a particular multi-

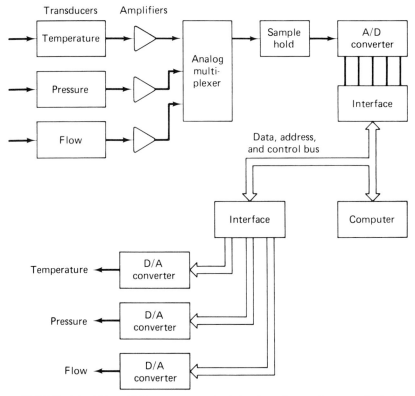

FIGURE 2.1 A/D and D/A converters are basic interface elements between physical variables and a microcomputer. [From Zuch, E. L. 1977. Where and when to use which data converter. IEEE Spectrum 14(6) : 39–42.]

plexed input for a fixed period of time sufficiently long for the A/D converter to encode the value of the voltage into a binary representation. By using multiplexing a number of analog channels share a single A/D converter. Each channel is periodically sampled at a fast enough rate to adequately represent the input signal. The interfaces and the microcomputer are discussed in Chapter 4. The interfaces provide for communication between the A/D and D/A converters and the microcomputer. The microcomputer accepts and processes the data from the A/D converter interface and sends binary data to the D/A interface. The D/A converters decode binary codes into analog voltages to control temperature, pressure, and flow, thereby forming a closed-loop system. This chapter presents each component of the analog–digital system in detail.

Binary codes

We first discuss binary codes, since the purpose of the A/D and D/A converters is to encode analog values into binary codes and to decode binary codes back into analog values. There are a number of different binary codes used in commercially available converter units. The two most common codes are ordinary binary and binary-coded decimal (BCD).

In an ordinary binary code having n bits, the most-significant bit (MSB) has a weight of 2^{n-1}, the second bit has a weight of 2^{n-2}, and so on until the least-significant bit (LSB), which has a weight of 2^0. We find the value of the number by adding up the weights of each of the nonzero bits. Figure 2.2 shows all 16 possible patterns

Decimal number	Decimal fraction	Code MSB ($\times 1/2$)	Bit 2 ($\times 1/4$)	Bit 3 ($\times 1/8$)	Bit 4 ($\times 1/16$)
0	0	0	0	0	0
1	$1/16 = 2^{-4}$ (LSB)	0	0	0	1
2	$2/16 = 1/8$	0	0	1	0
3	$3/16 = 1/8 + 1/16$	0	0	1	1
4	$4/16 = 1/4$	0	1	0	0
5	$5/16 = 1/4 + 1/16$	0	1	0	1
6	$6/16 = 1/4 + 1/8$	0	1	1	0
7	$7/16 = 1/4 + 1/8 + 1/16$	0	1	1	1
8	$8/16 = 1/2$ (MSB)	1	0	0	0
9	$9/16 = 1/2 + 1/16$	1	0	0	1
10	$10/16 = 1/2 + 1/8$	1	0	1	0
11	$11/16 = 1/2 + 1/8 + 1/16$	1	0	1	1
12	$12/16 = 1/2 + 1/4$	1	1	0	0
13	$13/16 = 1/2 + 1/4 + 1/16$	1	1	0	1
14	$14/16 = 1/2 + 1/4 + 1/8$	1	1	1	0
15	$15/16 = 1/2 + 1/4 + 1/8 + 1/16$	1	1	1	1

FIGURE 2.2 Ordinary binary codes. [From Sheingold, D. H. (ed.). 1977. Analog–digital conversion notes. Norwood, MA: Analog Devices, Inc.]

of 4 binary bits with their equivalent decimal fractions. The largest number that we can represent has all its bits equal to 1, which is a value of $2^n - 1$, or 15. The tabulated numbers are whole numbers, but in fact they represent fractions of full scale. To convert a binary code to the appropriate voltage equivalent, divide the code by 2^n and multiply the result by the full-scale voltage. Figure 2.3 shows the bit weights for up to 16 digits, but in most applications 8, 10, or 12 bits are used.

This binary code as given only represents unipolar values. To represent positive and negative values, bipolar coding is used. The most popular bipolar codes are 2's complement, offset binary, 1's complement, and sign magnitude. See Figure 2.4 for a summary of these codes.

Two's complement. In 2's-complement code, positive numbers are represented with a sign bit (MSB) of zero. Negative numbers are constructed by complementing each bit of a positive number and then adding one. For example, the 2's complement of 2 (0010) is its bit complement plus 1 (0001), or 1101 + 0001 = 1110.

One of the advantages of 2's-complement arithmetic is the negative-number representation, which provides for subtraction since it is simply the addition of a positive and a negative number. An example is 4 + (−1), or 0100 + 1111 = 0011 (the carry bit is ignored), or 3. Another advantage is an unambiguous code for zero. Also advantageous is the fact that many microprocessors perform 2's-complement arithmetic.

A disadvantage is that there is a large bit transition at zero (all bits change,

Bit	2^n	$1/2^n$ (decimal)	% Resolution	Parts per million
0	1	1.0	100.	1,000,000
1	2	0.5	50.	500,000
2	4	0.25	25.	250,000
3	8	0.125	12.5	125,000
4	16	0.0625	6.2	62,500
5	32	0.03125	3.1	31,250
6	64	0.015625	1.6	15,625
7	128	0.007812	0.8	7,812
8	256	0.003906	0.4	3,906
9	512	0.001953	0.2	1,953
10	1,024	0.0009766	0.1	977
11	2,048	0.00048828	0.05	488
12	4,096	0.00024414	0.024	244
13	8,192	0.00012207	0.012	122
14	16,384	0.000061035	0.006	61
15	32,768	0.0000305176	0.003	31
16	65,536	0.0000152588	0.0015	15

FIGURE 2.3 Binary bit weights or resolution. [From Sheingold, D. H. (ed.). 1977. Analog–digital conversion notes. Norwood, MA: Analog Devices, Inc.]

Number	Decimal fraction		Sign + magnitude	2's complement	Offset binary	1's complement
	Positive reference	Negative reference				
+7	+7/8	−7/8	0 1 1 1	0 1 1 1	1 1 1 1	0 1 1 1
+6	+6/8	−6/8	0 1 1 0	0 1 1 0	1 1 1 0	0 1 1 0
+5	+5/8	−5/8	0 1 0 1	0 1 0 1	1 1 0 1	0 1 0 1
+4	+4/8	−4/8	0 1 0 0	0 1 0 0	1 1 0 0	0 1 0 0
+3	+3/8	−3/8	0 0 1 1	0 0 1 1	1 0 1 1	0 0 1 1
+2	+2/8	−2/8	0 0 1 0	0 0 1 0	1 0 1 0	0 0 1 0
+1	+1/8	−1/8	0 0 0 1	0 0 0 1	1 0 0 1	0 0 0 1
0	0+	0−	0 0 0 0	0 0 0 0	0 0 0 0	0 0 0 0
0	0−	0+	1 0 0 0	(0 0 0 0)	(1 0 0 0)	1 1 1 1
−1	−1/8	+1/8	1 0 0 1	1 1 1 1	0 1 1 1	1 1 1 0
−2	−2/8	+2/8	1 0 1 0	1 1 1 0	0 1 1 0	1 1 0 1
−3	−3/8	+3/8	1 0 1 1	1 1 0 1	0 1 0 1	1 1 0 0
−4	−4/8	+4/8	1 1 0 0	1 1 0 0	0 1 0 0	1 0 1 1
−5	−5/8	+5/8	1 1 0 1	1 0 1 1	0 0 1 1	1 0 1 0
−6	−6/8	+6/8	1 1 1 0	1 0 1 0	0 0 1 0	1 0 0 1
−7	−7/8	+7/8	1 1 1 1	1 0 0 1	0 0 0 1	1 0 0 0
−8	−8/8	+8/8		(1 0 0 0)	(0 0 0 0)	

FIGURE 2.4 Commonly used bipolar codes. [From Sheingold, D. H. (ed.). 1977. Analog–digital conversion notes. Norwood, MA: Analog Devices, Inc.]

from 1111 to 0000) which can cause large transients because of speed differences in turning individual bits on and off. Nonlinearities also occur because of the major transitions at zero.

Offset binary. Offset binary is very similar to the 2's-complement code. It is a natural binary code with its zero at the negative full scale. The LSB is 2^{-n} of the whole bipolar range, and the MSB is turned on at analog zero. This code is similar to the 2's-complement code except that the MSBs are complements of each other. As in the 2's-complement code, there is a major transition at analog zero.

In a number of commercial converters special configurations are given to change to offset binary with minimum parts and skill. Figure 2.5(a) shows the voltage translation necessary to operate a D/A converter with an input range of 0 to 10 V from a signal source with a range of ±10 V. Figure 2.5(b) shows a circuit that performs the translation.

Sign magnitude. Sign magnitude uses two parts for the code, the magnitude and the sign bit. The code for a negative number is the same as the equivalent positive number except that the sign bit is set (0 for positive and 1 for negative). This code is particularly useful when the input signals vary around zero, because the bit transitions are small near zero. This minimizes large spikes due to bits changing at the same time.

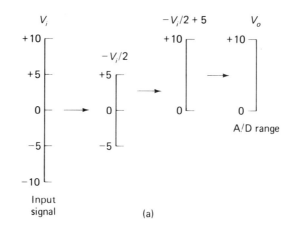

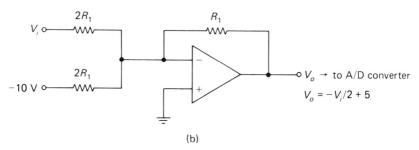

FIGURE 2.5 Translation of an input signal range to the proper range for an A/D converter. (a) The input signal range is halved and a dc offset is added. (b) Circuit to perform the range translation.

One problem with the sign-magnitude code is that these converters are comparatively expensive and difficult to use with 2's-complement microprocessors. Also, at zero there is a problem because there are two different binary codes for zero (negative and positive zero). Removing the ambiguity of the zeros requires hardware or software.

One's complement. One's-complement representation is sometimes used in computers, but 2's complement is predominant in microprocessors. The negative equivalent of a number is formed by complementing each bit of the number. An example is 3 (0011), which has a 1's complement of (1100). Subtraction is performed by adding numbers of opposite sign. Unlike 2's-complement arithmetic, where the carry bit is discarded, the carry bit in 1's complement is added to the total, an operation called "end-around carry." An example is $4 + (-3)$, or $0100 + 1100 = 0000 + 1 = 0001$ (or 1).

As in the case of the sign-magnitude code, there are two different representations for zero (0000 and 1111). Removal of the ambiguity of the zeros requires hardware or software. One's complement is not as easily implemented as is 2's complement. Usually, it is converted to 2's complement and then used on 2's-complement microcomputers.

Code conversion. Often one code must be converted to another code. Figure 2.6 shows relationships for converting among the four bipolar codes.

To Convert From ☞ To ↓ ☞	Sign Magnitude	2's Complement	Offset Binary	1's Complement
Sign Magnitude	NO CHANGE	If MSB = 1, complement other bits, add 00 .. 01	Complement MSB If new MSB = 1, complement other bits, add 00 .. 01	If MSB = 1, complement other bits
2's Complement	If MSB = 1, complement other bits, add 00 . . . 01	NO CHANGE	Complement MSB	If MSB = 1, add 00 . . . 01
Offset Binary	Complement MSB If new MSB = 0 complement other bits, add 00 . . . 01	Complement MSB	NO CHANGE	Complement MSB If new MSB = 0, add 00 . . . 01
1's Complement	If MSB = 1, complement other bits	If MSB = 1, add 11 . . . 11	Complement MSB If new MSB = 1, add 11 . . . 11	NO CHANGE

FIGURE 2.6 Relations among bipolar codes. [From Sheingold, D. H. (ed.). 1977. Analog–digital conversion notes. Norwood, MA: Analog Devices, Inc.]

Other codes. The four previous codes do not complete the list. Others include modified, complementary, and binary-coded-decimal codes. The primary advantage of other codes lies in their simplification of switching networks.

Sampling rates

A given signal must be sampled enough times per second to completely represent the data with an acceptable amount of error and yet not accumulate too many data points.

Sampling theorem. A primary tool for making sampling rate decisions is the sampling theorem, which is frequently misinterpreted. Properly stated, the sampling theorem says: If a continuous bandwidth-limited signal contains no frequency components higher than f_c, then the original signal can be completely recovered without distortion if it is sampled at the rate of at least $2f_c$ samples per second. Unfortunately, there seldom is a signal that contains no frequency components above any particular frequency. There is usually some sort of noise, or the transducer produces unwanted high frequencies while most of the desired information is in a small range of lower frequencies. Figure 2.7(a) shows the spectrum of ideal data after filtering with an ideal low-pass filter. Figure 2.7(b) shows the spectrum for this ideal case after sampling according to the sampling theorem. The spectrum for real data, however, looks more like Fig. 2.7(c). The frequency plot in Fig. 2.7(d) represents the spectrum of the real signal with frequency roll-off after sampling at $2f_c$ when f_c is the 3-dB point of the original signal.

We can see that the ideal sampled data of Fig. 2.7(b) do not have any overlap or "foldover" between the original signal and its sampled image, and thus there is no sampling error. However, the real data of Fig. 2.7(d) have overlap in the spectrum, which produces large sampling errors at the sampling frequency of $2f_c$. If the sampling frequency were higher, the overlap would be less because the tails of the original data and the sampling image would move farther apart and produce less overlap, hence less error. This error is called foldover or aliasing error. It is called "aliasing" because of the false frequencies that show up due to overlap.

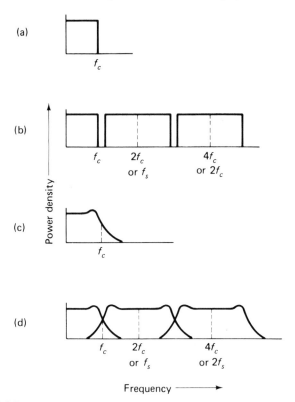

FIGURE 2.7 Frequency spectra. (a) Spectrum of ideal data and ideal filter response. (b) Spectrum of ideal sampled data. (c) Spectrum of actual data showing f_c at 3-dB corner frequency. (d) Spectrum of actual sampled data (overlap between two curves is part of the interpolation error). [From Gardenhire, L. W. 1964. Selecting sample rates. ISA J. 11 (4) : 59–64. Used with permission of ISA.]

This error shown in Fig. 2.8 is also called an error of commission. It can be reduced by placing a filter before the sampling process to attenuate the frequencies above f_c and reduce the amplitude of the overlap prior to sampling the signal.

Sometimes in the process of minimizing the errors of commission, the designer creates other errors, which can be greater. When a filter is added, there is a possibility of losing an important frequency component, an error of omission shown in Fig. 2.8.

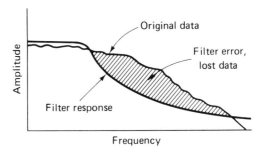

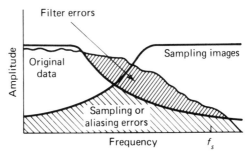

FIGURE 2.8 Filter errors (errors of omission) and sampling errors (errors of commission) for a hypothetical case. [From Macy, J., Jr. 1965. In R. W. Stacy and B. D. Waxman (eds.). Computers in biomedical research, Vol. 2. New York: Academic Press. Used with permission.]

Interpolation processes. In addition to the signal frequencies that dictate sampling rates at the input of an A/D system, we must also consider interpolation of the data at the D/A system output to reconstruct the digitized signal.

A common process is step or one-point interpolation, in which the value at the sample time is assumed to be the value of the function until the next sample time. This can cause severe errors, as shown in Fig. 2.9(a). The same signal is sampled by two channels, but at different times. The output of each of these channels is significantly different and loses some of the information content by a step interpolation. Instead of a step between each of the points we can use a straight-line or two-point interpolation to more closely approximate the original signal, as illustrated in Fig. 2.9(b).

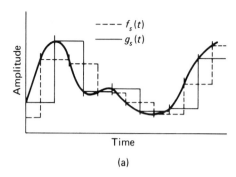

(a)

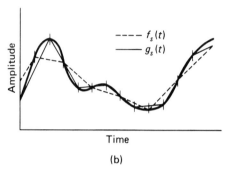

(b)

FIGURE 2.9 A continuous signal and its reconstructed approximations for samples at two different sampling times. (a) One-point interpolation. (b) Two-point interpolation. [From Macy, J., Jr. 1965. In R. W. Stacy and B. D. Waxman (eds.). Computers in biomedical research, Vol. 2. New York: Academic Press. Used with permission.]

There are also multipoint interpolation methods which compute secondary points to fill in between sampled points. Multipoint interpolation is also useful in digital filtering, if for example a value at a particular point in time is desired but sampling did not occur exactly at that point. In this case interpolation fills in blank spaces in data manipulation. Figure 2.10 shows equations for n-point interpolation. As an example of this technique, find a point V_r spaced three-fourths of the way from point $V_1 = 8$ to point $V_2 = 4$ using two-point interpolation. First compute the weighting factors:

$$W_1(t_r)|_{t_r=T_s/4} = \frac{1}{2} - \frac{T_s/4}{T_s} = \frac{1}{4}$$

$$W_2(t_r)|_{t_r=T_s/4} = \frac{1}{2} + \frac{T_s/4}{T_s} = \frac{3}{4}$$

Then multiply these weighting factors by the sampled data points:

$$V_r = W_1V_1 + W_2V_2 = (\tfrac{1}{4})8 + (\tfrac{3}{4})4 = 5$$

One Point

$W(t_r) = 1$

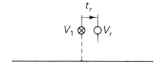

Two Points given

$W_1(t_r) = 1/2 - t_r/T_s$

$W_2(t_r) = 1/2 + t_r/T_s$

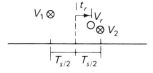

Three points given

$W_1(t_r) = -1/2(t_r/T_s) + 1/2(t_r/T_s)^2$

$W_2(t_r) = 1 - (t_r/T_s)^2$

$W_3(t_r) = 1/2(t_r/T_s) + 1/2(t_r/T_s)^2$

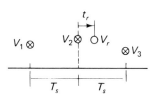

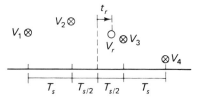

Four points given

$W_1(t_r) = -1/16 + 1/24(t_r/T_s) + 1/4(t_r/T_s)^2 - 1/6(t_r/T_s)^3$

$W_2(t_r) = 9/16 - 9/8(t_r/T_s) - 1/4(t_r/T_s)^2 + 1/2(t_r/T_s)^3$

$W_3(t_r) = 9/16 + 9/8(t_r/T_s) - 1/4(t_r/T_s)^2 - 1/2(t_r/T_s)^3$

$W_4(t_r) = -1/16 - 1/24(t_r/T_s) + 1/4(t_r/T_s)^2 + 1/6(t_r/T_s)^3$

Note: Weighting factors
       restricted to
          $-T_s/2 < t_r < T_s/2$

$V_r = \sum\limits_{i=1}^{n} W_i \cdot V_i$

FIGURE 2.10 Near-optimum weighting factors for digital multipoint interpolation. (From Gardenhire, L. W. 1970. Sampling and source encoding. Melbourne, FL: Consultant. Used with permission.)

This procedure can be expanded to more points and thus less errors, but the higher orders of interpolation require more number processing, hence more computer time.

Another method of signal reconstruction from sampled data is a combination of one-point interpolation and analog low-pass filtering. The D/A converter produces a step-function output as shown in Fig. 2.11. A filter then smoothes the converter's output to reconstruct the original continuous signal.

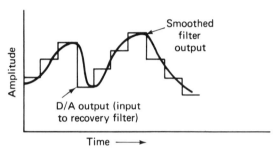

FIGURE 2.11 Smoothing the D/A converter's output in the recovery filter. (From Rockland Systems. 1976. The application of filters to analog and digital signal processing. Used with permission.)

2.2 DIGITAL-TO-ANALOG CONVERTERS

A block diagram of a D/A converter is given in Fig. 2.12. It has a register where the input binary code is held, a set of switches that are controlled by the register, and a resistor network in which different combinations of the resistors are selected by the switches. In the conversion process, a microcomputer supplies a parallel binary word to input lines I1 to I12 (I8 for an 8-bit converter) and issues a signal on

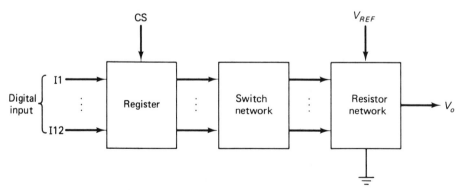

FIGURE 2.12 Block diagram of a 12-bit D/A converter.

the chip select (CS) line which latches the binary word into the register. This word controls the selection of resistors in the resistor network to hold the output voltage V_o constant until the next word is latched by a signal on CS. The resistor network has a user-supplied reference voltage V_{REF} which controls the range of the analog output voltage V_o.

D/A converter circuits

Figure 2.13 shows one type of D/A converter. Each resistor supplies a binary-weight increment of current $E_{\text{REF}}/(2^n \cdot 5 \text{ k}\Omega)$ to the summing junction of an operational amplifier. The output voltage is proportional to the current into this summing junction. In a 12-bit D/A converter, the range of resistors goes from $2^1 \cdot 5 \text{ k}\Omega$ or 10 kΩ to $2^{12} \cdot 5 \text{ k}\Omega$ or 20 MΩ, a range of 2048 : 1. Such a large range of resistor values is impractical in a monolithic integrated circuit.

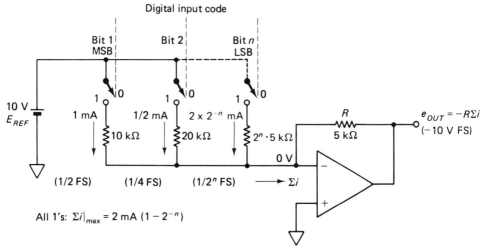

FIGURE 2.13 Simple D/A converter. [From Sheingold, D. H. (ed.). 1977. Analog–digital conversion notes. Norwood, MA: Analog Devices, Inc.]

Figure 2.14 shows another type of D/A converter which has a more limited range of resistor values in an *R–2R* ladder network. This type of network is very popular because it is not as sensitive to resistor tolerances as others, and it can be constructed out of two values of resistors. With the combination of resistors in this way, the Thèvenin equivalents of each bit are found to be binary-weighted. Figure 2.14(c) shows an example equivalent circuit for a binary input of 0100.

D/A conversion errors. Figure 2.15(a) shows the ideal relationship between the digital input and the analog output. This three-bit converter can have only eight

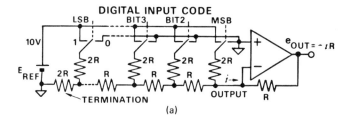

(a)

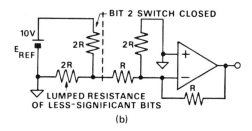

(b)

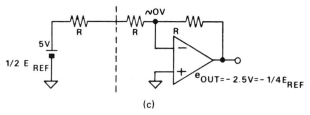

(c)

FIGURE 2.14   D/A converter using an *R–2R* ladder network in the current mode. (a) Basic circuit. (b) Example: Contribution of bit 2; all other bits "0." (c) Simplified equivalent circuit of (b). [From Sheingold, D. H. (ed.). 1977. Analog–digital conversion notes. Norwood, MA: Analog Devices, Inc.]

different voltage levels. These voltage levels are represented as bars to show that no other voltages can exist. This inability to represent any voltage desired is called resolution error. It is possible to represent a particular voltage to within $\pm\frac{1}{2}$ LSB of the full scale.

The D/A converter can have other errors, including offset error, scale factor error, nonlinearity, and nonmonotonicity. Figure 2.15(b) shows that offset error occurs when the D/A output is not zero for the digital code of zero. If the range does not go from zero to $2^n - 1$, then there is a scale-factor error, as shown in Fig. 2.15(c). Nonlinearity occurs when the differences between the bars is not uniform, as in Fig. 2.15(d). Figure 2.15(e) shows errors due to nonmonotonicity. Nonmonotonicity means that higher-weight binary codes produce lower analog output voltages than do lower-weight binary codes.

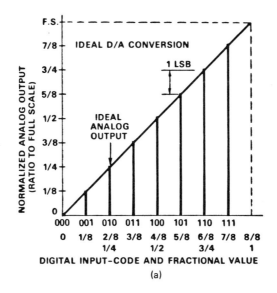

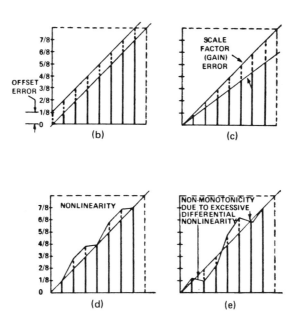

FIGURE 2.15 Conversion relationship in a 3-bit D/A converter and typical sources of error. (a) Ideal relationship. (b) Offset error. (c) Scale-factor error. (d) Linearity error. (e) Nonmonotonicity. [From Sheingold, D. H. (ed.). 1977. Analog–digital conversion notes. Norwood, MA: Analog Devices, Inc.]

2.3 ANALOG-TO-DIGITAL CONVERTERS

As in the case of D/A converters, this discussion describes the characteristics and limitations of A/D converters and is not intended to be a guide to the design of a converter. We anticipate that the user will select a commercially available unit.

In the A/D converter circuit of Fig. 2.16, the analog signal to be converted is connected to V_{IN}. A reference voltage V_{REF} provided by the user determines the range of the input voltage V_{IN}. A clock signal must be provided to control the internal circuitry of the converter. Typically, a microprocessor controls the conversion process by raising the START line from low to high. Since the conversion process does not occur instantaneously, the binary code for the input analog signal does not appear immediately on digital output lines 01 through 012 (08 in an 8-bit converter). The BUSY line is provided to signal the microprocessor when a conversion has been completed. BUSY stays low during the conversion process and goes high when valid data are available. Since there are more than eight output lines and the typical 8-bit processor can only access eight lines simultaneously, the output is divided into two segments. Output of the least-significant 8 bits (low byte) is controlled by the low-byte enable (LBE) line and the most-significant 4 bits (high byte) is controlled by the high-byte enable (HBE). When LBE and HBE are low, the output lines (01 to 012) are in a high-impedance state—in effect disconnected from the microcomputer system. By selectively raising LBE or HBE, the microprocessor removes the high-impedance state and connects to either the low or high byte, so that it can read the converted value. The control lines HBE, LBE, and BUSY permit the microprocessor to synchronize itself with the converter for data acquisition.

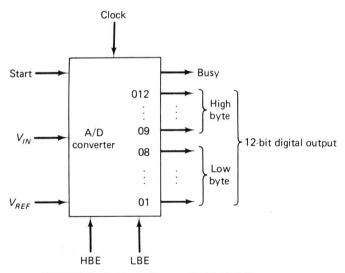

FIGURE 2.16 Block diagram of a 12-bit A/D converter.

Analog-to-digital converter circuits

Some A/D converter circuits contain a D/A converter. We discuss a number of different types of converters to illustrate the advantages of each.

Flash or parallel converter. The parallel converter shown in Fig. 2.17 is comparatively fast, with rates up to 25 MHz for 4-bit conversions. Comparators are biased 1 LSB apart by reference voltages. An input voltage is applied to all the comparators. The comparators biased above this input voltage are turned off while those below are turned on. The outputs of the comparators go to a decoder, which yields a binary number representing the analog input voltage.

This method uses $2^n - 1$ comparators in an n-bit converter. Thus 8-bit and 10-bit converters need 255 and 1023 comparators, respectively. Medical instrumentation does not use the parallel A/D converter because of the large number of

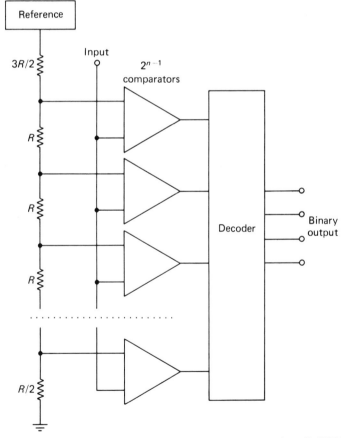

FIGURE 2.17 Parallel A/D converter. (Compliments of Datel-Intersil, 1978.)

comparators necessary and the lack of a requirement for such high-speed conversion.

Dual-slope integrating converter.　The dual-slope integrating converter converts the input voltage to a time interval which is then measured by a counter. This converter shown in Fig. 2.18 is widely used in digital voltmeters. The input is applied to an integrator. During the integration time T_1, a counter counts a clock frequency to a predetermined number, then resets the counter. Then the switch is thrown so that the circuit integrates a reference voltage until the integrator reaches zero. During this time T_2, the counter counts clock pulses and displays the count at the end of T_2. The counter then indicates the input voltage $E_i = (T_2/T_1)V_R$.

There are a number of advantages to this method. One advantage is the variable resolution obtainable. It is possible to have a larger counter and speed up the clock to achieve better resolution. Because of the integration process it is possible to get an excellent noise rejection by setting T_1 equal to a multiple of the period of the interfering noise. The obvious disadvantage is the long conversion time, making it suitable only for slowly changing signals such as temperatures.

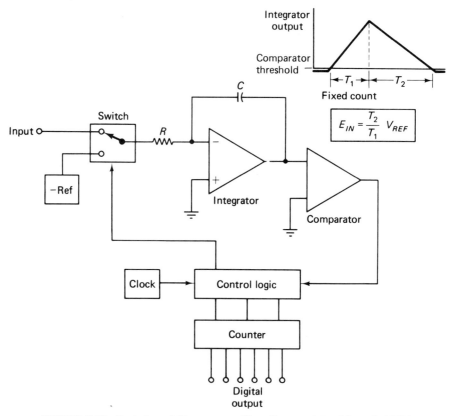

FIGURE 2.18　Dual-slope A/D converter. (Compliments of Datel-Intersil, 1978.)

Counter or servo converters. The counter converter is simple in principle and very inexpensive. Figure 2.19 shows that it includes a D/A converter which produces an analog output proportional to the contents of a counter. The conversion cycle starts by resetting the counter to zero. The digital counter then increments with each clock cycle, causing the output of the D/A converter to increase. When the D/A output is equal to or greater than the analog input voltage, the comparator signals the control logic to stop incrementing the counter. The output of the D/A converter shown in Fig. 2.20 is a step ramp which stops at the value of the input voltage.

Because the simple up-counter converter takes a long time for each conversion, an up-down counter can be used to track the input level, as shown in Fig. 2.21. Because of the counting process, counter converters are relatively slow and are not suitable for signals such as the ECG, EEG, and EMG, which have rapid amplitude transitions.

Voltage-to-frequency converter. A voltage-to-frequency converter (VFC), such as the LM331, provides an output train of pulses at a frequency proportional to input current or voltage (Pease, 1979). A counter accumulates the pulse count for a fixed period. High resolution is possible, since a 100-kHz converter counted for 2 s yields 18-bit resolution. Relative accuracy is good over a wide range of input voltages. VFCs require only two wires for transmission, because the two wires can carry both the excitation voltage and the output pulse train (Sheingold, 1977). However, VFCs are slow, they do not provide handshaking, and their asynchronous operation ties up the transmission line.

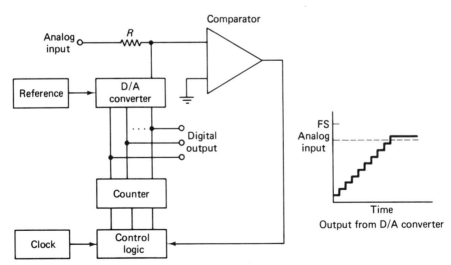

FIGURE 2.19 Counter or servo-type A/D converter. (Compliments of Datel-Intersil, 1978.)

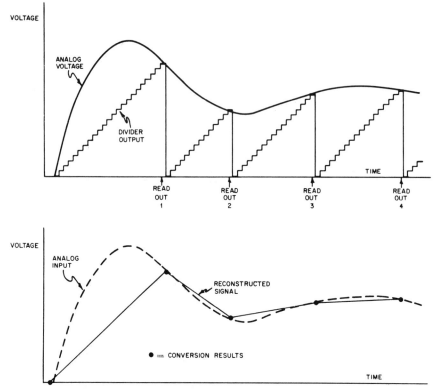

FIGURE 2.20 Counter converter output. (From Digital Equipment Corporation. 1964. Analog–digital conversion handbook. Maynard, MA. Used with permission.)

Successive approximation converter. The successive approximation converter shown in Fig. 2.22 is the most popular type of A/D converter for biomedical applications because it combines speed and simplicity and operates with a fixed conversion time which is independent of the amplitude of the analog input. It operates by approximating the analog input signal with a binary code and successively revising this code for each bit in the code until the best approximation is achieved. At each step in the approximation, the current estimate of the binary value of the analog input signal is saved in a special register called the successive approximation register. The contents of this register are converted to an analog signal by the D/A converter so that the comparator can determine whether the approximation is larger or smaller than the input signal. As shown in Fig. 2.23 for a 4-bit converter, the first approximation sets the MSB of the successive approximation register and resets all the other bits. If the D/A output is smaller than the input the MSB is left on and the next bit is tested. If the D/A output is larger, the MSB is turned off and the next bit tested. Each successive bit is similarly tested. After the LSB is tested, the conversion is complete and the output register contains the binary code. The same technique is used for 8, 10, or 12 bits.

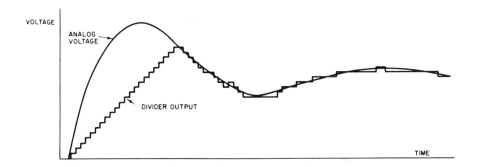

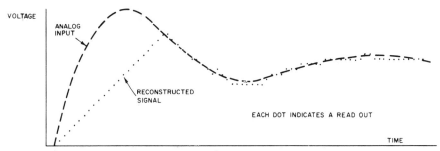

FIGURE 2.21 Up-down counter converter. (From Digital Equipment Corporation. 1964. Analog–digital conversion handbook. Maynard, MA. Used with permission.)

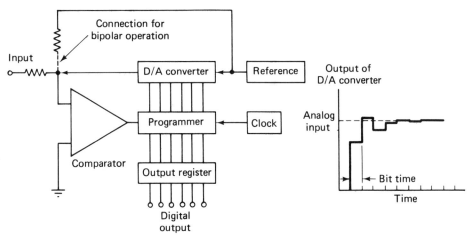

FIGURE 2.22 Successive approximation A/D converter. (Compliments of Datel-Intersil, 1978.)

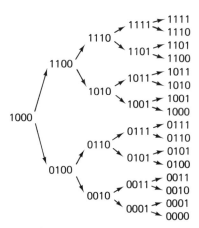

FIGURE 2.23   Operation diagram for a 4-bit successive approximation converter.

Because the bit decisions are made in serial order, some converters provide a serial output on a single line in addition to the parallel binary code. Some converters provide conversion rates up to 100 ns per bit. The input voltage must change very slowly to eliminate errors due to a changing signal during the conversion time. Therefore, a sample-and-hold circuit discussed later frequently precedes the A/D converter.

A/D conversion errors.   Figure 2.24(a) is a graph of the relationship between the analog input and the digital output for an ideal 3-bit A/D converter. We assume that all analog values exist, and we must quantize them by dividing the continuous analog range into eight discrete steps. The ideal analog value for a particular digital code is the center of the range which that code represents.

As in the D/A converter, the A/D converter has an error caused by the inability to represent any voltage exactly. In the conversion process, it is only possible to resolve to within a quantization uncertainty of $\pm\frac{1}{2}$ LSB of full scale. With a 12-bit converter we can resolve or quantize to 1 part in 4096, or 0.024% of full scale (see Fig. 2.3). A converter with a 10-V full scale could resolve a 2.4-mV input change. Resolution or quantization is a design parameter describing the precision of both D/A and A/D converters.

As in the case of the D/A converter, the A/D converter has offset, scale factor, nonlinearity, and nonmonotonicity errors. Figure 2.24(b) shows that offset error is present when the digital output transition from 000 to 001 occurs at an analog value other than $+\frac{1}{2}$ LSB of full scale. When a full-scale analog input signal does not produce the full range of digital output codes, there is a scale factor (or gain) error, as shown in Fig. 2.24(c). If the values between transitions are not equal, these errors, shown in Fig. 2.24(d), are called nonlinearities. Figure 2.24(e) shows that if the differential nonlinearity is excessive, it is possible to miss some codes. This last error is similar to nonmonotonicity error of D/A conversion. As

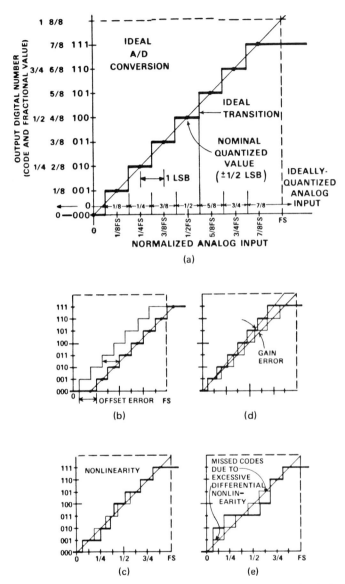

FIGURE 2.24 Conversion relationships in a 3-bit A/D converter and typical sources of error. (a) Ideal relationship. (b) Offset error. (c) Scale-factor error. (d) Linearity error. (e) Missed codes (due to excessive differential nonlinearity). [From Sheingold, D. H. (ed.). 1977. Analog-digital conversion notes. Norwood, MA : Analog Devices, Inc.]

the analog value increases, the code should change at the transition values, but does not and instead keeps the same code or jumps to the wrong code.

Shaft encoders. A shaft encoder is a mechanical device for converting shaft angle directly to a binary code. Angles of transducer arms in ultrasonic and radiological imaging devices were previously measured by potentiometers. Because of inaccuracy and unreliability caused by wear, potentiometers are being replaced by shaft encoders. Figure 2.25 shows that the encoding is done by a coding wheel and optical sensors. The light areas on the wheel are transparent and the dark areas are opaque. Thus the presence or absence of light generates the digital information.

If the edge of a shaded area is slightly misaligned, a false intermediate code can be generated when the shaft turns from one angle to the next. For example, the code 011 could become 111 momentarily if the MSB shading were misaligned. Since these patterns are diagonally opposite on the coding wheel, there is a transient error in output code of 180°. Such transition ambiguities are eliminated using the 3-bit Gray code wheel of Fig. 2.26. Since the Gray code has only one bit transition between angular codes, only codes for adjacent angles can be produced as the shaft rotates. Figure 2.27 compares bit changes for 4-bit Gray and binary encoders, and Fig. 2.28 lists the two codes.

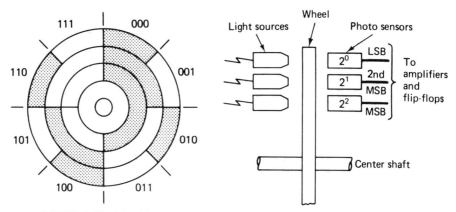

FIGURE 2.25 3-bit binary code wheel. (From Malvino, A. P., and Leach, D. P. 1981. Digital principles and applications, 3rd ed. © McGraw-Hill. Reproduced with permission.)

2.4 OTHER PARTS OF AN ANALOG-TO-DIGITAL SYSTEM

The data acquisition system usually includes parts other than the D/A converter and the A/D converter. As shown in Fig. 2.1, it also may include amplifiers, active filters, sample-and-hold circuits, and analog multiplexers.

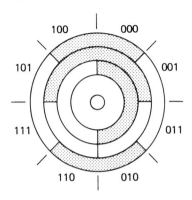

FIGURE 2.26 Gray code wheel. (From Malvino, A. P., and Leach, D. P., 1981. Digital principles and applications, 3rd ed. © McGraw-Hill. Reproduced with permission.)

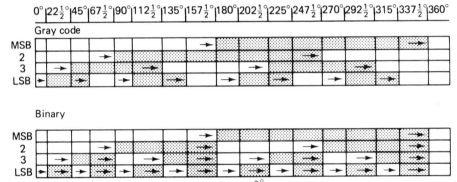

Note: Quantized angles are indicated value $\pm 11\frac{3}{4}^{\circ}$

FIGURE 2.27 Results of Gray versus binary encoder. [From Sheingold, D. H. (ed.). 1977. Analog–digital conversion notes. Norwood, MA: Analog Devices, Inc.]

Amplifiers

Amplifiers are usually necessary to translate small signals to the operating range of an A/D converter. A/D converters typically require an input of ± 10 V, ± 5 V, 0 to 10 V, or 0 to 20 V. Figure 1.9 shows a circuit that amplifies the ECG to a high-enough signal level to make use of the full operating range of an A/D converter. Instrumentation amplifiers also provide high rejection of common-mode voltages to minimize electrical interference.

Filters are used to limit the bandwidth of the processed signal in order to eliminate frequency folding and to reduce natural and man-made noise. Section 3.1 presents the design of several types of analog filters.

Decimal	Binary code	Gray code	Angle (degrees)
0	0 0 0 0	0 0 0 0	0.0
1	0 0 0 1	0 0 0 1	22.5
2	0 0 1 0	0 0 1 1	45.0
3	0 0 1 1	0 0 1 0	57.5
4	0 1 0 0	0 1 1 0	90.0
5	0 1 0 1	0 1 1 1	112.5
6	0 1 1 0	0 1 0 1	135.0
7	0 1 1 1	0 1 0 0	157.5
8	1 0 0 0	1 1 0 0	180.0
9	1 0 0 1	1 1 0 1	202.5
10	1 0 1 0	1 1 1 1	225.0
11	1 0 1 1	1 1 1 0	247.5
12	1 1 0 0	1 0 1 0	270.0
13	1 1 0 1	1 0 1 1	292.5
14	1 1 1 0	1 0 0 1	315.0
15	1 1 1 1	1 0 0 0	337.5

FIGURE 2.28 The Gray and binary codes. Underlines indicate the bits which change in sequential codes demonstrating the single bit transitions of the Gray code.

Analog multiplexers

Analog multiplexers are used to time share a single A/D converter among a number of analog channels. The multiplexer is a group of semiconductor switches (usually MOSFETs) arranged to provide a number of individual analog input channels and a single common output. The switches close one at a time to sequentially connect each input to the output. Each switch is controlled by a unique digital code.

With the cost of single-chip A/D converters decreasing, some system designs may benefit from the placement of an A/D converter at each analog input, which eliminates the need for a multiplexer. In this case, lower-speed A/D converters may be used.

There are a variety of multiplexers available with different characteristics such as operating speed and number of input channels. Some have special enable or inhibit lines to turn all the switches off so that they can be cascaded together. Because of nonideal transmission and open-circuit characteristics, analog multiplexers produce both static and dynamic errors. A multiplexer should be able to absorb line transients and overload conditions. A desirable feature is a break-before-make action to prevent shorting out channels.

There are a number of important parameters to look for in defining an analog multiplexer, including transfer accuracy, settling time, throughput rate, crosstalk, and input leakage current.

Transfer accuracy. Transfer accuracy is the percent error of the output compared to the input.

Settling time. Settling time is the time it takes for the output of the multiplexer to settle to within a defined error band after it has switched channels.

Throughput rate. Throughput rate is the highest rate that a multiplexer can switch from channel to channel and still maintain its specified accuracy. This rate is highly dependent upon the settling time.

Crosstalk. Crosstalk is caused by coupling between the off channels and the conducting channel. It is given as a percentage of full scale of the input signal on the conducting channel.

Input leakage current. Input leakage current is the current that flows into or out of an off channel input terminal due to nonideal switches.

Sample-and-hold circuit

A sample-and-hold circuit samples a signal upon command and holds the sampled value until the next command. It is used to hold the sampled value constant at the input of an A/D converter long enough so that it can be converted without error. This feature is particularly desirable on successive approximation converters, as the input should not change while the conversion is in process. For D/A conversion the sample and hold can hold the output constant to remove glitches that may appear between bit transitions.

An ideal sample-and-hold circuit consists of a switch and a capacitor, as shown in Fig. 2.29. When the switch is closed it is in the sampling mode. When the switch is open, the voltage is held at the output for a period of time. FET buffer amplifiers are used to limit the leakage from the capacitor. The switch is usually an FET to limit leakage during hold time.

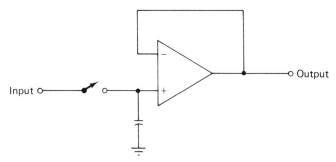

FIGURE 2.29 Schematic of ideal sample-and-hold circuit.

Each sample-and-hold circuit is characterized by a number of specifications, including acquisition time, aperture time, aperture uncertainty time, decay rate, and feed through.

Acquisition time.   Acquisition time is the time needed from the start of the sample command to charge the capacitor to the input voltage.

Aperture time.   Aperture time is the time delay (reaction time) from the start of the hold command until the time the output is actually held at the new value.

Aperture uncertainty time.   Aperture uncertainty time is the difference between maximum and minimum aperture time.

Decay rate.   Decay rate is a constant rate of change in the hold voltage caused by leakage from the storage capacitor.

Feed through.   In the hold mode, feed through is leakage from the input signal to the output. It varies with signal frequency and is expressed as a percentage of the input signal.

2.5   SYSTEMS AND SPECIFICATIONS

Data acquisition systems suitable for use with microcomputers are available in the form of modular hybrid circuits, single-chip integrated circuits, and single board systems. These systems may include multiplexers, sample-and-hold circuits, and A/D and D/A converter circuits to provide both analog input and output capabilities.

The modular hybrid circuits typically are designed for general application with several microcomputers. An A/D system in this type of technology typically includes a multiplexer, an A/D converter, and tristate output buffers for direct connection to a microcomputer bus.

Most single-chip integrated circuits include only the A/D or D/A converter itself or a multiplexer or a tristate buffer. However, there is at least one single-chip LSI data acquisition system on the market (National Semiconductor ADC0816/ADC0817) that includes an 8-bit A/D converter, a 16-channel multiplexer, and a tristate output buffer. More such LSI chips are being developed.

Single board systems are available, but they are generally designed specifically for use with only one microcomputer. Such systems generally include complete analog input/output capabilities with multiplexers, sample-and-hold circuits, A/D and D/A converters, and tristate buffers. They also include clock circuits for sampling-rate control and voltage translation circuits for adjusting A/D and D/A voltage levels for microcomputer compatibility. The general applicability of these systems make them useful for development of new applications. Since they are complete working systems, they frequently save design and troubleshooting time.

Sheingold (1977) provides factors for choosing data conversion components, application checklists, definitions of terms, and examples of converter selections.

REFERENCES

DATEL. 1978. Modules for data conversion. Bulletin CDA-J50807. Canton, MA.

DIGITAL EQUIPMENT. 1964. Analog-digital conversion handbook. Maynard, MA.

GARDENHIRE, L. W. 1964. Selecting sample rates. ISA J. 11(4): 59–64.

GARDENHIRE, L. W. 1970. Sampling and source encoding. Melbourne, FL: Radiation, Inc., Systems Div.

GARRETT, P. H. 1978. Analog systems for microprocessors and minicomputers. Reston, VA: Reston.

MACY, J., JR. 1965. In STACY, R. W., AND WAXMAN, B. D. (EDS.). Computers in bio-medical research, Vol. 2. New York: Academic Press.

MALVINO, A. P., AND LEACH, D. P. 1981. Digital principles and applications, 3rd ed. New York: McGraw-Hill.

PEASE, R. A. 1979. Designing V-f converters to handle bipolar signals. Electronics. 52: 139–145.

ROCKLAND SYSTEMS. 1976. The application of filters to analog and digital signal processing. West Nyack, NY.

SHEINGOLD, D. H. (ED.). 1977. Analog-digital conversion notes. Norwood, MA: Analog Devices, Inc.

ZUCH, E. L. 1977. Where and when to use which data converter. IEEE Spectrum 14(6): 39–42.

PROBLEMS

2.1 Give the decimal equivalent of these binary numbers.
  (a) 10001—2's complement
  (b) 00000—1's complement
  (c) 10000—offset binary
  (d) 10000—sign magnitude
  (e) 0011 0101—binary-coded decimal
  (f) 11111—ordinary binary
  (g) 11111—2's complement
  (h) 11111—offset binary

2.2 Give the voltage equivalents of the binary numbers in Problem 2.1 if the full-scale voltage range is ± 5 V.

2.3 Why is the successive approximation ADC faster than the counter converter for the same clock speeds?

2.4 What is the resolution of a 10-bit shaft encoder in degrees?

2.5 For an 8-bit counter ADC, what should be the clock rate for a conversion speed of 8 k samples/s?

2.6 Describe how the Gray code reduces ambiguity in an optical shaft encoder.

2.7 Design a 4-bit binary-ladder DAC with a 1-mA current in the MSB resistor and a 5-V full-scale output voltage.

2.8 Why is it not desirable to put the LSB on the innermost ring of an optical encoder?

2.9 Why is the sampling theorem alone not adequate to establish the proper sampling rate for a signal? What other considerations are involved?

2.10 What techniques can be used to reduce aliasing problems in a data acquisition system?

2.11 For an ADC with a full-scale input range of 5 V, how many bits are required to assure resolution of 0.5-mV signal levels?

3

Signal Processing—
Hardware versus Software

In analyzing physiological signals, we often must separate the signal from background noise such as 60-Hz interference. We may wish to extract some particular feature of a signal such as the QRS complex of the ECG. Filters are devices that perform these functions by attenuating unwanted frequencies. An analog filter processes the signal in analog form—the signal is always continuous. In a digital filter, the signal is sampled to convert it to a sequence of numbers so that it can be processed using a digital computer. We review in this chapter analog and digital approaches to common signal-processing techniques. These techniques are filtering, differentiation, integration, Fourier transformation, and peak and valley detection. We illustrate each technique with a biomedical application.

There are a number of books on analog and digital signal processing listed in the reference section of this chapter, each with its own strengths and weaknesses. The one that best expands on the concepts presented here is Lam (1979).

3.1 FILTERS*

This section presents the basic principles of analog and digital filters and shows how to design some of the more common types.

Analog filters

The term "analog filter" refers both to passive filters and electronic active filters. Active filters are used almost exclusively in signal processing because of the high performance and low cost of their active element, the operational amplifier. Therefore, we will not discuss passive filters.

First-order filters. Figure 3.1 shows three common first-order filters—low-pass, bandpass, and high-pass. For the low-pass filter the transfer function has the form

$$\frac{v_o}{v_i} = -\frac{R_f}{R_i(1 + j\omega\tau)}$$

where $\tau = R_f C_f$. The corner frequency is given by

$$f_2 = \frac{1}{2\pi\tau} = \frac{1}{2\pi R_f C_f}$$

Figure 3.2(a) shows the frequency response for this filter.

The high-pass transfer function has the form

$$\frac{v_o}{v_i} = -\frac{R_f}{R_i}\frac{j\omega\tau}{1 + j\omega\tau}$$

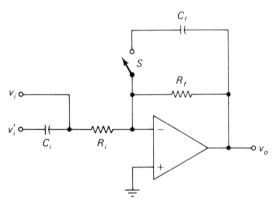

FIGURE 3.1 First-order active filter. With switch S open and input at v_i, the circuit is an inverter with the gain of $-R_f/R_i$. When S is closed, the circuit is a low-pass filter. When S is closed and the input is applied to v_i', the circuit is a bandpass filter. When S is open and the input is applied to v_i', the circuit is a high-pass filter.

---

*Section 3.1 written by Willis J. Tompkins and Hossein Baharestani.

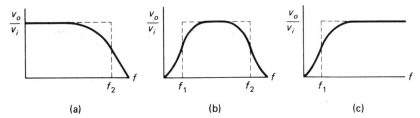

FIGURE 3.2 Frequency response of first-order filters. (a) Low-pass. (b) Bandpass. (c) High-pass.

where $\tau = R_i C_i$ and the corner frequency is $f_1 = 1/(2\pi\tau) = 1/(2\pi R_i C_i)$. Figure 3.2(c) shows the frequency response.

Combining the two filters into one yields the bandpass filter, with corner frequencies defined above and a frequency response shown in Fig. 3.2(b).

Higher-order filters. To obtain a higher rate of attenuation, higher-order filters should be used. We present here the two most common types of higher-order filters—Butterworth and Chebyshev. Johnson (1976) presents additional underlying theory, and Johnson and Hilburn (1975) present rapid design methods and tables.

Butterworth filters. The amplitude of the transfer function of a low-pass Butterworth filter is given by

$$|H(j\omega)| = \frac{G}{\sqrt{1 + (\omega/\omega_c)^{2n}}} \qquad n = 1, 2, 3, \ldots$$

where n is the order of the filter. This filter has an excellent flat response at low frequencies, but its rate of attenuation in the transition band is not as large as that of the Chebyshev type. Figure 3.3 shows the amplitude and phase responses of this filter.

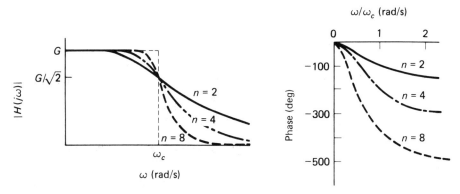

FIGURE 3.3 Butterworth amplitude and phase response. (From Johnson, D. E., and Hilburn, J. L. 1975. Rapid practical design of active filters. New York: Wiley. Used with permission.)

Chebyshev filter. For a Chebyshev low-pass filter, the amplitude is given by

$$|H(j\omega)| = \frac{A}{\sqrt{1 + \epsilon^2 C_n^2(\omega/\omega_c)}} \qquad n = 1, 2, 3, \ldots$$

where ϵ and A are constants and C_n is the Chebyshev polynomial of the first kind of degree n. Figure 3.4 shows a list of Chebyshev polynomials for $n = 0, 1, \ldots, 8$. Figure 3.5 shows examples of Chebyshev amplitude and phase responses for three values of n. The ripple width, a major drawback of Chebyshev filters, is given for $A = 1$ by

$$\mathrm{RW} = 1 - \frac{1}{\sqrt{1 + \epsilon^2}}$$

n	$C_n(\omega)$
0	1
1	ω
2	$2\omega^2 - 1$
3	$4\omega^3 - 3\omega$
4	$8\omega^4 - 8\omega^2 + 1$
5	$16\omega^5 - 20\omega^3 + 5\omega$
6	$32\omega^6 - 48\omega^4 + 18\omega^2 - 1$
7	$64\omega^7 - 112\omega^5 + 56\omega^3 - 7\omega$
8	$128\omega^8 - 256\omega^6 + 160\omega^4 - 32\omega^2 + 1$

FIGURE 3.4 Chebyshev polynomials of the first kind. (From Johnson, D. E. 1976. Introduction to filter theory. Reprinted by permission of Prentice-Hall, Inc.)

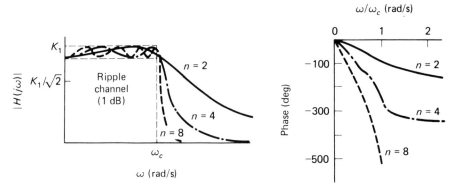

FIGURE 3.5 Chebyshev amplitude and phase responses. (From Johnson, D. E., and Hilburn, J. L. 1975. Rapid practical design of active filters. New York: Wiley. Used with permission.)

and in decibels by

$$RW_{dB} = 20 \log \sqrt{1 + \epsilon^2} = 10 \log (1 + \epsilon^2)$$

We determine ripple width by selecting ϵ, which characterizes the filter. Note that there is a trade-off in choosing one of these two filter types. Butterworth filters have a maximally flat response but a larger transition interval. Chebyshev filters have a very sharp transition from passband to stopband but have ripples in the passband. We must also consider phase response. In applications where phase response and amplitude response are both important, Chebyshev filters may not necessarily be better than Butterworth filters. In case phase response is the primary concern, a much better choice would be the Bessel filter (Johnson, 1976). Note that the same electrical circuit may serve as a Butterworth or Chebyshev filter, depending upon the selection of components.

Using frequency transformation techniques (Lindquist, 1977), a low-pass filter can be transformed to a high-pass, bandpass, or other filter. So all the theory developed for a low-pass filter prototype can also be used for other types. Figure 3.6 shows the frequency characteristics of second-order bandpass, high-pass, and bandstop filters.

Second-order low-pass filter. Figure 3.7(a) shows the Sallen and Key second-order low-pass circuit. Since the op amp and the resistors constitute a voltage-controlled voltage source (VCVS), the circuit is sometimes called a VCVS low-pass filter. The transfer function for this circuit is given by

$$\frac{v_o}{v_i} = \frac{Gb_0}{s^2 + b_1 s + b_0}$$

where

$$b_0 = \frac{1}{R_1 R_2 C_1 C} \quad \text{and} \quad b_1 = \frac{1}{R_2 C_1}(1 - \mu) + \frac{1}{R_1 C} + \frac{1}{R_2 C}$$

and $G = \mu = 1 + R_4/R_3$. Higher-order filters can be designed by cascading second-order ones. This is a popular low-pass filter with noninverting gain. It achieves a high gain, which can be adjusted by using a potentiometer for R_3 and R_4, and it has low output impedance. We can find the component values for a low-pass Butterworth filter as follows. First we select a standard value for the capacitor C. Next we find the K parameter from

$$K = \frac{10^{-4}}{f_c C}$$

We obtain the other component values from Fig. 3.7(b), given the corner frequency f_c, gain G, and order n. Since the tabulated values are for $K = 1$, we multiply each component value by K. Since some of the component values may not be

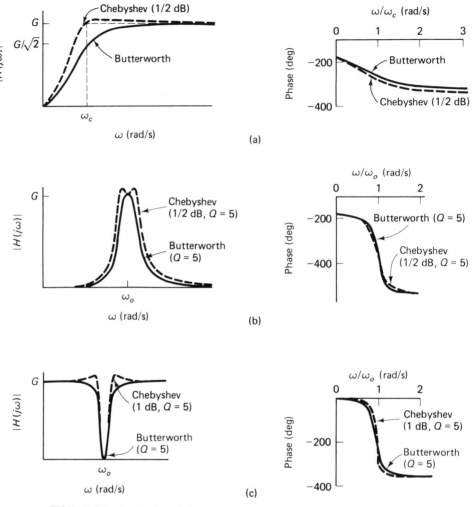

FIGURE 3.6 Amplitude and phase responses of second-order filters. (a) High-pass.
(b) Bandpass. (c) Bandstop. (From Johnson, D. E., and Hilburn, J. L. 1975. Rapid
practical design of active filters. New York: Wiley. Used with permission.)

standard, we construct the filter and check its characteristics. For higher-order
low-pass filters, as well as bandpass and high-pass, Chebyshev or Butterworth
filters, see Johnson (1976), Johnson and Hilburn (1975), and Lindquist (1977).

Twin-tee bandstop filter. We can realize a bandstop filter (also called a notch
filter) using the circuit of Fig. 3.8(a). This circuit, called a twin-tee, has a Q between
0.3 to 50 controlled by adjusting R_4. The lowest Q corresponds to the wiper of R_4
at ground. Figure 3.8(b) shows the range of adjustment of Q by changing R_4, for a
filter designed to reject 60-Hz interference. The transfer function of this filter has

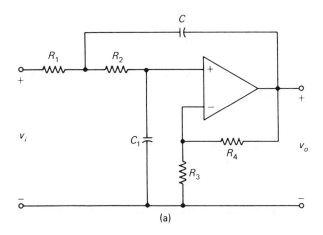

(a)

Circuit element values[a]

Gain	1	2	4	6	8	10
R_1	1.422	1.126	0.824	0.617	0.521	0.462
R_2	5.399	2.250	1.537	2.051	2.429	2.742
R_3	Open	6.752	3.148	3.203	3.372	3.560
R_4	0	6.752	9.444	16.012	23.602	32.038
C_1	0.33C	C	2C	2C	2C	2C

[a] Resistance in kilohms for a K parameter of 1.

(b)

FIGURE 3.7 Second-order low-pass Butterworth VCVS filters. (a) Gain can be adjusted by using a potentiometer for R_3 and R_4. (b) Circuit component design values. (From Johnson, D. E., and Hilburn, J. L. 1975. Rapid practical design of active filters. New York: Wiley. Used with permission.)

the form

$$\frac{v_o}{v_i} = \frac{s^3 + As^2 + Bs + C}{s^3 + Ds^2 + Es + C}$$

where the parameters A, B, C, D, and E depend upon the circuit components and can be found in Stout and Kaufman (1976). The gain is unity at both high and low frequencies and drops at the desired notch frequency. A practical way of designing this filter is as follows. Choose $R_1 = R_3$ equal to a standard value greater than 100 times the output resistance of the source. Set $R_2 = R_1/2$; C_1 and C_3 are found from

$$C_1 = C_3 = \frac{1}{4\pi f_0 R_2}$$

Set $C_2 = 2C_1$. Check f_0 for the values of the components chosen.

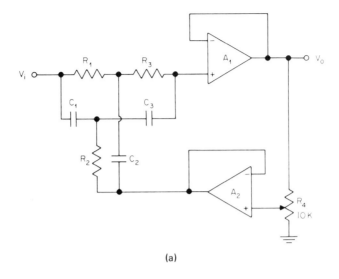

(a)

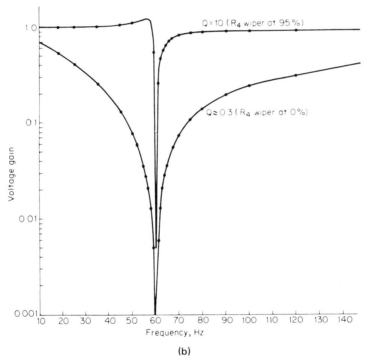

(b)

FIGURE 3.8 Twin-tee bandstop filter with adjustable Q. (a) Circuit diagram. (b) Plot of gain as a function of frequency. (From Stout, D. F., and Kaufman, M. 1976. Handbook of operational amplifier circuit design. New York: McGraw-Hill. Used with permission.)

As an example, the following values give a filter with the notch frequency of approximately 60 Hz:

$$R_1 = R_3 = 2\ \text{M}\Omega$$

$$R_2 = \frac{R_1}{2} = 1\ \text{M}\Omega$$

$$C_1 = C_3 = \frac{1}{4\pi(60)10^6} = 1320\ \text{pF}$$

$$C_2 = 2C_1 = 2640\ \text{pF}$$

$$f_0 = \frac{1}{2\pi}\left(\frac{C_1 + C_3}{C_1 C_2 C_3 R_1 R_3}\right)^{1/2} = 60.2\ \text{Hz}$$

Digital filters

A digital filter is either a digital electronic circuit or a computer program that processes samples of a signal to perform functions similar to analog filtering. Unlike the analog filter, the digital filter operates on a sequence of numbers rather than a continuous waveform. Each number in the sequence corresponds to a specific instant of time—a sampling instant when analog-to-digital (A/D) conversion occurs.

There are several advantages of digital filters over analog filters. First they have the high noise immunity of digital circuits. Second, the accuracy of a digital filter is dependent only on the roundoff error in the computer arithmetic. By appropriate programming this error can be made as small as required, whereas accuracy in analog circuits depends on component tolerances and circuit noise. Third, it is usually easier and cheaper to change the characteristics of a digital filter by changing the program or a section of it, or even entering the filter coefficients as data. Fourth, power supply and temperature variations and component aging have no effect on a program stored in a computer, so that the digital filter characteristics remain constant. This is especially important in medical applications, where most of the signals have low frequencies that might be distorted because of the drift in component values of an analog circuit. The constantly decreasing costs of minicomputers and microcomputers make it more economical to use them for filtering purposes rather than buying or building analog filters (Ackroyd, 1973).

The z transform. Chapter 2 presents the concept of sampling a continuous signal. For an A/D conversion clock period of T s/sample, we obtain a sequence of numbers, $(x(0), x(T), x(2T), x(3T), \ldots, x(kT))$. Each of these numbers corresponds to a discrete point in time; $x(0)$ occurs at $t = 0$, $x(T)$ at $t = T$, and $x(kT)$ at $t = kT$.

Without going into mathematical detail at this point, we can write what is known as the *z* transform of this sequence:

$$X(z) = x(0) + x(T)z^{-1} + x(2T)z^{-2} + \ldots + x(kT)z^{-k} \qquad (3.1)$$

or, in general,

$$X(z) = \sum_{n=0}^{\infty} x(nT)z^{-n}$$

Given any sequence such as

$$(\tfrac{1}{4}, \tfrac{1}{2}, \tfrac{1}{4})$$

we can immediately write its z transform:

$$H(z) = \tfrac{1}{4} + (\tfrac{1}{2})z^{-1} + (\tfrac{1}{4})z^{-2}$$

As we will see, the z transform is important in digital filtering because it describes the sampling process and plays a role in the digital domain similar to that of the Laplace transform in analog filtering.

In general, the z transform of any sequence

$$(f(0), f(T), f(2T), f(3T), \ldots, f(kT))$$

is

$$F(z) = f(0) + f(T)z^{-1} + f(2T)z^{-2} + \ldots + f(kT)z^{-k} = \sum_{n=0}^{\infty} f(nT)z^{-n} \qquad (3.2)$$

We can write the z transform for the discrete-time function analogous to a continuous-time function by substituting nT for t and finding $F(z)$ using eq. (3.2). Figure 3.9 shows examples of discrete-time signals analogous to common continuous-time signals. To find the z transform of the unit pulse of Fig. 3.9(a), which is analogous to a Dirac delta function, we note that it has a value only for $n = 0$. Therefore, we can see from the equation that its transform is $F(z) = f(0) = 1$. The unit step of Fig. 3.9(b) is unity for all positive integer values of n (n is always a positive integer in these discussions). Thus

$$F(z) = 1 + z^{-1} + z^{-2} + z^{-3} + \ldots$$

The z transform of a unit step is then a polynomial with an infinite number of terms. We can convert this polynomial to a more convenient form using the binomial theorem, which is

$$1 + v + v^2 + v^3 + \ldots = \frac{1}{1 - v}$$

If we let $v = z^{-1}$ in this equation, we see that the z transform of the unit step becomes

$$F(z) = \frac{1}{1 - z^{-1}}$$

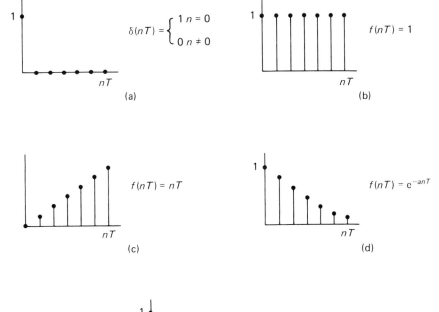

FIGURE 3.9 Discrete-time functions. All are equal to zero for $n < 0$. Variable n is an integer. (a) Unit impulse. (b) Unit step. (c) Ramp. (d) Decaying exponential. (e) Cosinusoid.

As a final example, let us find the z transform of the decaying exponential of Fig. 3.9(d). In this case

$$F(z) = 1 + e^{-aT}z^{-1} + e^{-2aT}z^{-2} + \cdots$$

Let us again apply the binomial theorem with $v = e^{-aT}z^{-1}$, giving the transform for the exponential

$$F(z) = \frac{1}{1 - e^{-aT}z^{-1}}$$

In general, we can use this technique to find the z transform analogous to any continuous-time function. The transforms that we have derived here and those of other common discrete-time functions are summarized in Fig. 3.10.

$f(t)$ for $t>0$	$F(s)$	$f(nT)$ for $nT>0$	$F(z)$
1 (unit step)	$\dfrac{1}{s}$	1	$\dfrac{1}{1-z^{-1}}$
t	$\dfrac{1}{s^2}$	nT	$\dfrac{Tz^{-1}}{(1-z^{-1})^2}$
e^{-at}	$\dfrac{1}{s+a}$	e^{-anT}	$\dfrac{1}{1-e^{-aT}z^{-1}}$
te^{-at}	$\dfrac{1}{(s+a)^2}$	nTe^{-anT}	$\dfrac{Te^{-aT}z^{-1}}{(1-e^{-aT}z^{-1})^2}$
$\sin \omega_c t$	$\dfrac{\omega_c}{s^2+\omega_c^2}$	$\sin n\omega_c T$	$\dfrac{(\sin \omega_c T)z^{-1}}{1-2(\cos \omega_c T)z^{-1}+z^{-2}}$
$\cos \omega_c t$	$\dfrac{s}{s^2+\omega_c^2}$	$\cos n\omega_c T$	$\dfrac{1-(\cos \omega_c T)z^{-1}}{1-2(\cos \omega_c T)z^{-1}+z^{-2}}$
$e^{-at}\sin \omega_c t$	$\dfrac{\omega_c}{(s+a)^2+\omega_c^2}$	$e^{-anT}\sin n\omega_c T$	$\dfrac{e^{-aT}(\sin \omega_c T)z^{-1}}{1-2e^{-aT}(\cos \omega_c T)z^{-1}+e^{-2aT}z^{-2}}$
$e^{-at}\cos \omega_c t$	$\dfrac{s+a}{(s+a)^2+\omega_c^2}$	$e^{-anT}\cos n\omega_c T$	$\dfrac{1-e^{-aT}(\cos \omega_c T)z^{-1}}{1-2e^{-aT}(\cos \omega_c T)z^{-1}+e^{-2aT}z^{-2}}$

FIGURE 3.10 Examples of continuous-time functions [$f(t)$] and analogous discrete-time functions [$f(nT)$] together with their Laplace transforms [$F(s)$] and z transforms [$F(z)$], respectively.

Elements of a digital filter. We use a microcomputer as a real-time digital filter if we program it to produce a number at its output for each number that it receives at the input. The rate at which it must handle the numbers is determined by the A/D conversion rate and is $1/T$ samples/s. We need only three types of operations to implement any linear digital filter: (1) storage, (2) multiplication by constants, and (3) addition. Figure 3.11 shows symbols used to represent these operations. If we apply to terminal A of the storage element of Fig. 3.11(a) our input sequence,

$$(x(0), x(T), x(2T), \ldots, x(nT))$$

which has the z transform

$$X(z) = x(0) + x(T)z^{-1} + x(2T)z^{-2} + \ldots + x(nT)z^{-n}$$

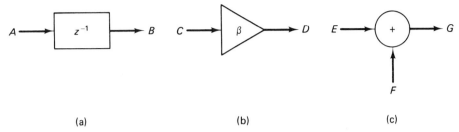

FIGURE 3.11 Digital filter operations. (a) Storage of a number for one clock period ($B = A$ in T seconds after the signal appears at A). (b) Multiplication by a constant ($D = \beta C$). (c) Addition ($G = E + F$).

we obtain at the output a new sequence,

$$(0, x(0), x(T), x(2T), \ldots, x(nT))$$

which has the z transform

$$Y(z) = 0 + x(0)z^{-1} + x(T)z^{-2} + \ldots + x(nT - T)z^{-n}$$

In this case, $x(0)$ enters the storage block at $t = 0$; simultaneously, the initialized contents of the block (which we always assume to be zero) are forced to the output. At $t = T$, $x(0)$ is forced out when $x(T)$ enters. Therefore, each ADC clock tick enters a new number into the storage element and forces the previously stored value (which is stored for exactly T s) to the output. The output sequence is identical to the input sequence except it has been delayed by T s.

It is apparent that the relationship between the output z transform $Y(z)$ from our storage block and the input transform $X(z)$ is

$$Y(z) = z^{-1}X(z)$$

Since $Y(z)$ and $X(z)$ are identical except for a T s delay, we see that the variable z^{-1} symbolizes this time shift. The z transform

$$A(z) = 1 + 2z^{-1} + 3z^{-4}$$

tells us that we received an initial data value of 1 followed by a value of 2 after T s and a value of 3 after $4T$ s. The corresponding sequence is

$$(1, 2, 0, 0, 3)$$

since no values occurred at clock ticks $2T$ and $3T$. A microcomputer system implements the storage function simply by placing data points in successive memory locations for later recall at appropriate clock times.

Figure 3.11(b) shows a second function necessary for implementing a digital filter—multiplication by a constant. For each number in the sequence of numbers that appears at the input of the multiplier, the product of the number and the constant appears instantaneously at the output. There is no storage or time delay in the multiplier. In any real system there is of course both some storage and some time delay because all arithmetic operations require finite time. Since very few general-purpose microprocessors have a multiply instruction, the multiply operation typically must be done by a slow successive addition algorithm. This is a primary factor which prevents real-time filtering for many applications.

The third and final operation necessary for digital filtering is addition of two numbers to produce a sum as shown in Fig. 3.11(c). At a clock tick the numbers from two different sequences are summed to produce an output number instantaneously—again we assume no storage or time delay in the addition operation. All microprocessors have addition capability.

In a practical system, the adders and multipliers do not have to produce their outputs immediately. Since their inputs are constant for the time interval between A/D converter clock ticks, they have actually almost T s to complete their operations before their inputs change.

All general-purpose microprocessors can perform the three operations necessary for digital filtering—storage, multiplication, and addition. Therefore, they all can implement basic digital filtering. If they are fast enough to do all the operations to produce an output value before the next input value appears (T s), we say they operate in real time. We can perform such operations as low-pass filtering of an ECG in a way similar to analog filtering in that the filtered version of the signal immediately appears at the output of the microcomputer-based digital filter as the signal is being input.

Transfer function. The z transforms of the input and output sequences of a digital filter, $X(z)$ and $Y(z)$, respectively, are related to each other by

$$Y(z) = H(z)X(z) \tag{3.3}$$

where $H(z)$ is called the transfer function of the filter.

There are two basic digital filter types—nonrecursive and recursive. For nonrecursive filters, the transfer function contains a finite number of elements and is in the form of a polynomial in the variable z^{-1}:

$$H(z) = \sum_{i=0}^{n} h_i z^{-i} = h_0 + h_1 z^{-1} + h_2 z^{-2} + \ldots + h_n z^{-n} \tag{3.4}$$

For recursive filters the transfer function is expressed as the ratio of two such polynomials:

$$H(z) = \frac{\sum_{i=0}^{n} a_i z^{-i}}{1 - \sum_{i=1}^{n} b_i z^{-i}} = \frac{a_0 + a_1 z^{-1} + a_2 z^{-2} + \ldots + a_n z^{-n}}{1 - b_1 z^{-1} - b_2 z^{-2} - \ldots - b_n z^{-n}} \tag{3.5}$$

The values of z for which $H(z)$ is zero are called zeros of the transfer function. For nonrecursive filters we find the zeros by setting the transfer function to zero and evaluating for z. For recursive filters we equate the numerator to zero and find z to obtain the zeros. The poles are defined as the values for which the transfer function becomes infinite. Nonrecursive filters have no poles. We find the pole locations for recursive filters by setting the denominator polynomial of the transfer function equal to zero and calculating the values of z. The locations of poles in the z plane, as seen later, determine the stability of a recursive filter. Since they have no poles, nonrecursive filters are always stable.

The z-plane pole–zero plot.   The mathematics of the z transform are based upon the definition

$$z = e^{sT} \tag{3.6}$$

where, as we know,

$$s = \sigma + j\omega$$

Therefore,

$$z = e^{\sigma T} e^{j\omega T} \tag{3.7}$$

By definition the magnitude of z is

$$|z| = e^{\sigma T}$$

and the phase angle is

$$\underline{/z} = \omega T$$

If we set $\sigma = 0$, the magnitude of z is 1 and we have

$$z = e^{j\omega T} = \cos \omega T + j \sin \omega T \tag{3.8}$$

This is the equation of a circle of unity radius called the unit circle in the z plane. Since the z plane is a direct mathematical mapping of the well-known s plane, let us consider the condition for stability of filters described by z-transform transfer functions.

The imaginary ($j\omega$) axis in the s plane ($\sigma = 0$) maps to points on the unit circle. Negative values of σ describe the left half of the s plane and map to the interior of the unit circle in the z plane. Positive σ values correspond to the right half of the s plane and map to points outside the unit circle in the z plane.

We know that all poles must lie either in the left-half of the s plane or on the imaginary axis for a continuous filter to be stable. Also, any poles on the imaginary axis must be simple. From our knowledge of the mapping between the s and z planes, we can now state the general rule for stability in the z plane. All poles must be either inside or on the unit circle. If they are on the unit circle, they must be simple. As in the s plane, zeros do not influence stability and can be anywhere in the plane. In a later section ("Simple Recursive Filter Example") we give an example of a stable single-pole filter that becomes unstable when its pole is moved from inside to outside the unit circle.

Figure 3.12 shows some of the important features of the z plane. Any angle ωT specifies a point on the unit circle. Since $\omega = 2\pi f$ and $T = 1/f_s$, this angle is

$$\omega T = \frac{2\pi f}{f_s} \qquad (3.9)$$

The angular location of any point on the unit circle is then designated by the ratio of a specified frequency f to the sampling frequency f_s. If $f = f_s$, $\omega T = 2\pi$; thus the sampling frequency corresponds to an angular location of 2π radians. For $f = 0$, $\omega T = 0$; hence dc is located at an angle of zero degrees.

Another important frequency is $f = f_s/2 = f_0$ at $\omega T = \pi$. This frequency, called the folding frequency, equals one-half the sampling rate. From Chapter 2 it is the maximum frequency that a digital filter can process properly. Recall that the sampling theorem establishes the constraint that the sampling rate must be at least twice the highest frequency in a sampled signal. We must bandlimit a signal, usually with an analog low-pass filter, to ensure that we are obeying the sampling theorem. We call such a filter an antialias filter because it excludes higher frequencies which could appear as lower-frequency aliases. Antialiasing cannot be accomplished with any digital filter process except by increasing the sampling rate to twice the highest frequency present. Since this is not usually practical, most digital signal processors have an analog front end—the antialias filter.

Figure 3.12 shows that we can refer to the angle designating a point on the unit circle in a number of ways based upon eq. (3.9). If we use the ratio f/f_s, this is called the normalized frequency. For $f = f_s$ this ratio is 1, and it corresponds to an angle of 2π rad. A ratio of $\frac{1}{4}$ designates a frequency of $f_s/4$ and the angle $\pi/2$. This approach has the advantage that we can discuss a general filter type such as low pass without defining specific frequencies. We can then assign any passband to this filter type simply by selecting an appropriate sampling frequency. This illustrates an important feature of a digital filter—the frequency-response characteristics are directly related to the sampling frequency.

If we have already established the sampling frequency, we can alternately specify the angular location of a point on the unit circle by frequency f. For example, if f_s is 180 samples/s, a frequency f of 60 Hz is at $\omega T = 2\pi/3$ rad.

Finally, we can use ωT as the angular location of a point. Angle $\omega T = 2\pi$ corresponds to f_s and π designates f_0. We choose to use ωT throughout this book, since it is the angle of variable z on the unit circle (i.e., $z = e^{j\omega T}$). Also, it is not frequency-specific; any frequency can be later selected as f_s.

For an analog filter we find the amplitude and phase responses by evaluating the transfer function on the imaginary axis of the s plane (i.e., $s = j\omega$). Since the imaginary s-plane axis maps to the z-plane unit circle, we evaluate the transfer function of a digital filter on the unit circle (i.e., $z = e^{j\omega T}$). In a manner analogous to the s-plane approach, we show in Fig. 3.13 a graphical solution for the response

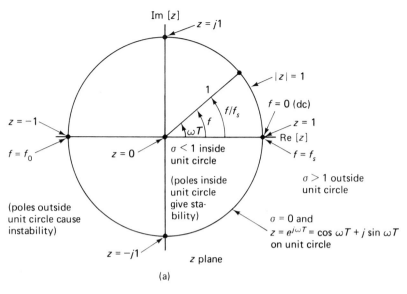

(a)

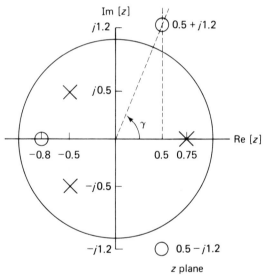

z plane

Complex conjugate poles at $z = -0.5 \pm j0.5$
Simple pole at $z = 0.75$
Complex conjugate zeros at $0.5 \pm j1.2$
Simple zero at $z = -0.8$
$\gamma = \tan^{-1}(1.2/0.5)$
z transform for the pole-zero pattern shown:

$$H(z) = \frac{(z + 0.8)(z - 0.5 + j1.2)(z - 0.5 - j1.2)}{(z - 0.75)(z + 0.5 + j0.5)(z + 0.5 - j0.5)}$$

(b)

FIGURE 3.12   Pole–zero plot in the z plane. (a) Definitions. (b) Example of a pole–zero plot.

of a digital filter. We evaluate the response at each of a number of points on the circle corresponding to different values of ωT by first drawing vectors from each of the poles and zeros to the point. The filter response at that point is the product of the vectors drawn from the zeros to the point divided by the product of the vectors from the poles, or

$$H(\omega T) = \frac{\bar{Z}_1 \cdot \bar{Z}_2}{\bar{P}_1 \cdot \bar{P}_2} \qquad (3.10)$$

The magnitude of $H(\omega T)$ is the amplitude response, and the angle is the phase

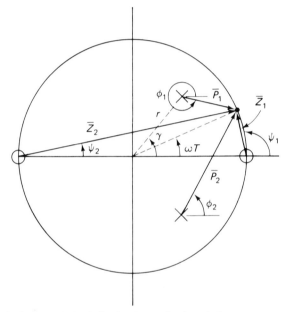

FIGURE 3.13 Graphical solution for the amplitude and phase responses of a digital filter.

response. Thus we can find the amplitude response by measuring the lengths of the vectors from the poles and zeros to the point on the unit circle and solving

$$|H(\omega T)| = \frac{|\bar{Z}_1| \cdot |\bar{Z}_2|}{|\bar{P}_1| \cdot |\bar{P}_2|} \qquad (3.11)$$

The phase response is

$$\underline{/H(\omega T)} = \psi_1 + \psi_2 - \phi_1 - \phi_2 \qquad (3.12)$$

Let us now find the response of the filter in Fig. 3.13. At $\omega T = 0$, the point of interest on the unit circle is coincident with the zero at $z = 1$ and $\bar{Z}_1 = 0$; the amplitude response $|H(\omega T)|$ is zero, since $|Z_1|$ is a multiplier in the numerator.

Also $\psi_1 = 0$, since $\bar{Z}_1 = 0$, $\psi_2 = 0$ and ϕ_1 and ϕ_2 are equal and opposite; thus the angle of $H(\omega T)$ is zero. As ωT increases and $\bar{Z}_1$ becomes finite in length, its angle ψ_1 becomes initially $\pi/2$ and increases as ωT increases to π, and its length $|Z_1|$ increases to a maximum of 2 at $\omega T = \pi$. Vector $\bar{Z}_2$ does the opposite; at $\omega T = 0$ its length is equal to 2 and decreases to zero at $\omega T = \pi$; its angle ψ_2 goes from 0 to $-\pi/2$. Since $|Z_2| = 0$ at $\omega T = \pi$, the amplitude response is zero again and the phase response is $\psi_2 = -\pi/2$. When $\omega T = \gamma$, the amplitude response is sensitive to the radial position of the pole. If it is very near the unit circle, length $|P_1|$ is very small. Since this length is in the denominator of the transfer function, the amplitude response gets very large. If the pole is near the origin, $|P_1|$ is larger and the overall amplitude response is smaller. The proximity of the pole to the unit circle controls the damping of the filter. When it is close, the filter is underdamped; when it is distant, it is overdamped; at some pole location along the radius it is critically damped. Since this pole controls filter damping, its angular location designates the critical frequency of the filter. Between $\omega T = 0$ and π, the phase response changes according to the summation of angles from $\pi/2$ to $-\pi/2$. The amplitude response increases from zero at $\omega T = 0$ (dc) to some peak at $\omega T = \gamma$ and decreases back to zero at $\omega T = \pi$. Therefore, this is a bandpass filter and γ is the center frequency.

Recall that f_s corresponds to 2π and f_0 to π. The sampling theorem restricts us to filter input frequencies of f_0 or smaller. Therefore, we need not go beyond $\omega T = \pi(f_0)$ to specify the response of any digital filter. This corresponds to the upper half of the unit circle. Because of the sampling process, increasing ωT beyond π results in repetition of the amplitude and phase responses folded around the folding frequency f_0. Figure 3.14 shows an example of the amplitude and phase characteristics of an ideal low-pass filter with linear phase response. Normally, we would only plot these characteristics to $\omega T = \pi$, since that is the only meaningful range for us.

The graphical solution is a powerful tool, especially for making an intuitive preliminary analysis of a new filter. Immediately, we can see the qualitative performance. For example, we now know that the amplitude response goes to zero wherever there is a zero on the unit circle. Also, poles near the circle cause an increase in amplitude at their angular frequencies. After some practice we can tell a great deal about a filter from inspection of the pole–zero plot.

For the exact amplitude and phase responses, we use an analytical approach. Since we desire the frequency response, we evaluate the transfer function on the unit circle by simply substituting $e^{j\omega T}$ for every occurrence of z. For example, for the recursive filter

$$H(z) = \frac{1 + z^{-1}}{1 - z^{-1}}$$

we obtain

$$H(\omega T) = \frac{1 + e^{-j\omega T}}{1 - e^{-j\omega T}} = \frac{e^{-j(\omega T/2)}\left(e^{j(\omega T/2)} + e^{-j(\omega T/2)}\right)}{e^{-j(\omega T/2)}\left(e^{j(\omega T/2)} - e^{-j(\omega T/2)}\right)} = \frac{2\cos(\omega T/2)}{2j\sin(\omega T/2)} = -j\cot\frac{\omega T}{2}$$

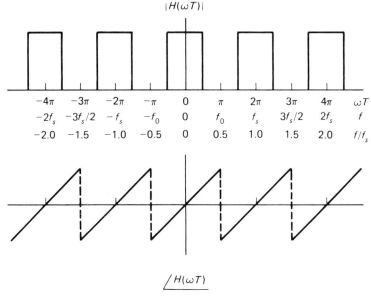

FIGURE 3.14 Amplitude and phase responses for a digital low-pass filter. The amplitude and phase characteristics repeat for every rotation around the unit circle. The pattern for the first π radians of each rotation repeats with a reversed frequency scale for the second π radians. Thus it is folded around frequency f_0.

The amplitude response is the magnitude of $H(\omega T)$,

$$|H(\omega T)| = \cot \frac{\omega T}{2}$$

and the phase response is

$$\underline{/H(\omega T)} = \frac{-\pi}{2}$$

We now have a set of powerful tools for analysis and design of digital filters.

Design of nonrecursive filters. With the theoretical background presented in the previous sections, we are ready to attack the main problem—designing the filter. The main advantage of a nonrecursive filter is that we can design it to have a completely linear phase response. This is especially important when we wish to minimize the distortion in the waveform, as in ECG analysis. We can also easily design nonrecursive filters to approximate arbitrarily specified amplitude responses.

Another feature of a nonrecursive filter is that its transfer function has a finite number of terms, as we have seen. Therefore, the effect of any switching transient or any other disturbance in the input will disappear after a period of time. We call this feature a finite impulse response (FIR). Also, as we mentioned previously, nonrecursive filters have only zeros in their transfer function, and therefore are always stable.

Unlike recursive filters, nonrecursive filters typically cannot approximate sharp cutoff filters. Although they have slow rolloff, they are quite popular because of ease of design, linear phase response, and guaranteed stability. Nonrecursive filter design usually starts with a numerical approximation which modifies the input sequence of numbers in such a way as to produce the desired filtering. We discuss two numerical methods called smoothing which approximate low-pass filters—the moving average and the polynomial fit.

Moving-average filter. Moving-average smoothing, also called the Hanning filter, is an algorithm that yields an output sequence given by

$$y(nT) = \tfrac{1}{4}[x(nT) + 2x(nT - T) + x(nT - 2T)] \tag{3.13}$$

This is a difference equation which states that the output value at any instant of time $y(nT)$ can be computed from one-fourth of the sum of $x(nT)$, the input value at that time, $x(nT - T)$, the previous input value T s ago scaled by a factor of 2 and $x(nT - 2T)$, the input value $2T$ s ago. For any input point, say $n = 5$, the output is

$$y(5T) = \tfrac{1}{4}[x(5T) + 2x(4T) + x(3T)]$$

This filter produces an output point which is a scaled average of three successive input points, with the center point of the three weighted twice as heavily as its two adjacent neighbors. Thus each output number is computed from a scaled average of three input points. The right-hand terms of the difference equation for this filter are points in the input array separated in time from each other by T s. We have previously used z^{-1} to indicate a T-s delay. Therefore, we can write the z transform of the difference equation by inspection:

$$Y(z) = \tfrac{1}{4}[X(z) + 2X(z)z^{-1} + X(z)z^{-2}]$$

To find the transfer function of this filter we apply the z transform of the unit impulse to its input and use the transfer function equation in a manner similar to finding the impulse response of a continuous filter. From Fig. 3.10, we see that $X(z) = 1$ for an impulse and the transfer function is

$$H(z) = \frac{Y(z)}{X(z)} = \frac{Y(z)}{1}$$

or

$$H(z) = \tfrac{1}{4} + \tfrac{1}{2}z^{-1} + \tfrac{1}{4}z^{-2} \tag{3.14}$$

Using our previously defined operation blocks, we can interpret this equation with the block diagram shown in Fig. 3.15(a). Such a block diagram is a useful summary

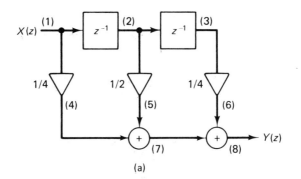

(a)

(1) $(1, 0, 0, 0, 0, \ldots)$
(2) $(0, 1, 0, 0, 0, \ldots)$
(3) $(0, 0, 1, 0, 0, \ldots)$
(4) $(1/4, 0, 0, 0, 0, \ldots)$
(5) $(0, 1/2, 0, 0, 0, \ldots)$
(6) $(0, 0, 1/4, 0, 0, \ldots)$
(7) $(1/4, 1/2, 0, 0, 0, \ldots)$
(8) $(1/4, 1/2, 1/4, 0, 0, \ldots)$

(b)

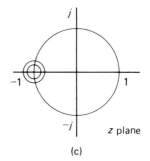

(c)

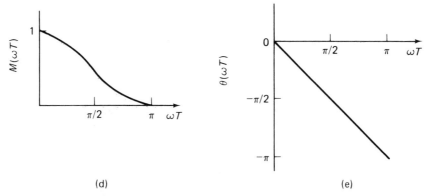

(d)

(e)

FIGURE 3.15 Moving-average (Hanning) filter. (a) Block diagram. (b) Responses to a unit impulse for points in the filter. (c) Pole–zero plot. (d) Amplitude response. (e) Phase response.

of the transfer function equation because it shows graphically all the functions that we must perform to implement the filter with either hardware or software.

We can study a filter by applying number sequences at its input and observing the response. If we apply a unit impulse to the input of our block diagram, we obtain the sequences shown in Fig. 3.15(b). Sequence (1) is the unit impulse. Sequence (2) at the output of the first storage element is simply the input sequence delayed by one clock time. The initial zero in sequence (2) comes from the initial stored value in the storage element, which we always set to zero. Sequence (3) is the same as (2) again, delayed by the second storage block. Sequences (4), (5), and (6) are sequences (1), (2), and (3), respectively, after modification by the multipliers in the pathways. Sequence (7) comes from adding (4) and (5) point by point for equivalent clock times. Summation of (6) and (7) produces sequence (8), which is the response of the filter for a unit impulse input. All but the first three terms are zero; hence we say that this filter has a finite impulse response (FIR). Unlike a recursive filter, which has an infinite number of terms in its transfer function and hence has an infinite impulse response (IIR), the Hanning filter only processes three data points at a time. Typical of a nonrecursive filter, it only remembers a limited number of points (two in this case); thus transients and other fast events disappear from its output quickly. Since its transfer function is a simple polynomial, this filter has no poles. We find its zeros by setting the transfer function to zero and evaluating for z:

$$H(z) = \tfrac{1}{4}(1 + 2z^{-1} + z^{-2}) = 0$$
$$z^2 + 2z + 1 = 0$$
$$z = -1, -1$$

There are two zeros both located at -1 in the z plane. Figure 3.15(c) shows the pole–zero plot. We can find the amplitude and phase response either analytically or graphically from the pole–zero plot. For the analytical approach, we substitute for z in the transfer function, $z = e^{j\omega T}$:

$$H(z) = \tfrac{1}{4}(1 + 2z^{-1} + z^{-2})$$
$$H(e^{j\omega T}) = \tfrac{1}{4}(1 + 2e^{-j\omega T} + e^{-j2\omega T})$$
$$H(e^{j\omega T}) = [\tfrac{1}{2}(1 + \cos \omega T)]e^{-j\omega T}$$

The amplitude response of the filter is the magnitude of this expression, and the phase response is the phase angle.

$$M(\omega T) = |H(e^{j\omega T})| = \tfrac{1}{2}(1 + \cos \omega T) \qquad (3.15a)$$
$$\Theta(\omega T) = \underline{/H(e^{j\omega T})} = -\omega T \qquad (3.15b)$$

Figure 3.15(d) and (e) shows plots of these functions. We see that the passband is characteristic of a low-pass filter. The amplitude response is unity at dc and rolls off to zero at the folding frequency (i.e., the folding frequency occurs at $\omega T = \pi$, since $2\pi f T = \pi$ or $f = 1/2T$). As we desire for most biomedical applications, the phase response is linear.

Smoothing by least-squares polynomial fitting. This algorithm implements a low-pass nonrecursive filter by approximating sets of points in the input sequence by a parabolic polynomial. We can select any odd number of points to be fit by each parabola. In the following discussion we fit a parabola to every group of five points in the input sequence using a least-squares error criterion. As each new sample point appears, we make a parabolic approximation to this new point, together with the four most recently sampled input points. Thus we find a new five-point parabola for every new point in the input sequence. As we will see, the output sequence of this filter is the set of center points of the five-point parabolas which we calculate. The polynomial for a parabola is

$$p(nT + kT) = s_0(nT) + ks_1(nT) + k^2s_2(nT) \tag{3.16}$$

where $p(nT + kT)$ is the value of the parabola evaluated at each of the five possible values of k $(-2, -1, 0, -1, 2)$. The variables $s_0(nT)$, $s_1(nT)$, and $s_2(nT)$ are the variables that we must find to fit each of the parabolas to five input data points. Figure 3.16(a) shows the input data sequence and a parabolic fit to five data points.

We achieve the fit by finding a parabola (coefficients s_0, s_1, and s_2) which best approximates the five data points as measured by the least-squares error. This error is

$$\epsilon(s_0, s_1, s_2) = \sum_{k=-2}^{2} \{x(nT - kT) - [s_0(nT) + ks_1(nT) + k^2s_2(nT)]\}^2$$

We minimize this least-squares error by setting the partial derivatives with respect to the parabola variables equal to zero:

$$\frac{\delta\epsilon}{\delta s_0} = 0 \qquad \frac{\delta\epsilon}{\delta s_1} = 0 \qquad \frac{\delta\epsilon}{\delta s_2} = 0$$

We obtain a set of simultaneous equations from these partial derivatives.

$$5s_0(nT) + \quad 0 \quad + 10s_2(nT) = \sum_{k=-2}^{2} x(nT - kT) \tag{3.17a}$$

$$0 \quad + 10s_1(nT) + \quad 0 \quad = \sum_{k=-2}^{2} kx(nT - kT) \tag{3.17b}$$

$$10s_0(nT) + \quad 0 \quad + 34s_2(nT) = \sum_{k=-2}^{2} k^2x(nT - kT) \tag{3.17c}$$

Solving these equations gives

$$s_0(nT) = \tfrac{1}{35}[-3x(nT - 2T) + 12x(nT - T) + 17x(nT)$$
$$+ 12x(nT + T) - 3x(nT + 2T)] \tag{3.18a}$$

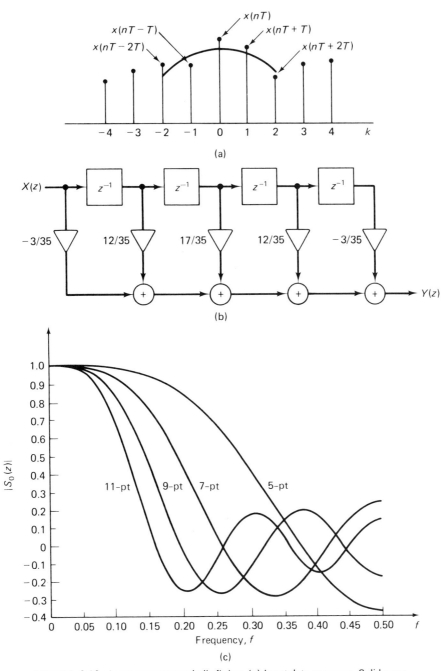

FIGURE 3.16 Least-squares parabolic fitting. (a) Input data sequence. Solid curve shows parabola computed from 5 points of the sequence. The center point of the parabola is $s_0(nT)$ in the output sequence. (b) Block diagram for low-pass nonrecursive filter based on a 5-point fit. (c) Amplitude responses for 5-, 7-, 9-, and 11-point fits. [Frame (c) from Hamming, R. W. 1977. Digital filters. Reprinted by permission of Prentice-Hall, Inc.]

$$s_1(nT) = \tfrac{1}{10}[-2x(nT - 2T) - x(nT - T) + x(nT + T)$$
$$+ 2x(nT + 2T)] \tag{3.18b}$$
$$s_2(nT) = \tfrac{1}{14}[2x(nT - 2T) - x(nT - T) - 2x(nT)$$
$$- x(nT + T) + 2x(nT + 2T)] \tag{3.18c}$$

Recalling that we only want to save the center points of the parabolas [i.e., $p(nT)$ or $k = 0$] as the output sequence, we evaluate eq. (3.16) at $k = 0$, to obtain

$$p(nT + kT) = s_0(nT) + ks_1(nT) + k^2 s_2(nT)|_{k=0} = s_0(nT)$$

Thus the parabola coefficient $s_0(nT)$ given in eq. (3.18a) is the output sequence number calculated from a set of five input sequence points. The output sequence so obtained is similar to the input sequence but with less noise (i.e., low-pass-filtered) because the parabolic fitting provides a smoothed approximation to each set of five data points in the input sequence.

Each of the right-hand terms in eq. (3.18a) corresponds to one number in the input sequence displaced by T s from adjacent terms. Thus we can write the z transform for our low-pass filter:

$$S_0(z) = \tfrac{1}{35}(-3 + 12z^{-1} + 17z^{-2} + 12z^{-3} - 3z^{-4})$$

Figure 3.16(b) shows the block diagram. As in the Hanning filter, there is no feedback from the output or intermediate stages to the input. Lack of such feedback is a characteristic of nonrecursive filters which distinguishes them from recursive types.

To find the frequency response of this filter, we replace z in the transfer function by $e^{j\omega T}$ and obtain

$$|S_0(\omega T)| = \tfrac{1}{35}(17 + 24 \cos \omega T - 6 \cos 2\omega T)$$

Figure 3.16(c) shows this amplitude response for the 5-point parabolic filter and also responses for filters based upon smoothing using groups of 7, 9, and 11 points for each fitted parabola. We list here the transfer function coefficients of these filters (Hamming, 1977).

$$\tfrac{1}{35}(-3, 12, 17, 12, -3) \qquad\qquad \text{(5-point fit)} \quad (3.19a)$$
$$\tfrac{1}{21}(-2, 3, 6, 7, 6, 3, -2) \qquad\qquad \text{(7-point fit)} \quad (3.19b)$$
$$\tfrac{1}{231}(-21, 14, 39, 54, 59, 54, 39, 14, -21) \qquad \text{(9-point fit)} \quad (3.19c)$$
$$\tfrac{1}{429}(-36, 9, 44, 69, 84, 89, 84, 69, 44, 9, -36) \quad \text{(11-point fit)} \quad (3.19d)$$

Figure 3.16(c) shows that the larger the number of points in the fit, the faster the rolloff. Unfortunately, the 11-point fit has more than twice as many multiplications and additions as a 5-point fit. Thus it may not be practical in a particular application because of time constraints.

Before leaving this filter, consider the following interesting point about this algorithm. If we differentiate eq. (3.16) and evaluate the result at the center point of the parabola ($k = 0$), we get

$$\frac{dp(nT - kT)}{dk} = s_1(nT) + 2ks_2(nT)|_{k=0} = s_1(nT) \qquad (3.20)$$

Thus s_1 is an output sequence that approximates the derivative of the input sequence. Instead of saving the value of the center point of the parabola, we save the slope of the parabola at the center point. We discuss this filter later in this chapter in the derivative section.

We can design nonrecursive low-pass filters of this symmetric type. We start with a 5-point numerical definition:

$$y(nT) = ax(nT - 2T) + bx(nT - T) + cx(nT) + bx(nT + T)$$
$$+ ax(nT + 2T) \qquad (3.21)$$

The transfer function is

$$H(z) = a + bz^{-1} + cz^{-2} + bz^{-3} + az^{-4}$$

By substituting $z = e^{j\omega T}$ we can find the amplitude response:

$$|H(\omega T)| = 2a \cos 2\omega T + 2b \cos \omega T + c \qquad (3.22)$$

This is an even function of ω because the filter is symmetric; otherwise, the frequency response would also have sine terms. Our design problem, now, is to find the parameters a, b, and c to match our needs. As an example, let us assume that we need a filter with the following characteristics:

$$|H(0)| = 1 \quad \text{and} \quad |H(\pi)| = 0$$

These conditions simply mean that we want to pass the low frequencies and stop the high ones. Substituting these values in eq. (3.22) and solving for a, b, and c yields

$$b = \tfrac{1}{4}$$
$$c = \tfrac{1}{2} - 2a$$

Equation (3.22) is reduced to

$$|H(\omega T)| = 2a \cos 2\omega T + \tfrac{1}{2} \cos \omega T + \tfrac{1}{2} - 2a \qquad (3.23)$$
$$|H(\omega T)| = 4a\{1 + \cos \omega T[\cos \omega T - (1 - \tfrac{1}{8}a)]\} \qquad (3.24)$$

This equation describes a family of curves that are shown in Fig. 3.17 for some values of the parameter a. These curves are all even and periodic. From Fig. 3.17 we can decide what filter (or what value of a) meets our requirements. Suppose that we want to balance the two halves of the filter by requiring that

$$\left| H\left(\frac{\pi}{2}\right) \right| = \frac{1}{2}$$

From eq. (3.23) we get

$$\left| H\left(\frac{\pi}{2}\right) \right| = -2a + \frac{1}{2} - 2a = \frac{1}{2}$$

Thus

$$a = 0 \qquad c = \tfrac{1}{2}$$

Hence, from eq. (3.21),

$$y(nT) = \tfrac{1}{4}[x(nT - T) + 2x(nT) + x(nT + T)]$$

The transfer function is

$$H(z) = \tfrac{1}{4}(1 + 2z^{-1} + z^{-2})$$

and

$$|H(\omega T)| = \tfrac{1}{2}(1 + \cos \omega T)$$

which is the Hanning filter discussed earlier.

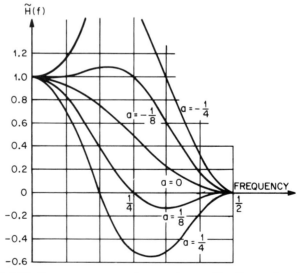

FIGURE 3.17 Frequency response of symmetric smoothing filter as a function of the parameter a. (From Hamming, R. W. 1977. Digital filters. Reprinted by permission of Prentice-Hall, Inc.)

We could have assumed the following conditions on the filter:

$$|H(0)| = 1$$

$$\frac{d|H(0)|}{d\omega T} = 0$$

$$\frac{d^2|H(0)|}{d\omega T^2} = 0$$

These conditions state that we wish the frequency response to be as tangent at $\omega T = 0$ as possible. Continuing as before, we obtain

$$a = \tfrac{1}{16}$$

$$y(nT) = \tfrac{1}{16}[-x(nT - 2T) + 4x(nT - T) + 10x(nT) + 4x(nT + T)$$
$$- x(nT + 2T)]$$

and

$$|H(\omega T)| = -\tfrac{1}{8}\cos 2\omega T + \tfrac{1}{2}\cos \omega T + \tfrac{5}{8}$$

Nonrecursive notch filter. We can design a filter that completely rejects a single frequency using the difference equation

$$y(nT) = \tfrac{1}{3}[x(nT) + x(nT - T) + x(nT - 2T)] \tag{3.25}$$

The transfer function is

$$H(z) = \tfrac{1}{3}(1 + z^{-1} + z^{-2}) \tag{3.26}$$

Solving for the zeros, we obtain

$$z^2 + z + 1 = 0$$

$$z = -0.5 \pm j0.866$$

The two zeros are located on the unit circle at $\omega T = \pm 2\pi/3$, as shown in Fig. 3.18(a). A zero located on the unit circle completely eliminates the frequency corresponding to that point. Suppose that we desire to eliminate 60-Hz interference. We select a sampling frequency of 180 samples/s. Since the sampling frequency corresponds to the unit circle angle 2π, 60 Hz is located at $(60/180)2\pi = 2\pi/3$, or exactly at the location of the zero. We find the amplitude and phase response as before by substituting $z = e^{j\omega T}$:

$$|H(\omega T)| = \tfrac{1}{3}(1 + 2\cos \omega T)$$

$$\underline{/H(\omega T)} = -\omega T$$

Figure 3.18(b) shows the amplitude response of this notch filter.

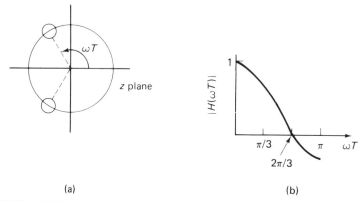

(a)   (b)

FIGURE 3.18 Nonrecursive 60-Hz notch filter. (a) Pole–zero plot. $f_s = 180$ samples/s; $\omega T = 2\pi/3$. (b) Amplitude response for $T = 1/180$ s. 60 Hz corresponds to $\omega T = 2\pi/3$.

Design of recursive filters.   Recursive filters have the potential for sharp rolloffs. Unlike the design of a nonrecursive filter which frequently is based upon approximating an input sequence numerically, recursive-filter design frequently starts with an analog filter that we would like to approximate. Their transfer functions can be represented by an infinite sum of terms or ratio of polynomials. Since they use feedback, they may be unstable if improperly designed. Also, they typically do not have linear phase response.

Simple recursive filter example.   Let us consider the simple filter of Fig. 3.19(a). We find the transfer function by applying a unit pulse at $X(z)$. Figure 3.19(b) shows the sequences at various points in the filter. Sequence (1) defines the unit pulse. From the output sequence (2), we write the transfer function:

$$H(z) = 1 + \tfrac{1}{2}z^{-1} + \tfrac{1}{4}z^{-2} + \tfrac{1}{8}z^{-3} + \ldots \tag{3.27}$$

Using the binomial theorem, we can write the infinite sum as a ratio of polynomials:

$$H(z) = \frac{Y(z)}{X(z)} = \frac{1}{1 - \tfrac{1}{2}z^{-1}} \tag{3.28}$$

We can write the difference equation corresponding to this function by first multiplying terms to give

$$X(z) = Y(z) - \tfrac{1}{2}Y(z)z^{-1}$$

We then write the difference equation by inspection:

$$x(nT) = y(nT) - \tfrac{1}{2}y(nT - T)$$

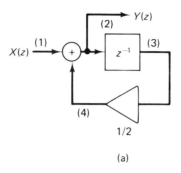

(a)

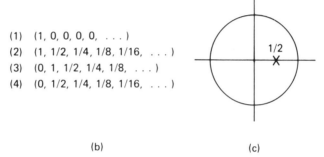

(1) (1, 0, 0, 0, 0, ...)
(2) (1, 1/2, 1/4, 1/8, 1/16, ...)
(3) (0, 1, 1/2, 1/4, 1/8, ...)
(4) (0, 1/2, 1/4, 1/8, 1/16, ...)

(b)   (c)

FIGURE 3.19 Simple recursive filter. (a) Block diagram. (b) Response to a unit pulse. (c) Pole–zero plot.

Rearranging terms gives

$$y(nT) = x(nT) + \tfrac{1}{2}y(nT - T) \tag{3.29}$$

Unlike the nonrecursive case where the current output point $[y(nT)]$ is dependent only upon current and past values of x, this recursive filter requires not only the current value of the input $[x(nT)]$ but the previous value of the output itself $[y(nT - T)]$. Since past history of the output influences the next output value, which in turn influences the next successive output value, a transient requires a large number of sample points before it disappears from an output signal. As we have mentioned, this is not a problem in a nonrecursive filter because it has no feedback.

This sample filter has no zeros because there is no z term in the numerator of the transfer function. We find the poles by setting the denominator equal to zero.

$$1 - \tfrac{1}{2}z^{-1} = 0$$
$$z - \tfrac{1}{2} = 0$$
$$z = \tfrac{1}{2}$$

The pole–zero plot for this single-pole filter is in Fig. 3.19(c). Again we could substitute $z = e^{j\omega T}$ and find the amplitude and phase response. This is a low-pass filter.

If we replace the multiplier constant of $\frac{1}{2}$ in this filter by 2, the output response to a unit impulse is (1, 2, 4, 8, 16, . . .). The filter is unstable, as indicated by the increase in the size of the output sequence with each successive sample. The response to a unit pulse input not only does not disappear with time, it increases by a factor of 2 each T s. We desire a unit pulse response that decays toward zero. Calculating the location of the pole with the multiplier of 2, we find that the pole is at $z = 2$. It is outside the unit circle, and the filter is unstable, as expected.

Design of second-order recursive filters.   Figure 3.20 shows the pole–zero plots for the four types of filters—low pass, bandpass, high pass, and band reject. The general design equation in Fig. 3.20(e) has a standard recursive form for each of the filters.

We start the design by selecting the sampling frequency f_s, which must be at least twice the highest frequency contained in the input signal. Next we choose the critical frequency f_c. This is the cutoff frequency for low- and high-pass filters, the resonant frequency for a bandpass filter and the notch frequency for a band-reject filter. These two choices establish θ, the angular location of the poles.

We then select r, the distance of the poles from the origin. This is the damping factor, given by

$$r = e^{-aT} \tag{3.30}$$

See the table of Fig. 3.10 for the relationship between this variable and continuous-time functions. We have seen from the graphical solution for the amplitude response that underdamping occurs as the poles approach the unit circle (i.e., $r \rightarrow 1$ or $a \rightarrow 0$) and overdamping results for poles near the origin (i.e., $r \rightarrow 0$ or $a \rightarrow \infty$). For these filters, critical damping occurs at $r = \frac{1}{2}$ and $\theta = \pi/8$. Moving the poles by increasing r or θ causes underdamping, and decreasing either variable causes overdamping (Soderstrand, 1972). As we have done in other designs, we find the frequency response by substituting $e^{j\omega T}$ for z in the final transfer function.

These second-order filters have operational characteristics similar to second-order analog filters. The rolloff is slow, but we can cascade several identical sections to improve it. Of course, we may have time constraints in a real-time system which limit the number of sections that can be cascaded in software implementations. In these cases we design higher-order filters.

Recursive filter design by bilinear transformation.   We can design a recursive filter that functions approximately the same way as a model analog filter. We start with the s-plane transfer function of the filter that we desire to mimic. We accomplish the basic digital design by replacing all the occurrences of the variable s by the approximation

$$s \simeq \frac{2}{T} \frac{1 - z^{-1}}{1 + z^{-1}} \tag{3.31}$$

This substitution does a nonlinear translation of the frequencies of the s plane to

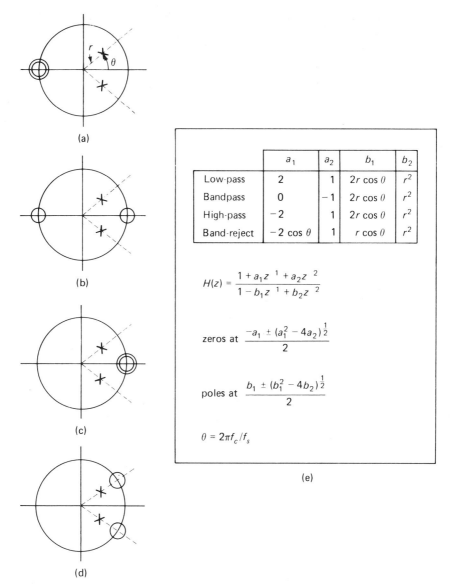

The table and equations within figure (e):

	a_1	a_2	b_1	b_2
Low-pass	2	1	$2r \cos \theta$	r^2
Bandpass	0	-1	$2r \cos \theta$	r^2
High-pass	-2	1	$2r \cos \theta$	r^2
Band-reject	$-2 \cos \theta$	1	$r \cos \theta$	r^2

$$H(z) = \frac{1 + a_1 z^{-1} + a_2 z^{-2}}{1 - b_1 z^{-1} + b_2 z^{-2}}$$

$$\text{zeros at} \quad \frac{-a_1 \pm (a_1^2 - 4a_2)^{\frac{1}{2}}}{2}$$

$$\text{poles at} \quad \frac{b_1 \pm (b_1^2 - 4b_2)^{\frac{1}{2}}}{2}$$

$$\theta = 2\pi f_c / f_s$$

FIGURE 3.20 Elementary two-pole recursive digital filters. (a) Low-pass. (b) Bandpass. (c) High-pass. (d) Band reject (notch). (e) General equation.

those of the z plane. This warping of the frequency axis is defined by

$$\omega' = \frac{2}{T} \tan \frac{\omega T}{2} \tag{3.32}$$

where ω' is the analog domain frequency corresponding to the digital domain frequency ω. To do a bilinear transform, we first prewarp the frequency axis by substituting the relation for ω' for all the critical frequencies in the Laplace transform of the filter. We then replace s in the transform by its z-plane equivalent. Suppose that we have the transfer function

$$H(s) = \frac{\omega'_c}{s^2 + \omega'^2_c}$$

We substitute for ω'_c using eq. (3.32) and for s with eq. (3.31), to obtain

$$H(z) = \frac{\dfrac{2}{T} \tan \dfrac{\omega T}{2}}{\left(\dfrac{2}{T} \dfrac{1 - z^{-1}}{1 + z^{-1}}\right)^2 + \left(\dfrac{2}{T} \tan \dfrac{\omega T}{2}\right)^2}$$

This z transform is the description of a digital filter that performs approximately the same as the model analog filter. We can design high-order filters with this technique.

Recursive filter design using transform tables. We can design digital filters to approximate analog filters of any order with transform tables such as those in Stearns (1975). These tables give the Laplace and z-transform equivalents for corresponding continuous- and discrete-time functions. We have already introduced such a table in Fig. 3.10. To illustrate the design procedure, let us consider the second-order filter of Fig. 3.21(a), The analog transfer function of this filter is

$$H(s) = \frac{A}{LC} \frac{1}{s^2 + (R/L)s + 1/LC} \tag{3.33}$$

Solving for the poles, we obtain

$$s = -a \pm j\omega_c$$

where $a = R/2L$

$\omega_c = [(1/LC) - (R^2/4L^2)]^{1/2}$

We can rewrite the transfer function as

$$H(s) = \frac{A}{LC} \frac{1}{(s + a)^2 + \omega_c^2}$$

Figure 3.21(b) shows the s-plane pole–zero plot. We now note the similarity between this transform and the one listed in Fig. 3.10 for the continuous-time function $e^{-at} \sin \omega_c t$. The z transform for the corresponding discrete-time function, $e^{-anT} \sin n\omega_c T$, is in the form

$$H(z) = \frac{Gz^{-1}}{1 - b_1 z^{-1} - b_2 z^{-2}}$$

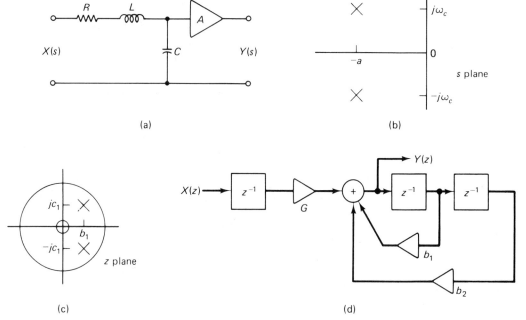

FIGURE 3.21 Second-order filter. (a) Analog filter circuit. (b) Transfer function pole–zero plot for the analog filter. (c) Pole–zero plot for digital version of the second-order filter. (d) Block diagram of the digital filter.

where $b_1 = 2e^{-aT} \cos \omega_c T$

$b_2 = -e^{-2aT}$

$G = (1/\omega_c)(A/LC)e^{-aT} \sin \omega_c T$

Variables a, ω_c, A, L, and C come from the analog filter design. This transfer function has one zero at $z = 0$ and two poles at

$$z = b_1 \pm j(b_1^2 + 4b_2)^{1/2} = b_1 \pm jc_1$$

Figure 3.21(c) shows the z-plane pole–zero plot. We can find the block diagram by substituting for $H(z)$ the ratio $Y(z)/X(z)$ and collecting terms.

$$GX(z)z^{-1} = Y(z) - b_1 Y(z)z^{-1} - b_2 Y(z)z^{-2}$$

The difference equation is

$$y(nT) = Gx(nT - T) + b_1 y(nT - T) + b_2 y(nT - 2T)$$

From this difference equation we can write a program in a straightforward manner to implement the filter. We can also construct the block diagram as shown in Fig. 3.21(d).

This transform-table design procedure provides a technique for quickly designing digital filters that are close approximations to analog filter models. If we have the transfer function of an analog filter, we still usually must make a substantial effort to implement the filter with hardware. However, once we have the z transform, we have the complete filter design specified and only need to write a straightforward program to implement the filter.

A microcomputer for signal processing.   The Intel 2920 is a single-chip, programmable microcomputer designed for real-time digital signal processing. A general-purpose microcomputer only does one operation per instruction, such as adding two numbers together. In contrast, this device shown in Fig. 3.22 does several operations per instruction cycle, such as inputting from the A/D converter, multiplying the number from the input by a constant, and storing the new value in its own internal memory until the next ADC clock tick. Thus this microcomputer has the three operations necessary to implement a digital filter—storage, multiplication by a constant, and addition. Furthermore, it has its own reprogrammable memory with enough space to store commands to implement a number of filters (up to about 44 total poles) operating in real time on signals with several-kHz bandwidths. We can process four analog input signals with the on-chip-multiplexed A/D converter. We can simultaneously output processed analog signals through the eight-channel D/A converter.

Once we know the z transform of the filter that we would like to program, we can directly implement the design using the specialized instruction set of this microcomputer. Of course, like the support required for all microcomputers we need significant hardware and software developmental resources to accomplish meaningful filtering tasks with this device. In time, this microcomputer and others like it will have a significant impact on the field of signal processing—a field that has been largely an analog domain up to the present time.

3.2 DERIVATIVE*

In engineering, we must often find the rate of change of a function with respect to time—the derivative of the function. Differentiators can be used to find positive- or negative-going slopes, maxima or minima, or point of greatest slope. In these cases, the differentiated output is compared with a positive or negative value, a zero value, or greatest value, respectively. Differentiators are also useful in changing waveshapes and generation of waveforms. This section describes both analog and digital approaches to differentiation as well as problems associated with these two methods. Two problems in analog differentiators are instability and increasing gain with frequency that causes high-frequency noise amplification. Digital systems suffer from errors in approximation and sampling insufficiencies that intro-

---

*Section 3.2 written by James D. Woodburn and Willis J. Tompkins.

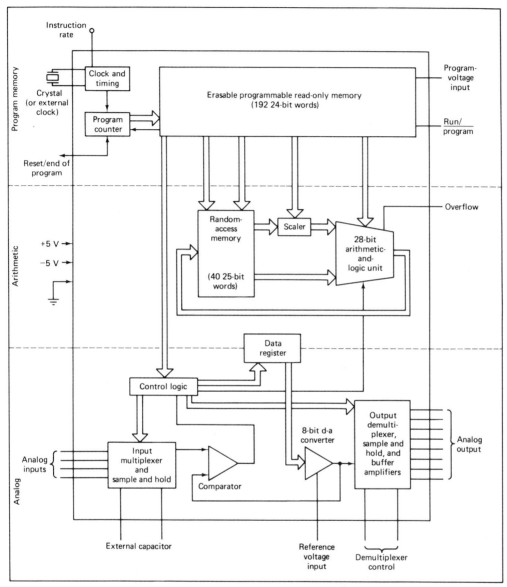

FIGURE 3.22 Intel 2920 single-chip microcomputer for real-time signal processing. (Reprinted by permission of Intel Corporation, copyright 1979.)

duce numerical error. First, we review the concept of differentiation to help clarify the analog and digital approaches. Then we examine a practical example that uses differentiation.

Definition of a derivative

Figure 3.23 shows that the slope m between any two points of a function is

$$m = \frac{\Delta y}{\Delta t} = \frac{f(t_1 + \Delta t) - f(t_1)}{t_1 + \Delta t - t_1} = \frac{f(t_1 + \Delta t) - f(t_1)}{\Delta t} \tag{3.34}$$

The instantaneous slope at P is approximated as Δt approaches zero.

$$f'(t) = m_p = \lim_{\Delta t \to 0} \frac{\Delta y}{\Delta t} = \lim_{\Delta t \to 0} \frac{f(t_1 + \Delta t) - f(t_1)}{\Delta t} \tag{3.35}$$

This is the definition of a derivative. The Δt value has important consequences in digital differentiation, since it represents one of the limiting factors in the accuracy of the process, as we will show later.

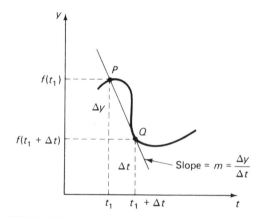

FIGURE 3.23   Curve showing calculation of slope for line PQ.

Analog approach to differentiation

The simplest form of a differentiator is the RC network shown in Fig. 3.24(a). It has an output that approximates the derivative of the input function as long as v_o is small relative to v_i. The circuit is a differentiator because of the mathematical properties relating current and voltage across the capacitor.

$$v_0 = Ri = RC\frac{d(v_i - v_o)}{dt} \simeq RC\frac{dv_i}{dt} \qquad \text{if } v_o \ll v_i$$

A small RC time constant keeps the output proportional to the differentiated input by maintaining v_o small. Figure 3.24(b) shows that this is a very useful circuit as a first approximation to differentiation. Discontinuities in the waveform, which theoretically produce an infinite derivative amplitude, cause sharp peaks in the output of the real circuit. This simple circuit has distortion and is accurate only over a limited low-frequency range.

We use operational amplifier (op amp) circuits to better approximate ideal differentiators. The circuit shown in Fig. 3.25(a) separates the differentiating components C_i and R_f so that voltage changes across R_f do not reduce the voltage applied to C_i. This circuit also provides for the precise corner frequencies necessary for reduction of high-frequency noise and instability inherent in op-amp differentiators.

Figure 3.25(b) shows the frequency response of the op-amp differentiator. The instability of the circuit is due to the intersection of the ideal gain curve (dashed) with the operational amplifier open-loop gain curve. The curves must cross with a rate of closure of less than 12 dB/octave for stability (Stout and Kaufman, 1976). In order to reduce the rate of closure, R_i and C_f are provided to modify the solid curve by holding the gain constant at frequencies above f_1. This

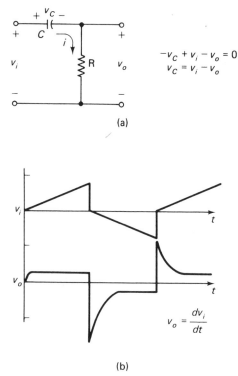

(a)

$$-v_C + v_i - v_o = 0$$
$$v_C = v_i - v_o$$

(b)

$$v_o = \frac{dv_i}{dt}$$

FIGURE 3.24 Passive analog differentiator. (a) Simple RC circuit. (b) Circuit input v_i and resulting output v_o.

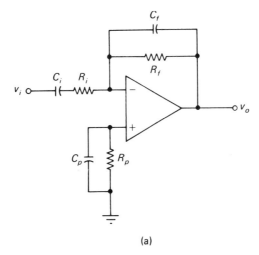

(a)

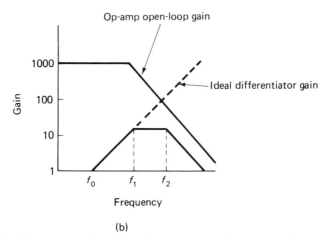

(b)

FIGURE 3.25 Active analog differentiator. (a) Low-noise op-amp circuit with good stability.(b) Bode plot. f_0 is unity-gain crossover frequency; f_1 and f_2 are first- and second-corner frequencies of closed-loop circuit.

gain control assures stable circuit operation. The corner frequencies provided by these two components also reduce the high-frequency noise problems that develop due to the increased gain at higher frequencies. This noise can sometimes be great enough to completely obscure a low-voltage input signal. We choose the components by using the following design formulas:

$$v_o = -R_f C_i \frac{dv_i}{dt}$$

$$f_0 = \frac{1}{2\pi R_f C_i}$$

$$f_1 = \frac{1}{2\pi R_i C_i}$$

$$f_2 = \frac{1}{2\pi R_f C_f}$$

$$R_p = R_f$$

$$C_p = \frac{10}{2\pi f_0 R_p}$$

The resistor values should be kept between 1 kΩ and 10 MΩ to reduce noise and drift. A dc bias current flows through R_f into the negative input of the op amp. This produces an offset voltage at the output. R_p is added to compensate for this offset voltage. Typical bias current values for bipolar monolithic operational amplifiers run from 10 to 1000 nA. If $R_f = 1$ MΩ and bias current $I_b = 100$ nA, the voltage offset produced will be (100 nA)(1 MΩ) $= 100$ mV. R_p will not exactly eliminate this problem, because the two input bias currents are not exactly equal. C_p bypasses the thermal noise generated by R_f to ground but is only needed if R_p is greater than 5 to 10 kΩ. The values for R_p and C_p come from the design formulas as well as values that define the corner frequencies on the Bode plot in Fig. 3.25(b).

Digital differentiation

There are a number of different methods available for differentiating an input signal digitally. Some of the methods are differentiation by secant-line approximations, two- or three-point forward-difference approximations, and interpolating or smoothing polynomials. These methods involve differing amounts of numerical calculation with the trade-offs of greater accuracy and resolution versus increased memory needs and computing time. Since the input waveforms are usually continuous and differentiation is a continuous function, a numerical derivative only approximates the ideal derivative. Each method contains its own margin of error that decreases as the interval between points decreases. This corresponds to sliding point Q closer to point P in Fig. 3.23 and obtaining the value of the slope nearer and nearer to the instantaneous slope at P.

We know that the Laplace transform for a differentiator is

$$H(s) = s$$

Thus the continuous-time amplitude response is linear with frequency and has a constant phase shift of $\pi/2$ rad, as given by

$$H(j\omega) = j\omega$$

A digital filter cannot increase in amplitude indefinitely with frequency because the frequency response must fold over at a frequency equal to one-half the sampling rate. Thus the amplitude response of an ideal digital differentiator increases with frequency only to f_0, where it goes to zero and the folding pattern repeats. We review here three algorithms for differentiation—the 2-point difference, the 3-point central difference, and the least-squares polynomial fit.

Two-point difference. The simplest differentiation algorithm uses the sampled data from an A/D converter with Δt equal to the sampling interval, T. It forms a crude approximation of the derivative by subtracting from the newest sample the one just before it. Since this process only involves one subtraction, it requires at most only a few instructions. The speed and memory-size problems are therefore insignificant and it calculates this derivative in real time.

The difference equation for this algorithm is

$$y(nT) = \frac{1}{T}[x(nT) - x(nT - T)]$$

The z transform of this equation is

$$Y(z) = \frac{1}{T}[X(z) - X(z)z^{-1}]$$

The transfer function is

$$H(z) = \frac{1}{T}(1 - z^{-1})$$

This is a nonrecursive filter with a single zero at $z = 1$. Figure 3.26(a) shows a block diagram and pole–zero plot. We find the amplitude response by substituting $z = e^{j\omega T}$.

$$H(\omega T) = \frac{1}{T}(1 - e^{-j\omega T}) = \frac{1}{T}[e^{j(\omega T/2)} - e^{-j(\omega T/2)}]e^{-j(\omega T/2)}$$

giving

$$H(\omega T) = \frac{1}{T}\left(2j \sin \frac{\omega T}{2}\right)e^{-j(\omega T/2)}$$

Thus the amplitude and phase responses are

$$|H(\omega T)| = \frac{2}{T} \sin \frac{\omega T}{2}$$

$$\underline{/H(\omega T)} = \frac{\pi}{2} - \frac{\omega T}{2}$$

Figure 3.27 gives a plot of the amplitude response. To achieve proper amplitude scaling, we must multiply the input sequence by $1/T$. Note that the gain at f_0 does

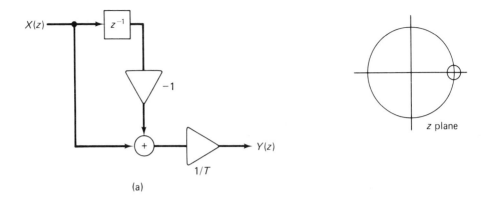

(a)

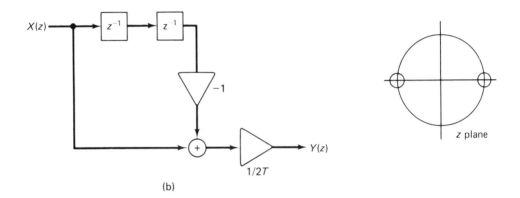

(b)

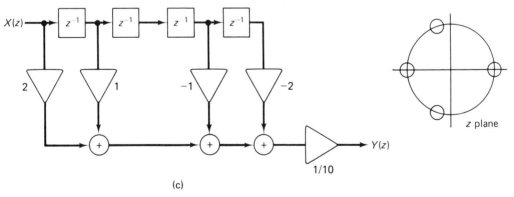

(c)

FIGURE 3.26 Block diagrams and pole–zero plots of nonrecursive digital filters for differentiation. (a) 2-point difference. (b) 3-point central difference. (c) 5-point polynomial fit.

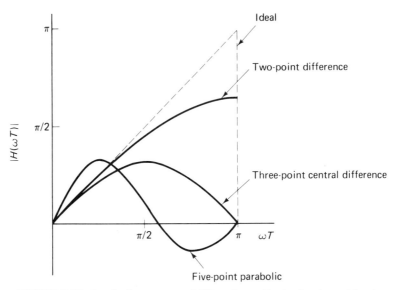

FIGURE 3.27 Amplitude responses of differentiators. For the 2-point and 3-point difference filters, the sampling period T is set to 1.

not go to zero as we indicated it should for an ideal differentiator. This amplification of the higher frequencies tends to emphasize noise at the expense of the lower-frequency signal of interest. Although simple to implement, this algorithm is a poor approximation to the ideal derivative and hence is not useful for many applications.

Three-point central difference. In this approach, we select an equation describing the desired approximation and then compare it to the Taylor expansion. For a 3-point central difference approximation of $f'(t_i)$, the equation is

$$f'(t_i) = \alpha f(t_i) + \beta f(t_{i+1}) + \gamma f(t_{i-1})$$

The Taylor expansion for the derivative is

$$
\begin{aligned}
f'(t_i) = \alpha f(t_i) &+ \beta\left[f(t_i) + (\Delta t)f'(t_i) + \frac{(\Delta t)^2}{2!}f''(t_i) + \frac{(\Delta t)^3}{3!}f'''(\xi_1)\right] \\
&+ \gamma\left[f(t_i) - (\Delta t)f'(t_i) + \frac{(\Delta t)^2}{2!}f''(t_i) - \frac{(\Delta t)^3}{3!}f'''(\xi_2)\right]
\end{aligned}
\tag{3.36}
$$

where $t_i < \xi_1 < t_{i+1}$ and $t_{i-1} < \xi_2 < t_i$. By setting the coefficients on the right side of eq. (3.36) so as to eliminate terms, including variables $f(t_i)$, $f''(t_i)$, and

$f'''(\xi)$, which do not appear on the left side, we get

$$\alpha + \beta + \gamma = 0$$

$$\beta - \gamma = \frac{1}{\Delta t}$$

$$\beta + \gamma = 0$$

Solving these three equations gives $\alpha = 0$, $\beta = 1/(2\Delta t)$, $\gamma = -1/(2\Delta t)$. Substituting these variables into eq. (3.36) gives

$$f'(t_i) \simeq \frac{1}{2\Delta t}[f(t_{i+1}) - f(t_{i-1})]$$

The difference equation for this derivative is

$$y(nT) = \frac{1}{2T}[x(nT) - x(nT - 2T)] \tag{3.37}$$

The transfer function is

$$H(z) = \frac{1}{2T}(1 - z^{-2})$$

By substituting $z = e^{j\omega T}$, we obtain the amplitude and phase response:

$$|H(\omega T)| = \frac{1}{T}\sin \omega T$$

$$\underline{/H(\omega T)} = \frac{\pi}{2} - \omega T$$

Figure 3.26(b) shows the block diagram and pole–zero plot for this filter. Figure 3.27 shows that the amplitude response goes to zero at f_0, as we desire. However, it only approximates the linear portion of the ideal curve over a small range—up to about $\pi/6$ rad. As an example of its performance, for a sampling rate of 600 samples/s, this filter only differentiates well for frequencies below 50 Hz [i.e., $(\pi/6)f_s/2\pi = f_s/12$]. Note the similarity between this response and that of the practical analog differentiator of Fig. 3.25.

Least-squares polynomial fit. Section 3.1 shows that we can approximate the derivative using a polynomial-fitting technique. Equations (3.18b) and (3.20) summarize the results of this analysis for a 5-point fit, giving for the derivative of a function p,

$$y(nT) = p'(nT) = s_1(nT) = \tfrac{1}{10}[2x(nT + 2T) + x(nT + T) \atop - x(nT - T) - 2x(nT - 2T)] \tag{3.38}$$

where $x(nT)$ is the center point of a 5-point parabolic fit. This equation calculates the slope of a 5-point parabola at its center point from the input data sequence. The transfer function is

$$H(z) = \tfrac{1}{10}(2 + z^{-1} - z^{-3} - 2z^{-4})$$

Substituting $z = e^{j\omega T}$ to find the frequency response gives

$$H(\omega T) = \tfrac{2}{10}(j2 \sin 2\omega T + j \sin \omega T)e^{-j2\omega T}$$

The amplitude response is

$$|H(\omega T)| = \tfrac{2}{10}(2 \sin 2\omega T + \sin \omega T)$$

and the phase response is

$$\underline{/H(\omega T)} = \frac{\pi}{2} - 2\omega T$$

Figure 3.26(b) shows the block diagram and pole–zero plot for this filter. In addition to the two zeros at $z = \pm 1$ identical to the 3-point central difference filter, there are two additional zeros at $z = -0.25 \pm j0.968$. These serve to low-pass-filter the signal more than the other two filters, as shown in Fig. 3.27. Although its approximation to the ideal derivative is not as good as the others at low frequencies, this filter has the advantage that its gain is not a function of sampling period like the 2-point and 3-point filters.

If we use more than 5 points for each parabola, the approximation to the derivative improves with a penalty of additional computing time required. The coefficients for 5-, 7-, 9-, and 11-point fitting are

$\tfrac{1}{10}(-2, -1, 1, 2)$	(5-point)	(3.39a)
$\tfrac{1}{28}(-3, -2, -1, 1, 2, 3)$	(7-point)	(3.39b)
$\tfrac{1}{60}(-4, -3, -2, -1, 1, 2, 3, 4)$	(9-point)	(3.39c)
$\tfrac{1}{110}(-5, -4, -3, -2, -1, 1, 2, 3, 4, 5)$	(11-point)	(3.39d)

This derivative algorithm has the advantage that some of the high-frequency noise normally associated with the process of differentiation is attenuated because of the inherent smoothing character of the polynomial fitting approach.

A differentiator application—ECG analysis

Hospitals and research facilities monitor many physiological parameters every day. Most of them either change very slowly or occur with such regularity that constant observation yields little benefit. But often, these small or irregular changes are of extreme importance, and valuable personnel time must be spent keeping a close watch on the parameter values. For example, a person who has suffered a heart attack and is in the intensive-care unit (ICU) has his or her ECG monitored as often as possible to detect changing rhythm or waveform morphologies while the slower-developing conditions of electrolyte imbalance are monitored less often.

One of the solutions to continuous monitoring lies in an analog or digital system that detects and alarms on important changes in parameters. In ECG monitoring, for example, waveform morphology and rhythm change are two classes of parameters that are of interest in analyzing the functioning of the heart. Section 1.2 goes into detail about the parameters that must be considered in developing an automatic monitoring system and also describes a cardiotachometer that monitors rhythm changes, more specifically, the heart rate. Chapter 6 illustrates a very advanced ECG waveform arrhythmia monitor which uses both analog and digital techniques. This section examines a small portion of this waveform analyzer, the use of differentiation to detect the QRS wave of an ECG. We can also extend this method to any variable that can be detected by finding a velocity threshold. We can also use peak detectors to find the R wave, subject to such errors as amplitude distortion from noise and electrode-skin offset potential changes.

Analog method. Figure 3.28(a) shows a basic block diagram of an analog R-wave detector. Figure 3.28(b) shows the resulting waveforms. Section 1.2 describes the ECG amplifier and Section 3.1 the operation of filters. The filter here eliminates high-frequency noise above 100 Hz that would distort the ECG waveform and possibly cause errors by producing velocity changes resembling those of the QRS. The comparator produces an output that indicates the relative difference between its input signal and the reference voltage v_r. When its input exceeds the reference voltage, it generates a positive pulse that indicates the occurrence of an R wave. We can adjust v_r to produce a pulse only for the R wave by applying the ECG signal to one oscilloscope channel and the comparator output to the other channel. We can observe the correlation between the two to show when the reference voltage is properly set.

The advantage of this system, as with all analog systems, lies in the simplicity of assembling the components, lack of required programming experience, real-time processing of the signal (no storage of data necessary), and small expense. The problems involved, however, are those of stability and bandwidth limitations, as discussed earlier.

Digital method. Computer analysis of ECGs provides much more powerful processing than analog techniques as shown in Fig. 3.29(a). After the lead selection, signal amplification and transmission are completed, the ECG signal undergoes A/D conversion. To maintain frequency resolution better than the 100 Hz that is the highest useful frequency in ECGs, the Committee on Electrocardiography of the American Heart Association recommends a sampling rate of 500 samples/s with 9-bit amplitude resolution. The next step involves waveform recognition, called feature extraction, which usually necessitates finding the QRS wave using a

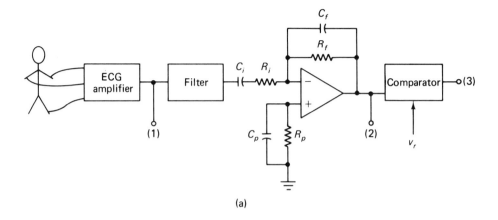

(a)

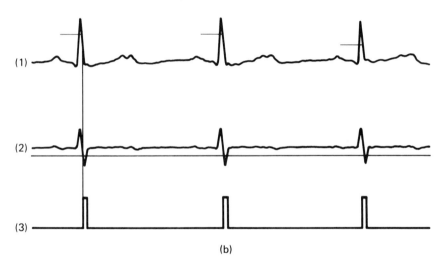

(b)

FIGURE 3.28 Analog QRS detection. (a) Block diagram of differentiation circuit. (b) Signals at circuit nodes. (1) is the amplified ECG. (2) is the derivative of the ECG. (3) is the pulse train produced when the derivative exceeds a negative threshold set by v_r.

differentiation technique. The choice of derivative algorithm depends on what amount of error is acceptable, how much memory is available, and the time proportioned to these calculations. Both difference and parabolic-fit techniques reduce the high-frequency noise that might confuse the pattern extraction routines. The computer compares the output of the routine to a preset value (analogous to v_r) and, when it is exceeded, sets a flag or enables an interrupt to indicate the presence of an R wave. Figure 3.29(b) shows the results of this system.

The advantages of a digital system include the ability to change parameters in software, the stability inherent in the numerical algorithms, the noise suppression through smoothing of data points, and the possibility of using very powerful manipulations, such as signal averaging. The disadvantages are cost, required programming experience, and accuracy, limited by the amount of time and memory space allocated to the program.

The problems with R-wave detection and ECG signal analysis in general are that many pathological conditions and artifacts exist that can mask, distort, or eliminate the parameters being observed and make automatic analysis very difficult.

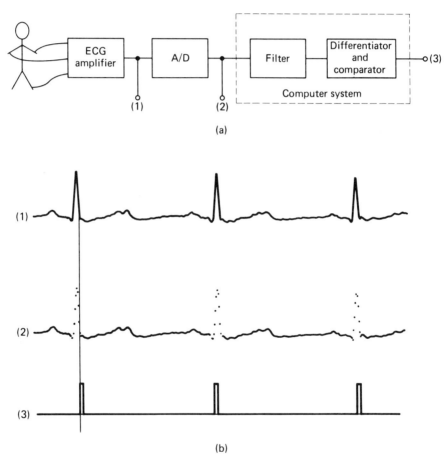

FIGURE 3.29 Digital QRS detection. (a) Block diagram of differentiator system. (b) Signals at circuit nodes. (1) is the amplified analog ECG. (2) is the discrete-time signal which represents the ECG after A/D conversion. (3) is the pulse train produced by the digital computer program, which implements the differentiation and thresholding algorithm.

3.3 INTEGRATION*

The general form of the integral is

$$A = \int_{t_1}^{t_2} f(t) \, dt \tag{3.40}$$

A is the area under the function between the limits t_1 to t_2. The evaluation of the integral can be accomplished analytically. This method lends itself quite readily to integral solutions by electronic analog techniques. A second technique for the determination of integral solutions is by approximating the function via curve-fitting techniques at a finite number of points, where

$$A = \sum_{n=t_1}^{t_2} f(n) \, \Delta t \tag{3.41}$$

The Laplace transform of an integrator is

$$H(s) = \frac{1}{s}$$

Thus the continuous-time response is inversely proportional to frequency and the phase is a constant $-\pi/2$ as given by

$$H(j\omega) = \frac{1}{j\omega}$$

A number of numerical techniques exist that can be programmed to provide digital integration.

Analog integrator

Figure 3.30 shows a simple analog integrator. We solve for v_o by summing currents at node 1, assuming that op amp A_1 has infinite input resistance and zero input current. Using Laplace transforms, we have

$$\frac{v_i - 0}{R} + \frac{v_o - 0}{1/sC} = 0$$

$$-\frac{v_i}{sRC} = v_o$$

$$v_o = -\frac{1}{RC} \int_{t_1}^{t_2} v_i \, dt + v_{ic} \tag{3.42}$$

Thus the electronic integrator output is equal to the negative integral of the input voltage scaled by a factor of $1/RC$.

The integrator will eventually saturate, causing v_o to remain constant even if v_i is still increasing. This occurs when C is completely charged, at which time v_o equals v_C. The saturation is not necessarily a consequence of the input v_i. The

---

*Section 3.3 written by Willis J. Tompkins and Stephen L. Paugh.

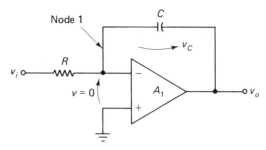

FIGURE 3.30 Simple integrator.

integrator can still saturate when v_i equals zero, since our op amp is not ideal and a finite current flows into the input terminals to supply the base current of the input transistors.

The three-mode integrator shown in Fig. 3.31 is useful for setting initial conditions, integrating, and holding. With S_2 open and S_1 closed we have the standard inverter circuit. Since the input resistance is equal to the feedback resistance, the inverter gain is -1 and v_o equals v_{ic}. We adjust v_{ic} for the desired initial condition. Once the desired initial condition is reached, we open S_1. We close S_2 to initiate the integration. We hold S_2 closed for a duration equal to $t_2 - t_1$ and then open it. With both switches open, the output voltage, v_o, is held constant, a useful feature, since the output indicator is often a voltmeter.

Frequently, the various switches are relay contacts with all switches having the same subscript (e.g., all the S_1's) controlled by the same relay. This simplifies setting initial conditions and initiating integration when a number of integrators are used in the solution of complex integrals. The current trend is to replace the relays with solid-state switches.

The electronic integrator is simple and can be hardwired to fit a particular solution. Integrators are a basic component in analog computers with plug-in

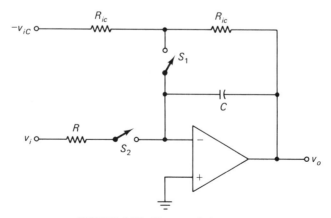

FIGURE 3.31 Three-mode integrator.

sockets for various resistor and capacitor combinations so that the user can program a particular solution.

The electronic integrator is prone to drift, which requires that reset switches be periodically closed to remove residual charges on the feedback capacitors. The initial condition applied to the feedback capacitor may have to be scaled down, as most solid-state integrators work with ± 15-V supplies. These low power-supply voltages also limit the maximum output voltage that can be obtained before saturation.

Digital integrator

With the advent of microprocessor-based instruments the technique of digital integration is becoming available to more users. Unlike the analog integrator a digital integrator does not have drift problems because the process is a computer program, which is not influenced in performance by residual charge on capacitors. We discuss here three popular digital integration techniques—rectangular summation, trapezoidal summation, and Simpson's rule.

Rectangular integration. This algorithm performs the simplest integration. It approximates the integral as a sum of rectangular areas. Figure 3.32(a) shows that each rectangle has a base equal in length to one sample period T and in height to the value of the most recently sampled input $x(nT - T)$. The area of each rectangle is $Tx(nT - T)$. The difference equation is

$$y(nT) = y(nT - T) + Tx(nT - T) \qquad (3.43)$$

where $y(nT - T)$ represents the sum of all the rectangular areas prior to adding the most recent one. The error in this approximation is the difference between the area of the rectangle and the actual signal represented by the sampled data. The z transform of eq. (3.43) is

$$Y(z) = Y(z)z^{-1} + TX(z)z^{-1}$$

and

$$H(z) = \frac{Y(z)}{X(z)} = T\frac{z^{-1}}{1 - z^{-1}} \qquad (3.44)$$

This transfer function has a pole at $z = 1$ and a zero at $z = 0$, as shown in Fig. 3.32(a). The amplitude and phase responses are

$$|H(\omega T)| = \frac{T}{2\sin(\omega T/2)}$$

and

$$\underline{/H(\omega T)} = -\frac{\pi}{2} - \frac{\omega T}{2}$$

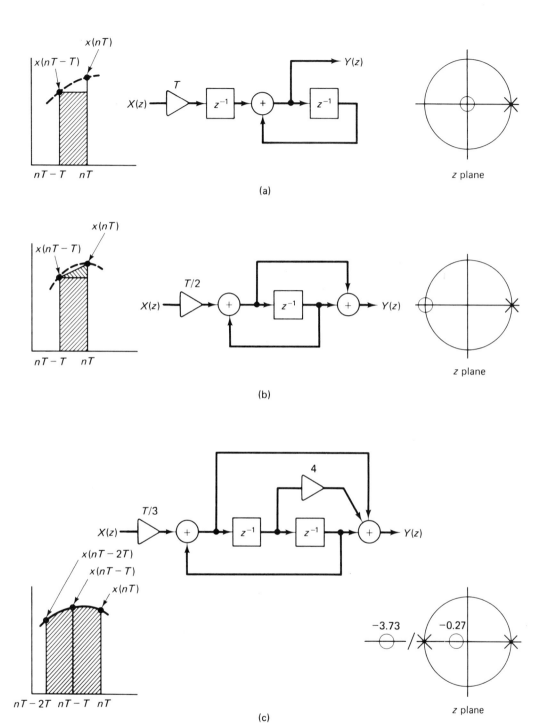

FIGURE 3.32 Digital integrators. Summation areas, block diagrams, and pole–zero plots. (a) Rectangular integration. (b) Trapezoidal integration. (c) Simpson's rule for integration.

Figure 3.33 shows the amplitude response. We can reduce the error of this filter by increasing the sampling rate significantly higher than the highest frequency present in the signal that we are integrating. This has the effect of making the width of each rectangle small compared to the rate of change of the signal, so that the area of each rectangle better approximates the input data. Increasing the sampling rate also corresponds to using only the portion of the amplitude response at the lower frequencies, where the rectangular response better approximates the ideal response. Unfortunately, higher than necessary sampling rates increase computation time and waste memory space by giving us more sampled data than are necessary to characterize a signal. Therefore, we select other digital integrators for problems where higher performance is desirable.

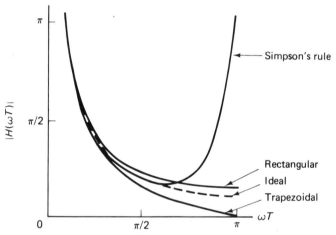

FIGURE 3.33 Amplitude responses for digital integrators. The sampling period T is set equal to 1.

Trapezoidal integration. This filter improves upon rectangular integration by adding a triangular element to the rectangular approximation, as shown in Fig. 3.32(b). The difference equation is the same as for rectangular integration except that we add the triangular element to give

$$y(nT) = y(nT - T) + Tx(nT - T) + \frac{T}{2}[x(nT) - x(nT - T)] \quad (3.45)$$

This gives the transfer function

$$H(z) = \frac{T}{2}\frac{1 + z^{-1}}{1 - z^{-1}} \quad (3.46)$$

The block diagram and pole–zero plot are in Fig. 3.32(b). Like the rectangular approach, this function still has a pole at $z = 1$, but the zero is moved to $z = -1$, the location of the folding frequency, giving us zero amplitude response at f_0. The amplitude and phase response are

$$|H(\omega T)| = \frac{T}{2} \cot \frac{\omega T}{2}$$

and

$$\underline{/H(\omega T)} = -\frac{\pi}{2}$$

The amplitude response approximates that of the ideal integrator much better than the rectangular filter and the phase response is exactly equal to that of the ideal response. The trapezoidal technique provides a very simple, effective nonrecursive integrator.

Simpson's rule. This numerical technique is the most widely used integration algorithm. Figure 3.32(c) shows that this approach approximates the signal corresponding to three input sequence points by a polynomial fit. The incremental area added for each new input point is the area under this polynomial. The difference equation is

$$y(nT) = y(nT - 2T) + \frac{T}{3}[x(nT) + 4x(nT - T) + x(nT - 2T)] \quad (3.47)$$

The transfer function is

$$H(z) = \frac{T}{3} \frac{1 + 4z^{-1} + z^{-2}}{1 - z^{-2}} \quad (3.48)$$

Figure 3.32(c) shows the block diagram and pole–zero plot for this filter. The amplitude and phase response are

$$|H(\omega T)| = \frac{T}{3} \frac{2 + \cos \omega T}{\sin \omega T}$$

and

$$\underline{/H(\omega T)} = -\frac{\pi}{2}$$

Figure 3.33 shows the amplitude response. Like the trapezoidal technique, the phase response is the ideal $-\pi/2$. Simpson's rule approximates the ideal integrator for frequencies less than about $f_s/4$ better than the other techniques. However, it amplifies high-frequency noise near the folding frequency. Therefore, it is a good approximation to the integral but is dangerous to use in the presence of noise. Integration of noisy signals can be accomplished better with trapezoidal integration.

An integrator application—cardiac output

Cardiac output is the volume of blood pumped by the heart per unit time. Normal human cardiac output is about 5 liters/min. During cardiac catheterization, cardiac output is normally measured by the dye-dilution technique described here. During surgery, cardiac output is sometimes measured by thermodilution, as described in Section 1.4. The principle is the same for both techniques, the indicator differs.

Figure 3.34(a) shows that the dye-dilution technique is an invasive procedure. It requires the insertion of two catheters, one into an artery and one into a vein, under local anesthetic. The patient is sedated but awake during the process.

A quantity of dye is rapidly injected into the patient's right atrium, where it becomes thoroughly mixed with the blood entering the pulmonary circulation. The concentration of the dye is measured as it leaves the left ventricle. Figure 3.34(b) shows a plot of the concentration of the dye observed in the artery as a function of time.

To calculate cardiac output, we need to make two assumptions. First, that for the long-time average, left ventricular output is equal to right ventricular output, and second, that all of the right ventricular output goes to the lungs. These assumptions are quite valid, and the determination of cardiac output exhibits good reproducibility. In addition, the dye used must be inert, harmless, measurable, economical, and must remain intravascular. Indocyanine green (cardiogreen) meets these requirements. The optical absorption peak of indocyanine green is at 805 nm. This particular wavelength is desirable since the optical absorption of the blood is independent of the oxygen concentration at this wavelength. The concentration of the dye in the left ventricular output is monitored by an absorption photometer whose detector is centered at 805 nm.

Once we have a dye-dilution curve like that of Fig. 3.34(b), we need to compensate for the dye recirculation occurring at t_r. This is done by exponentially extrapolating the curve from time t_r to the abscissa under the dye-dilution curve. The shaded area is then integrated to find the integrated area. Dividing this integral into the total quantity of dye injected gives the cardiac output over the duration of the curve:

$$F = \frac{m}{\int_0^{t_f} c(t)\, dt}$$

where F = flow (cardiac output)
$\quad\quad m$ = quantity injected
$\quad c(t)$ = instantaneous concentration

EXAMPLE

If 5 mg of injected dye results in an area under the curve of 50 mg·s/liter, then flow

$$F = \frac{5 \text{ mg}}{50 \text{ mg·s/liter}} = 0.1 \text{ liter/s}$$

$$= (0.1)(60 \text{ s/min}) = 6 \text{ liters/min}$$

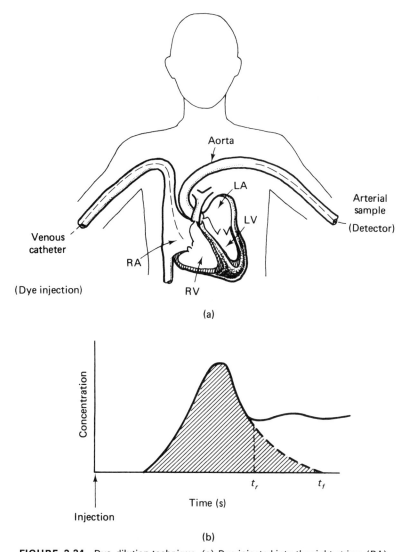

FIGURE 3.34 Dye-dilution technique. (a) Dye injected into the right atrium (RA), passes through the right ventricle (RV), through the lungs, and into the left atrium (LA). It then enters the left ventricle (LV) and is pumped into the aorta and to the detector. (b) Dye-dilution curve.

The entire process can be computerized. An A/D converter changes the analog signal from the absorption photometer to a digital signal that can be stored in the memory of a computer. Programs implement algorithms to extrapolate the curve, calculate the area, and convert the results to liters/min. The amount of dye originally injected is entered using a keyboard. The output can be a digital readout, cathode-ray tube, or hard-copy printer.

An advantage of the digital integrator is its ability to perform recirculation compensation using software. The digital integrator also provides versatility in output presentation, allowing the display of the dye concentration curve along with the cardiac output calculation, if desired.

3.4 FOURIER ANALYSIS*

In this section we discuss the Fourier spectrum representation of signals and the fast Fourier transform. We then give an example of the application of the fast Fourier transform in biomedical signal processing.

Spectrum representation

In biomedical engineering, we frequently deal with time-varying signals. We may represent such a signal as a plot of amplitude versus time. We call this representation a function in the time domain. Another way we may represent a signal is a plot of amplitude versus frequency. We call this representation a function in the frequency domain or a spectrum representation. If we pick any arbitrary function in the time domain, we can find a corresponding unique function in the frequency domain.

Continuous Fourier transform

The Fourier transform states that any function in the time domain can be expressed in the frequency domain as a sum of a dc component and a number (possibly infinite) of sinusoidal components of varying amplitude, frequency, and phase such that at every instant the sum corresponds to the time-domain function. The time- and frequency-domain representations of a signal are equivalent. Either representation alone is sufficient to characterize the signal, and given one representation, we can convert or transform to the other. We retain this dual representation because we may be able to visualize the signal more easily in one domain than in the other. Also, as we shall see later, we are able to perform some mathematical operations easier in one or the other of the domains.

The functional transformation between the time and frequency domains, called the continuous Fourier transform (CFT), is

$$F(\omega) = \int_{-\infty}^{\infty} x(t)e^{-j\omega t}\, dt \qquad (3.49)$$

where $x(t)$ is the time-domain function and $F(\omega)$ the frequency-domain function. To transform from the frequency domain to the time domain, we use an expression,

---

*Section 3.4 written by Handayani Tjandrasa and Gregory S. Furno.

called the inverse Fourier transform (IFT):

$$x(t) = \frac{1}{2\pi} \int_{-\infty}^{\infty} F(\omega)e^{j\omega t}\, d\omega \tag{3.50}$$

Note that these transformations require analytic solutions; that is, we must find a mathematical formulation for our $x(t)$ and then compute $F(\omega)$ by performing the integration. For simple functions of $x(t)$, this method is practical, but for more complicated applications, both determining $x(t)$ and performing the integration may be difficult.

Discrete Fourier transform

A practical method exists for transforming functions between the time and frequency domains if we approximate the functions by a set of sampled data points such as those collected with an analog-to-digital converter. We gather N time-domain samples of the function (signal) spaced at equal time intervals T. We now represent the time-domain function by $x(m)$, for $m = 0, 1, \ldots, N - 1$. Thus we have fixed a block of data whose duration is NT seconds long. The frequency-domain function then becomes a set of discrete equally spaced samples rather than a continuous function. We represent it by $X(k)$ for $k = 0, 1, \ldots, N - 1$. We call this approximation to the continuous Fourier transform the discrete Fourier transform (DFT), and define it as

$$X(k) = \frac{1}{N} \sum_{m=0}^{N-1} x(m)W^{mk} \qquad \text{for } k = 0, 1, \ldots, N - 1 \tag{3.51}$$

where

$$W = e^{-j2\pi/N} \tag{3.52}$$

Essentially, the DFT takes a time-domain function represented by a set of samples and transforms it into a set of frequency-domain points through a large number of complex (i.e., real and imaginary) multiplications and additions. To go from the frequency to the time domain, we use the inverse discrete Fourier transform (IDFT), defined as

$$x(m) = \sum_{k=0}^{N-1} X(k)W^{-mk} \qquad \text{for } m = 0, 1, \ldots, N - 1 \tag{3.53}$$

The DFT assumes that the time-domain function $x(m)$ is periodic, with a period NT. Therefore, when we transform $X(k)$ into $x(m)$ with the IDFT we obtain one cycle of $x(m)$, and it is implicit that this cycle repeats itself. Also, because the DFT uses sampled data, the function $X(k)$ produced from $x(m)$ is periodic in the frequency domain with N points in each period, but only $N/2$ points are unique.

Figure 3.35 helps point out the differences between the DFT and the CFT. The time function in Fig. 3.35(c) is the result of multiplying the cosine function of Fig. 3.35(a) together with the rectangular window function of Fig. 3.35(b). The

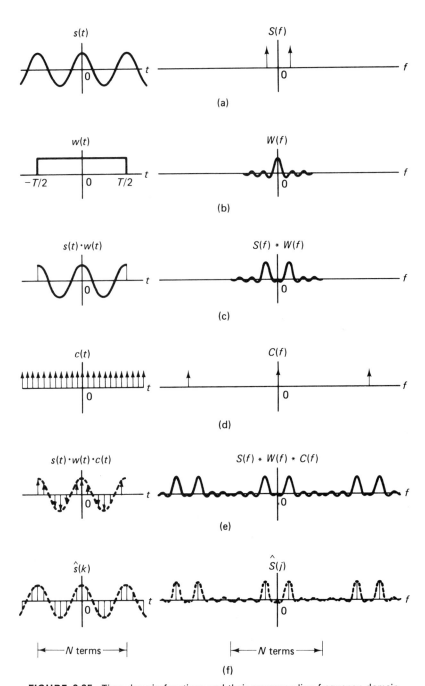

FIGURE 3.35 Time-domain functions and their corresponding frequency-domain equivalents. The time-domain functions are (a) cosine function, (b) rectangular window function, (c) product of functions (a) and (b), (d) set of impulses, (e) product of (c) and (d), and (f) assumed periodic function from which (e) was obtained. [From Bergland, G. D. 1969. A guided tour of the fast Fourier transform. IEEE Spectrum 6(7): 41–52.]

CFT of each of these functions is shown on the right. Let us consider this product in Fig. 3.35(c) to be the time function $x(m)$ we want to transform using the DFT. We must first sample $x(m)$ by multiplying by the set of impulses shown in Fig. 3.35(d). The result of the multiplication in Fig. 3.35(e) is a single set of data in the time domain with the CFT shown to its right. Note how sampling has caused the spectrum to repeat itself. To complete the DFT, we must assume that the time-domain function in Fig. 3.35(e) is periodic, as shown in Fig. 3.35(f), and the frequency-domain function becomes discrete, as required by the DFT. Observe in Fig. 3.35(f) that only $N/2$ of the N terms indicated in the frequency-domain function are unique. The other $N/2$ terms are mirror images. This means that for the frequency-domain representation to be valid over a frequency range of $N/2$ terms, the time-domain representation will contain N sample points. Now, should the CFT in Fig. 3.35(c) contain frequencies in a range greater than the $N/2$ range in Fig. 3.35(f) because of too low a sampling rate set in Fig. 3.35(d), then those frequencies above $N/2$ would overlap into the next $N/2$ interval. Aliasing would result, where these overlapping frequencies falsely represent the time-domain function, as discussed in Chapter 2. Therefore, we must either eliminate using an analog filter frequencies in our signal that extend beyond the $N/2$ limit (which is one-half the sampling frequency f_s), or we must increase the sampling rate to at least twice the highest so that there is no overlap.

Fast Fourier transform

If we choose N and f_s carefully, the DFT can closely approximate the CFT. However, such an approximation usually requires a large value for N (256 or more), and the total number of calculations required is of the order of N^2. This many computations make real-time DFT analysis impossible even with the fastest digital computers. Fortunately, an algorithm developed by Cooley and Tukey (1965), called the fast Fourier transform (FFT), calculates the DFT, taking advantage of the fact that many of the terms created by substituting integral values of m and k into eqs. (3.52) and (3.53) are identical, since the expression $e^{(-j2\pi/N)(mk)}$ generates cyclically repetitive results. By combining in an orderly fashion predictably identical terms, the FFT reduces the number of calculations to the order of $N \log_2 N$. For $N = 500$, the DFT requires about a 250,000 calculations, while the FFT needs only 4500, or about 2% as many as the DFT. Yet the two methods give identical results.

Figure 3.36(a) is a flow diagram that indicates the computations involved in a simple eight-point FFT. This diagram is simply a graphical interpretation of eq. (3.51) for $N = 8$. It shows how to generate the individual equations that transform the time-domain function $x(m)$ for $m = 0, 1, \ldots, 7$, into the frequency-domain function $X(k)$ for $k = 0, 1, \ldots, 7$. The $x(m)$ values are arranged in vertical columns to the left in the figure, while the $X(k)$ values are on the right. To use the diagram, start at the $x(m)$ nodes on the left and move to the right, adding and multiplying terms along the way until you reach the $X(k)$ nodes. If you are traveling

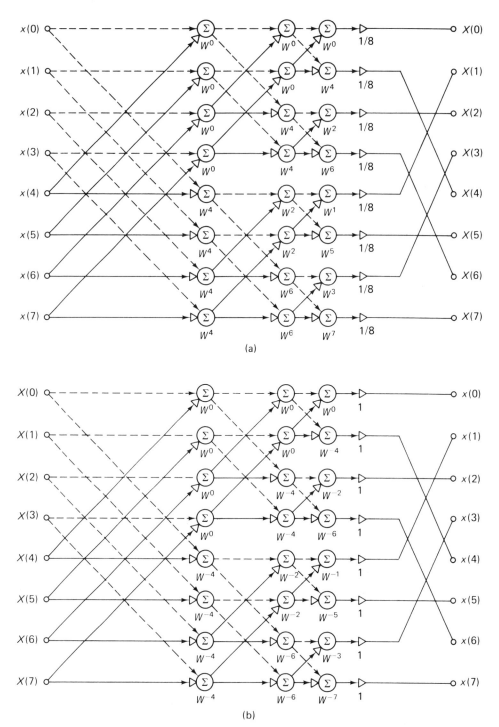

FIGURE 3.36 Flow diagrams for 8-point transforms. (a) Fast Fourier transform. (b) Inverse fast Fourier transform.

on a dashed line, you reach a summer (circle), where you add the starting $x(m)$ term to one other entering term. If you are traveling on a solid line you encounter a multiplier (triangle). Each multiplier is some power of W that multiplies the $x(m)$ term before it goes to a summer to be added to another term. You continue in this fashion until you reach the $X(k)$ nodes on the right. As an example, starting in the upper left corner with $x(0)$ and moving right, we come to a summer circle and form $[x(0) + x(4)W^0]$. Continuing right, we form $\{[x(0) + x(4)W^0] + [x(2) + x(6)W^0]W^0\}$. We keep up this process until all the $X(k)$ terms are found. To get the DFT values $X(k)$, we multiply the final terms by $\frac{1}{8}$ before ending at the $X(k)$ nodes.

Note that the time-domain term $x(i)$ on the left does not produce frequency-domain term $X(i)$ on the right. If the time-domain data points are in order [i.e., $x(0)$, $x(1)$, $x(2)$, . . .], the frequency-domain data points will be out of order. In order to properly sequence the $X(k)$ array, the points are sorted by subscript. The subscripts are expressed as binary numbers, and sorting is accomplished by a bit-reversal algorithm. Note, for example, that $x(3)$ produces $X(6)$ and $x(6)$ produces $X(3)$. In binary notation $x(3)$ is $x(011)$ and $X(6)$ is $X(110)$. The bit patterns in the subscripts are exactly reversed—the most significant bit in one pattern is the least significant in the other. A bit-reversal algorithm is thus used to shuffle each $X(k)$ into its proper array location as the final step in the FFT process.

To use the FFT procedure to compute an IFFT, we replace W with its complex conjugate $\bar{W}$ (or change the sign of the exponent) and eliminate the final $\frac{1}{8}$ multipliers [see eq. (3.53)]. A flow diagram of the IFFT is given in Fig. 3.36(b).

FFT subroutine

Figure 3.37 shows an FFT subroutine in FORTRAN which may be used to compute the DFT or the IDFT based upon eq. (3.52) or (3.53).

Applications

The FFT algorithm saves computation time and makes digital signal processing in real time practical for many research areas. Some types of digital analysis that can be done by FFT algorithms include the computation of harmonic analysis and synthesis, spectral analysis, convolution sequences, cross correlation, Fourier integrals, Fourier series and convolution integrals, and numerical solutions to partial differential equations.

An FFT example—EEG compressed spectral array

In the compressed spectral array (CSA) method, the resulting spectra are plotted in time sequence (each power spectrum is plotted slightly above the previous spectrum) in order to produce a three-dimensional effect, so that the resultant plots can be interpreted easily. The CSA technique compresses spectral information about the voluminous EEG tracings into a small space. This method is useful for neurological diagnosis, monitoring of depth of anesthesia, and sleep staging. Figure 3.38 shows the CSA during various sleep stages. The frequency changes for

```
        SUBROUTINE FFT(X,N,INV)
C **********************************************************************
C
C       THIS PROGRAM IMPLEMENTS THE FFT ALGORITHM TO COMPUTE THE DISCRETE
C       FOURIER COEFFICIENTS OF A DATA SEQUENCE OF N POINTS
C
C       CALLING SEQUENCE FROM THE MAIN PROGRAM:
C       CALL FFT(X,N,INV)
C           N:  NUMBER OF DATA POINTS
C           X:  COMPLEX ARRAY CONTAINING THE DATA SEQUENCE.  IN THE END DFT
C               COEFFS. ARE RETURNED IN THE ARRAY, MAIN PROGRAM SHOULD
C               DECLARE II AS --  COMPLEX X(512)
C           INV:  FLAG FOR INVERSE
C               INV=0  FOR FORWARD TRANSFORM
C               INV=1  FOR INVERSE TRANSFORM
C
C **********************************************************************

        COMPLEX X(512),W,T,CMPLX
C
C       CALCULATE THE # OF ITERATIONS (LOG. N TO THE BASE 2)
C
        ITER=0
        IREM=N
10      IREM=IREM/2
        IF (IREM.EQ.0) GO TO 20
        ITER=ITER+1
        GO TO 10
20      CONTINUE
        SIGN=-1
        IF (INV.EQ.1) SIGN=1.
        NXP2=N
        DO 50 IT=1,ITER
C
C       COMPUTATION FOR EACH ITERATION
C       NXP:  NUMBER OF POINTS IN A PARTITION
C       NSP2:  NXP/2
C
        NXP=NXP2                                    C
        NXP2=NXP/2                                      N2=N/2
        WPWR=3.141592/FLOAT(NXP2)                       N1=N-1
        DO 40 M=1,NXP2                                  J=1
C                                                       DO 65 I=1,N1
C       CALCULATE THE MULTIPLIER                        IF (I.GE.J) GO TO 55
C                                                       T=X(J)
        ARG=FLOAT(M-1)*WPWR                             X(J)=X(I)
        W=CMPLX(COS(ARG),SIGN*SIN(ARG))                 X(I)=T
        DO 40 MXP=NXP,N,NXP                     55      K=N2
C                                               60      IF (K.GE.J) GO TO 65
C       COMPUTATION FOR EACH PARTITION                  J=J-K
C                                                       K=K/2
        J1=MXP-NXP+M                                     GO TO 60
        J2=J1+NXP2                              65      J=J+K
        T=X(J1)-X(J2)                                   IF (INV.EQ.1) GO TO 75
        X(J1)=X(J1)+X(J2)                               DO 70 I=1,N
40      X(J2)=T*W                               70      X(I)=X(I)/FLOAT(N)
50      CONTINUE                                75      CONTINUE
C                                                       RETURN
C       UNSCRAMBLE THE BIT-REVERSED DFT COEFFS'         END
```

FIGURE 3.37 Subroutine for computing the FFT and the IFFT. (From Ahmed, N.,
and Rao, K. R. 1975. Orthogonal transforms for digital signal processing. New York:
Springer-Verlag. Used with permission.)

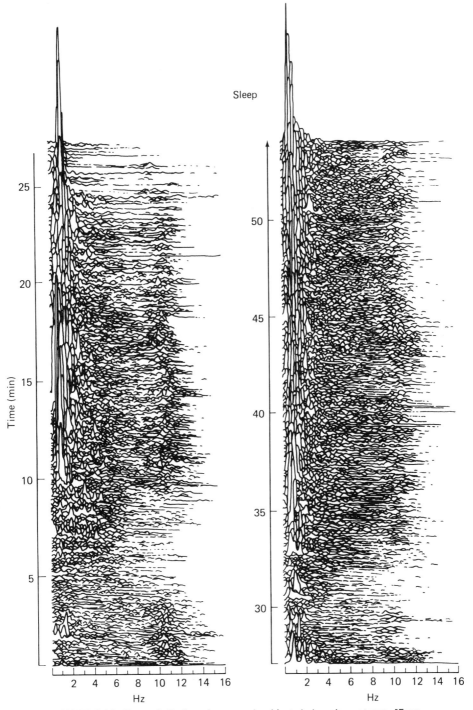

Sleep

Time (min)

25

20

15

10

5

2 4 6 8 10 12 14 16
Hz

50

45

40

35

30

2 4 6 8 10 12 14 16
Hz

FIGURE 3.38 Spectral display of a normal subject during sleep stages. [From Bickford, R. G., et al. 1972. The compressed spectral array (CSA)—a pictorial EEG. Proc. San Diego Biomed. Symp. 11 : 365–370.]

different levels of sleep can be easily read from the spectral display. These plots were obtained by sampling the EEG signal at a rate of 128 samples/s on a PDP-12 computer with 8 kwords of memory. The frequency range of the power spectra is between 0.25 and 16 Hz with a frequency resolution of 0.25 Hz.

3.5 PEAK AND VALLEY DETECTION*

Analog circuit

Figure 3.39(a) shows a basic positive peak detector circuit. Placing a diode in the op-amp feedback loop causes the circuit to act as an ideal diode. Let us consider the sinusoidal input signal v_i shown in Fig. 3.39(b). As v_i increases in the positive direction, the capacitor is charged until v_i reaches its peak value. When v_i decreases, the diode is reverse-biased. Then the capacitor discharges through the negative input of the op amp or the loading resistor R if it is present. The decay rate of v_o is minimized by using an FET amplifier for the input amplifier and keeping R high. The output rise time is determined by the short-circuit current I_m of the op amp. Provided that the op-amp slew rate does not limit the circuit, the maximum slew

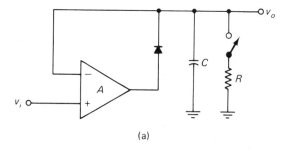

(a)

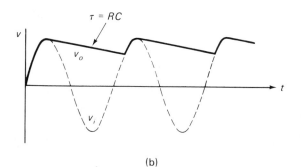

(b)

FIGURE 3.39 Basic positive peak detector. (a) Circuit diagram. (b) Output signal for a sine-wave input.

*Section 3.5 written by Handayani Tjandrasa.

rate of the circuit is

$$\frac{\Delta v_o}{\Delta t} = \frac{I_m}{C}$$

Figure 3.40 shows that a second op amp can isolate any load resistance R. In this case the voltage discharge rate is the input current of the follower divided by the value of C.

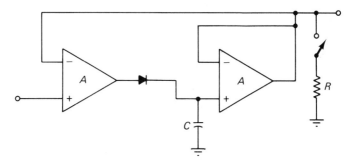

FIGURE 3.40 Simple buffered peak detector.

Peak and valley detector

We can detect peaks and valleys by using two positive peak detectors. Figure 3.41 shows the block diagram of this peak and valley detector. The output of the first positive peak detector gives the peak value of v_i. Subtracting v_i from the peak of this signal gives the peak-to-valley value. We obtain the valley output v_{o2} by subtracting the output of the second peak detector from v_{o1}. We select the capacitor values to give a desired decay rate. Too high a decay rate results in a high ripple output, while too low a decay rate prevents the detector from following rapidly changing waveforms.

Figure 3.42 shows the complete circuit for a simple peak and valley detector.

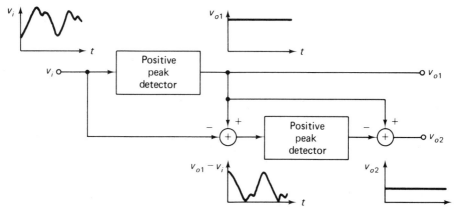

FIGURE 3.41 Block diagram of a peak and valley detector.

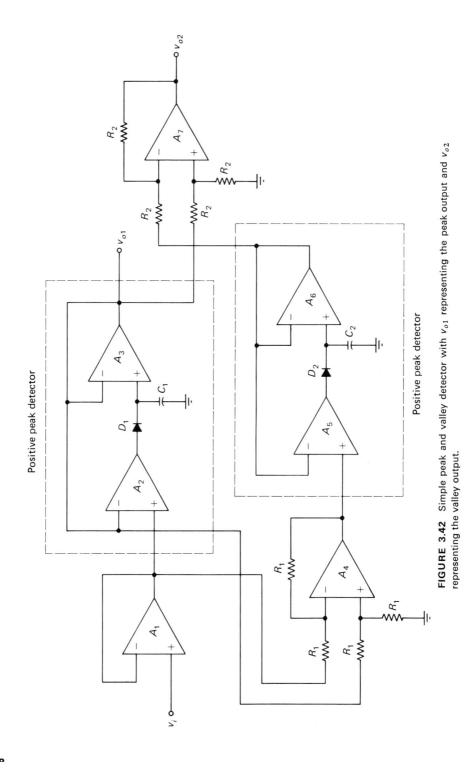

FIGURE 3.42 Simple peak and valley detector with v_{o1} representing the peak output and v_{o2} representing the valley output.

The input signal enters the input of a buffer amplifier A_1. Amplifiers A_2 and A_3, A_5 and A_6 operate as positive peak detectors. The output of A_3 gives the peak value. Amplifiers A_4 and A_7 operate as differential amplifiers with a gain of 1.

Mathematical methods for finding the peak and valley of a signal

Newton's method. We may determine the maximum, minimum, and zero of a function from a gradient descent technique such as Newton's method. Figure 3.43 shows that we may obtain the zero of a function by drawing a tangent line at the approximation t_i and then performing the next approximation. We repeat this process until we find the zero. The next approximation is given by

$$t_{i+1} = t_i - \frac{f(t_i)}{f'(t_i)}$$

We can only perform this method for a well-behaved function. To find the maximum and minimum values of a function, we can adapt this method by obtaining the values as the zeros of the differential function of $f(t)$. The approximation equation is given by

$$t_{i+1} = t_i - \frac{f'(t_i)}{f''(t_i)}$$

Derivative method. We can calculate the maximum and minimum values of a function $f(t)$ by finding points where its first derivative is equal to zero. We may determine these extreme values as a maximum or a minimum by computing the function's second derivative. For $f''(t) < 0$, the value gives a maximum, whereas for $f''(t) > 0$, the value represents a minimum.

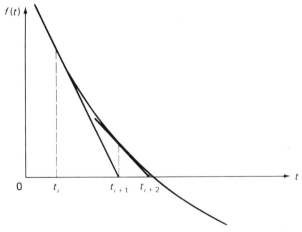

FIGURE 3.43 Newton's method to find the zero of a function.

Algorithms

To find the peak and valley values of a signal using digital processing, we should smooth the raw data by a low-pass digital filter to minimize high-frequency noise before processing. Section 3.1 discusses methods of low-pass filtering used in digital processing. We can obtain maximum and minimum points by searching the changes of the first differences between consecutive data points. Section 3.2 summarizes derivative algorithms that can be used for peak and valley detection. We can obtain a maximum or minimum by recognizing a point at which there is a change of sign, so that the two slopes on the right and left sides of a point are of opposite sign.

The application of algorithms to identify the important events of the blood-pressure wave. The measurement of blood pressure is an important tool for diagnosing hemodynamic dysfunction. The direct measurement of pressure is important for the critically ill patient. In addition to analog techniques, computer techniques have been introduced to monitor the arterial pressure of critically ill patients. The important events to be identified in the blood-pressure waveform are the end-diastolic pressure, the peak systolic pressure, and the end of systolic ejection (dicrotic notch). The pressure minimum represents the end of one cardiac cycle and the beginning of the next. The rapid upstroke of the pressure waveform indicates pumping of the blood from the left ventricle of the heart into the aorta and the trunk of the arterial tree. The blood pressure reaches its maximum value during systole and decreases as the ventricle relaxes. The dicrotic notch represents the end of systolic ejection. The sampling rate used in pressure analysis is 50 to 250 Hz. Some algorithms determine the important events of pressure data using the QRS complex for time identification.

Fozzard et al. (1974) have described a multiple-sample, serial-difference method to scan the data and to filter out high-frequency artifacts. They detect the extreme values by chord minimum selection. Figure 3.44 shows that the iteration starts by selecting a chord that spans eight time intervals. The algorithm tries various starting times of $s \pm n$ and selects the interval span that yields the chord of shortest length (C_{s-1}^8). It then repeats the selection for the chords that span four time intervals in the interval terminated by C_{s-1}^8. The selection of the chord of shortest length yields C_{s+1}^4. The iteration repeats with chords spanning time intervals of length 2 and then 1, which determines the extreme value. The dicrotic notch is sought in a predetermined interval between the end-diastolic pressure and the peak systolic pressure. Other investigators have used digital filters to locate the dicrotic notch using a matched filter.

Starmer et al. (1973) used a series of algorithms to detect the dicrotic notch. First they used ECG R-wave detection to locate the pressure-data segment to be analyzed. They determined R-wave location by obtaining a data point where the absolute value of the first derivative exceeded a preset threshold (see Section 3.2 for a summary of this approach). They determined the end-diastolic pressure as a data point that is followed by four first derivatives greater than 10 mm Hg/s. They

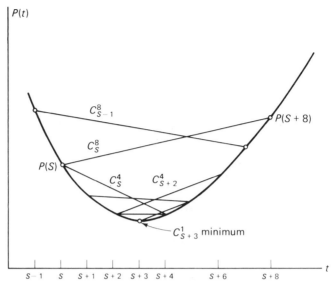

FIGURE 3.44 Determining the minimum value by successive approximation. (From Fozzard, H. A., et al. 1974. Algorithms for analysis of on-line pressure signals. Conf. Comput. Cardiol., pp. 77–83.)

determined the peak systolic pressure by seeking the maximum filtered pressure. Using a moving-average filter similar to the one described in Section 3.1, they removed high-frequency noise.

The dicrotic notch is defined as a local minimum pressure occurring in the region of maximum second derivative. It is found in a predetermined interval between peak systolic pressure and end-diastolic pressure. The second derivative of pressure may be obtained using a least-squares estimate based on the parabolic filter derivative in Section 3.2.

Nygards et al. (1976) used a derivative method to detect the important events of the arterial pressure wave. They examined the pressure wave from QRS reference points. They determined the onset of ejection by finding the point that has its first derivative exceeding the threshold value (the threshold value is given as one-half of the maximum difference during the first 5 s of recording). They determined the onset of ejection by the point where the second derivative is maximum (see Fig. 3.45). They obtained the dicrotic notch by determining the point that has a maximum second derivative after the peak systolic pressure.

Other investigators apply the AZTEC preprocessing technique to the pressure data. This technique is a zero-order interpolator and it produces amplitude-dependent and frequency-independent filtering. The advantages offered by this technique are time and program space savings. Using an AZTEC program, an important event may be determined by searching for a data point that has a slope exceeding a threshold value. Figure 3.46 shows the resulting AZTEC representation. We discuss AZTEC in depth in Chapter 6.

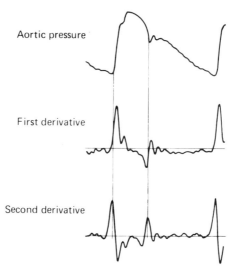

FIGURE 3.45 Recognition of critical points in an arterial pressure wave. (From Nygards, M. E., et al. 1976. On-line computer preprocessing of pressure data from cardiac catheterizations. Comput. Programs Biomed. 5 : 272–282. Used with permission.)

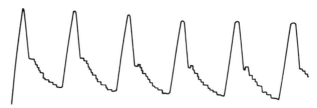

FIGURE 3.46 Resulting AZTEC representation of arterial blood pressure. (From Fozzard, H. A., et al. 1974. Algorithms for analysis of on-line pressure signals. Conf. Comput. Cardiol., pp. 77–83.)

Evaluation

The results of manual and automatically computed pressure values show little difference if the signals processed are of normal quality. With a good measuring instrument, an automatic pressure monitoring system gives better results for very low diastolic pressures and pulsus alternans, which cannot be indicated correctly by an analog monitor.

The other advantage of an automatic system is the objectivity of the analysis, which is independent of the trained eye of the physician. The primary problem encountered in automatic systems is the occurrence of artifacts, which must be separated from the signal of interest. Also, catheter frequency response affects the result of the algorithm. Using a catheter with inadequate frequency response causes smoothing of the pressure signal, including the dicrotic notch. Therefore, the catheter should be selected to provide a signal whose fidelity high enough to meet the requirements of the algorithm.

REFERENCES

ACKROYD, M. H. 1973. Digital filters. London: Butterworth.

AHMED, N., AND RAO, K. R. 1975. Orthogonal transforms for digital signal processing. New York: Springer-Verlag.

ANTONIOU, A. 1979. Digital filters: analysis and design. New York: McGraw-Hill.

BENSON, D. W., JR. 1971. An algorithm for defining the cardiac cycle using ascending aortic blood flow. Comput. Biomed. Res. 4: 216–223.

BERGLAND, G. D. 1969. A guided tour of the fast Fourier transform. IEEE Spectrum 6(7): 41–52.

BICKFORD, R. G., BILLINGER, T. W., FLEMING, N. I., AND STEWART, L. 1972. The compressed spectral array (CSA)—a pictorial EEG. Proc. San Diego Biomed. Symp. 11: 365–370.

BUTLER, L. A. 1976. A real-time software system on the PDP-11 for two-channel EEG spectral analysis during surgery. Comput. Progr. Biomed. 6: 1–10.

COCHRAN, W. T., ET AL. 1976. What is the fast Fourier transform? IEEE Trans. Audio Electroacoust. AU-15: 45–55.

COOLEY, J. W., AND TUKEY J. W. 1965. An algorithm for the machine calculation of complex Fourier series. Math. Comput. 19: 297–301.

COOLEY, J. W., LEWIS, P. A. W., AND WELCH, P. D. 1967. Application of the fast Fourier transform to computation of Fourier integrals, Fourier series, and convolution integrals. IEEE Trans. Audio Electroacoust. AU-15: 79–84.

CORINTHIOS, M. J. 1971a. The design of a class of fast Fourier transform computers. IEEE Trans. Comput. C-20: 617–623.

CORINTHIOS, M. J. 1971b. A fast Fourier transform for high-speed signal processing. IEEE Trans. Comput. C-20: 843–846.

CORINTHIOS, M. J. 1975. A parallel radix-y fast Fourier transform computer. IEEE Trans. Comput. C-24: 80–92.

COX, J. R., NOLLE, F. M., FOZZARD, H. A., AND OLIVER, G. C., JR. 1968. AZTEC, a preprocessing program for real-time ECG rhythm analysis. IEEE Trans. Biomed. Eng. BME-15: 128–129.

COX, J. R., JR., NOLLE, F. M., AND ARTHUR, R. M. 1972. Digital analysis of the electroencephalogram, the blood pressure wave, and the electrocardiogram. Proc. IEEE 60: 1137–1164.

DOEBELIN, E. O. 1975. Measurement systems: application and design, 2nd ed. New York: McGraw-Hill.

FOZZARD, H. A., KINIAS, P., AND PAI, A. L. 1974. Algorithms for analysis of on-line pressure signals. Conf. Comput. Cardiol., pp. 77–83.

FRANCIS, G. R. 1974. An improved systolic–diastolic pulse separator. Med. Biol. Eng. 12: 105–108.

GENTLEMAN, W. M. 1966. Fast Fourier transforms—for fun and profit. AFIPS Proc. Fall Joint Comput. Conf. 29:563–578.

GREENFIELD, J. C., JR., STARMER, C. F., AND WALSTON, A. 1971. Measurement of aortic blood flow in man by the computed pressure derivative method. J. Appl. Physiol. 31:792–795.

HAMMING, R. W. 1977. Digital filters. Englewood Cliffs, NJ: Prentice-Hall.

HOFF, M. E., AND TOWNSEND, M. E. 1979. Single-chip *n*-MOS microcomputer processes signals in real time. Electronics 52:105–110.

HUBER, F. 1975. EEG spectral analysis for Nova computers. Comput. Progr. Biomed. 4:175–179.

JOHNSON, D. E., AND HILBURN, J. L. 1975. Rapid practical design of active filters. New York: Wiley.

JOHNSON, D. E., 1976. Introduction to filter theory. Englewood Cliffs, NJ: Prentice-Hall.

JUNG, W. G. 1974. IC op-amp cookbook. Indianapolis, IN: Sams.

LaFARA, R. L. 1973. Computer methods for science and engineering. Rochelle Park, NJ: Hayden.

LAM, H. Y-F. 1979. Analog and digital filters: design and realization. Englewood Cliffs, NJ: Prentice-Hall.

LANCASTER, D. 1978. Active-filter cookbook. Indianapolis, IN: Sams.

LINDQUIST, C. S. 1977. Active network design with signal filtering applications. Long Beach, CA: Steward & Sons.

NAYLOR, W. S. 1971. An analog preprocessor for use in monitoring arterial pressure. Biomed. Eng. 6(2):77–80.

NYGARDS, M. E., TRANESJÖ, J., ATTERHÖG, J. H., BLOMQUIST, P., EKELUND, L. G., AND WIGERTZ, O. 1976. On-line computer preprocessing of pressure data from cardiac catheterizations. Comput. Progr. Biomed. 5:272–282.

PINSON, L. J., AND CHILDERS, D. G. 1974. Frequency-wave number spectrum analysis of EEG multielectrode array data. IEEE. Trans. Biomed. Eng. BME-21:192–206.

RABINER, L. R., AND GOLD, B. 1975. Theory and application of digital signal processing. Englewood Cliffs, NJ: Prentice-Hall.

ROCKLAND SYSTEMS CORP. 1976. The application of filters to analog and digital signal processing. West Nyack, NY.

ROCKLAND SYSTEMS CORP. 1977. Spectrum analysis—theory, implementation and applications. West Nyack, NY.

ROTHCHILD, R. S. 1971. Real time signal analysis. Med. Electron. Data 2(2):110–125.

SABAH, N. H., AND SARHAN, A. 1977. Peak-detecting window discriminator. Med. Biol. Eng. Comput. 15:205–206.

SODERSTRAND, M. A. 1972. On-line digital filtering using PDP-8 or PDP-12. In Computers in the neurophysiology laboratory, Vol. 1, pp. 31–49. Maynard, MA: Digital Equipment Corporation.

STANLEY, W. D. 1975. Digital signal processing. Reston, VA: Reston.

STARMER, C. F., McHALE, P. A., AND GREENFIELD, J. C., JR. 1973. Processing of arterial pressure waves with a digital computer. Comput. Biomed. Res. 6:90–96.

STEARNS, S. D. 1975. Digital signal analysis. Rochelle Park, NJ: Hayden.

STOCKHAM, T. G. 1966. High speed convolution and correlation. AFIPS Proc. Spring Joint Comput. Conf. 28:229–233.

STOUT, D. F., AND KAUFMAN, M. 1976. Handbook of operational amplifier circuit design. New York: McGraw-Hill.

STRAUSS, L. 1970. Wave generation and shaping. New York: McGraw-Hill.

STREMLER, F. G. 1977. Introduction to communication systems. Reading, MA: Addison-Wesley.

TOBEY, G. E., HUELSMAN, L. P., AND GRAEME, G. G. 1971. Operational amplifiers design and application. New York: McGraw-Hill.

WARNER, H. R., SWAN, H. J. C., CONNOLLY, D. C., TOMPKINS, R. G., AND WOOD, E. H. 1953. Quantitation of beat-to-beat changes in stroke volume from the aortic pulse contour in man. J. Appl. Physiol. 5:495–507.

WARTAK, J., MILLIKEN, J. A., AND KARCHMAR, J. 1970. Computer program for pattern recognition of electrocardiograms. Comput. Biomed. Res. 4:344–374.

WEAVER, C. S., VON DER GROBEN, J., MANTEY, P. E., TOOLE, J. G., COLE, C. A., JR., FITZGERALD, J. W., AND LAWRENCE, R. W. 1968. Digital filtering with applications to electrocardiogram processing. IEEE Trans. Audio Electroacoust. AU-16: 350–387.

PROBLEMS

3.1 Design a second-order low-pass Butterworth VCVS filter with a corner frequency of 100 Hz and gain of 10.

3.2 The filter of Fig. 3.8 is to be used to eliminate 60-Hz interference from a signal. The designer uses ac coupling through a capacitor. Will this filter work properly? Why?

3.3 What are the advantages of digital filters?

3.4 What are the advantages and disadvantages of recursive and nonrecursive filters?

3.5 Design a nonrecursive smoothing filter that is as flat in its passband as possible, and meets the following requirements: $H(0) = 1$, $H(\pi/2) = 0$.

3.6 Design a low-pass digital filter with a sampling rate of 200 Hz and a 3-dB frequency of 40 Hz. At 60 Hz the attenuation must be greater than 40 dB and a flat passband response is required.

3.7 Using the schematic of a differentiation circuit [Fig. 3.25(a)], design an analog system to differentiate and detect certain unipolar EEG γ-wave changes. Find the values for R_i, R_p, R_f, C_i, C_p, and C_f. Assume an output of ± 5 V and a maximum input slope of 0.1 V/100 μs.

3.8 Compare the differentiation techniques of 2-point difference and 5-point least-squares polynomial fitting by finding and graphing the derivative of the QRS complex given in Fig. P3.1 using the two different techniques.

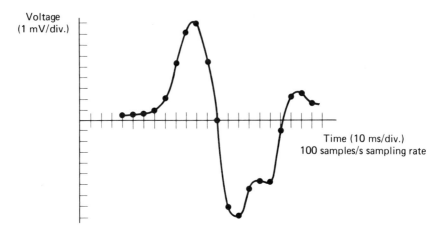

FIGURE P3.1 ECG QRS complex.

3.9 Draw a flowchart implementing the derivative using a 5-point least-squares polynomial fit. Assume that data to be differentiated are stored in memory locations 0100_{16} through $01FF_{16}$ and the answer is to be stored beginning at 0200_{16}.

3.10 Assume that a 7-point least-squares polynomial-fit differentiation routine takes 100 instructions, a subtraction differentiation routine takes 20 instructions, and each instruction takes an average of 5 μs. What is the maximum sampling rate for real-time differentiation using each technique?

3.11 If 5 mg of dye were injected at $t = 0$, and the average concentration of dye on the arterial side were 1.7 mg/liter during the interval from $t = 0$ to $t = 40$ s, what would be the cardiac output?

3.12 The compressed spectral array displays information in the form of a frequency, time, and amplitude plot. Present techniques give a plot of the frequency spectrum over a discrete-time interval. Is it theoretically possible to find the spectrum for all values of time? Why or why not? (*Hint:* Consider the constraints of the Fourier transform.)

3.13 Using Newton's method, calculate the square root x of a given number n, represented by equation $x^2 - n = 0$ by finding the zero of the quadratic function $f(x) = x^2 - n$. Find the square-root value of 2 with an accuracy of six decimal places. (*Hint:* Start the iteration with the first approximating value $x_0 = 1.4$.)

4

Microcomputer
Design

4.1 INTRODUCTION TO THE MICROCOMPUTER SYSTEM*

In 1971 Intel Corporation introduced the microprocessor, which has created a revolution in the electronics and data-processing industries. Use of the microprocessor is spreading to many fields because of its low cost, small size, and powerful computing capability (Toong, 1977).

Basic microcomputer architecture

Figure 4.1 shows the major units of a microcomputer. The central processing unit (CPU) performs arithmetic and logical operations and includes the processor control unit. The read-only memory (ROM) stores a set of instructions or program and fixed information that need not be modified as the program runs. The contents of random-access memory (RAM) can be read and changed. RAM is used for

---

*Section 4.1 written by Yongmin Kim.

167

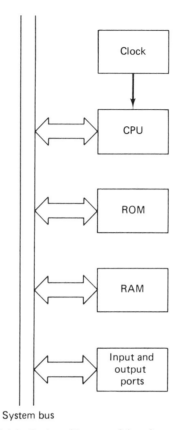

System bus

FIGURE 4.1   Basic architecture of the microcomputer.

storing temporary data. Input and output ports provide paths for transferring information between the computer and the outside world. The clock generates timing pulses to synchronize actions inside the computer. One important fact is that all units communicate with one another over the system bus one at a time. This system bus consists of an address bus, a data bus, and a control bus.

We now define the difference between microprocessor and microcomputer because these terms are used interchangeably in the literature. The microprocessor is usually a chip that performs the functions of the CPU of a traditional computer. The microcomputer is a computer system that makes use of a microprocessor chip together with other supporting chips, as shown in Fig. 4.1. Microcomputer systems can also be constructed that employ several bit-slice microprocessor chips. These bit-slice systems are used in high-speed, high-performance applications and require significant developmental hardware and software aids. They are not generally used in medical instruments because single-chip, 8-bit processors are adequate for most applications. At the other end of the spectrum are single-chip microcomputers, which have all the elements of a computer, including memory and input/output ports on the LSI chip. In this book we concentrate on the single-chip, 8-bit micro-processor.

Figure 4.2 shows a simplified block diagram of a microprocessor, which includes internal registers, an arithmetic logic unit (ALU), a control unit, status flags, and clock logic. A sequence of instructions (program) is stored in ROM. The program counter always specifies the location in the program memory, which is usually in ROM, of the next instruction to be performed. After the current instruction is completed, the control unit fetches the next instruction from the memory through the system bus, stores it in the instruction register, and decodes it, thus generating the control signals that cause the instruction to be executed. Then the control unit fetches and executes the next instruction. A typical microcomputer is able to do several hundred thousand instructions per second.

The accumulator stores temporary data and is the source of one of the operands used by the ALU in an arithmetic or logical operation. The stack pointer is used for stack management and will be discussed later in this chapter. Status flags are set (logic 1) or cleared (logic 0), depending upon the result of an ALU operation. These flags usually include carry, zero, sign, and overflow.

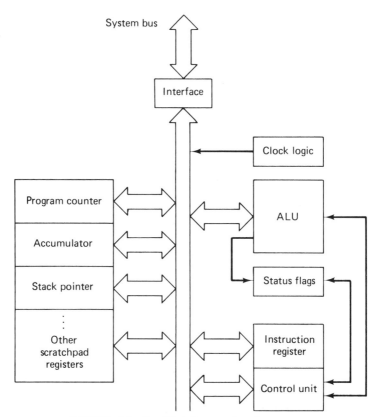

FIGURE 4.2 Simplified diagram of a microprocessor.

Large-scale-integration technologies

A microprocessor chip contains several thousand transistors. Without LSI (large-scale-integration) technology, the microprocessor could not have been developed. Figure 4.3 shows speed versus power dissipation and speed versus relative packing density for the main LSI technologies. There are two broad groups: bipolar and metal-oxide semiconductor (MOS). The bipolar group includes transistor-transistor logic (TTL), emitter-coupled logic (ECL), and integrated-injection logic (I²L). Bipolar devices are fast but consume more power and space than MOS (except I²L) devices. The MOS group includes n-channel MOS (NMOS), p-channel MOS-

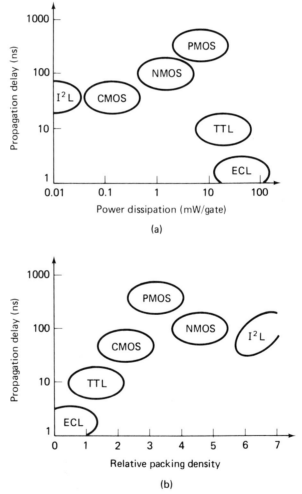

FIGURE 4.3 LSI technology comparisons. (a) Propagation delay versus power dissipation. (b) Propagation delay versus relative packing density.

(PMOS), and complementary symmetry MOS (CMOS). MOS devices are relatively slow but save power and space. One popular version of TTL is Schottky TTL. It is faster and a low-power version consumes less power than does standard TTL. Another recent technology is silicon on sapphire (SOS). It reduces the capacitive coupling between devices, which yields faster operation than does MOS. I²L is the most recent and promising LSI technology. It has lower power dissipation and higher packing density than the MOS group while operating at speeds in the bipolar range.

Early microprocessors employed PMOS technology. Recent microprocessors employ NMOS for low cost and medium speed, CMOS for extremely low power, and TTL for high speed. It is likely that I²L will be able to replace many of the technologies described above while retaining their good features.

Advantages of the microcomputer

As the complexity of hardwired logic increases beyond a certain point the microcomputer becomes advantageous because of its low cost, flexibility, reliability, and decision-making capability. Its cost includes not only hardware but also design and programming cost. Flexibility means that we can modify the system function later by changing the software or program contained in ROM without a hardware change. This cannot be done with hardwired logic. Employing a microcomputer reduces the number of components in a complex design, thereby increasing reliability. The microcomputer can make decisions and perform proper actions under program control, so the microcomputer seems to be intelligent. Small size, accuracy, and the ability to store and manipulate bulk data are other advantages. A major potential disadvantage is speed. For some high-speed applications, hardwired logic is still desirable.

After deciding that a microcomputer is desirable and feasible in a particular application, we must select a particular microprocessor. In this step we must consider total cost to meet specification, including supporting chips, speed, software support, and power consumption. After development, the hardware and software are integrated and tested. Finally, the microcomputer system is implemented and a new instrument is born.

4.2 MICROPROCESSOR HARDWARE DESIGN*

In this section we discuss digital system fundamentals and basic hardware attributes of microprocessors.

Design considerations for digital devices

In designing and implementing the microcomputer, we must give special consideration to the characteristics of digital circuits and compatibility, especially when using components from different logic families. In small-scale-integration (SSI) and

---

*Section 4.2 written by Yongmin Kim.

medium-scale-integration (MSI) circuits, TTL has been a leading logic family and includes a variety of devices, while CMOS is rapidly encroaching on TTL.

Propagation delay.   The propagation delay is the time difference between input and output logic level changes. The system speed is usually determined by the propagation delay, so that TTL with its small delay is good for the high-performance system whereas PMOS is not (see Fig. 4.3).

Transfer characteristic.   Figure 4.4(a) shows a CMOS inverter. The input voltage v_i drives both gates and v_o is the drain voltage. Figure 4.4(b) shows the ideal input/output voltage transfer characteristic of an inverter. When the input voltage v_i is less than $V_{DD}/2$, the output is logic 1. When v_i is greater than $V_{DD}/2$, the output is logic 0. Here V_{DD} is called the threshold voltage. Figure 4.4(c) shows the transfer characteristic of a CMOS inverter with a 5-V power supply. When v_i is less than 2 V, the p transistor is turned on and the n transistor is turned off. Therefore, the output voltage is about 5 V. When v_i is greater than 3 V, the n transistor is turned on and the p transistor is turned off, making the output voltage approach 0 V. When v_i is 2.5 V, the output voltage is indeterminate. Therefore, for reliability we must avoid the input voltage range between 2 and 3 V except during switching. One of the two transistors is always off, so there is no current path in the quiescent state. Figure 4.4(d) shows that CMOS draws significant power only during switching. Figure 4.4(e) shows power dissipation versus input frequency. At higher frequencies, CMOS loses its low-power advantage.

Figure 4.5(a) shows a standard TTL inverter. The power-supply voltage is fixed at 5 V and only a 5% variation (from 4.75 to 5.25 V) is permitted. Figure 4.5(b) shows the transfer characteristic of a TTL inverter. This characteristic changes with temperature and power-supply voltage. When v_i is low, Q_1 is saturated, Q_2 and Q_3 are turned off and Q_4 is turned on. Therefore, the output voltage v_o is logic 1 (high). When v_i is high, Q_1 is active in the reverse mode, thus turning Q_2 and Q_3 on and Q_4 off. The output voltage becomes logic 0 (low). Manufacturers guarantee that even under the worst operating conditions shown in Fig. 4.5(c), the output voltage is greater than 2.4 V and less than 0.4 V if the input voltage is less than 0.8 V and greater than 2.0 V, respectively.

Comparing CMOS with TTL, CMOS has the advantages of low power, a more ideal transfer characteristic and a power-supply voltage from 3 to 18 V. In speed, however, TTL is superior.

Fan-in.   The fan-in is the maximum number of inputs to one gate. In practice, fan-in is limited only by the number of pins available on a chip.

Fan-out.   Fan-out is the number of input gates that one gate output can drive. It is usually limited by loading. Figure 4.5(c) shows the worst-case TTL gate-loading rule. A standard TTL output can supply current to at least 10 gates when it is at logic 1 and can sink current from 10 gates when it is at logic 0. The fan-out of standard TTL therefore is 10.

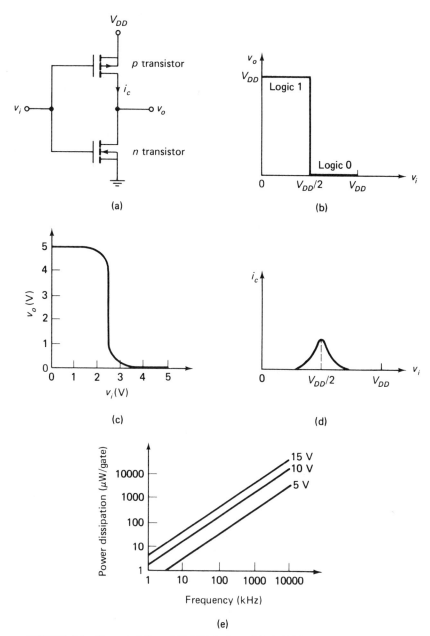

FIGURE 4.4 Characteristics of CMOS devices. (a) A CMOS inverter, where the drains of each transistor are connected to each other to yield v_o. (b) Ideal characteristic of a CMOS inverter. (c) Transfer characteristic of a CMOS inverter when V_{DD} is 5 V. (d) CMOS current versus input voltage. Note the near-zero current in the quiescent state. (e) Power dissipation versus input frequency. As the power-supply voltage increases, propagation delay decreases, but more power is consumed.

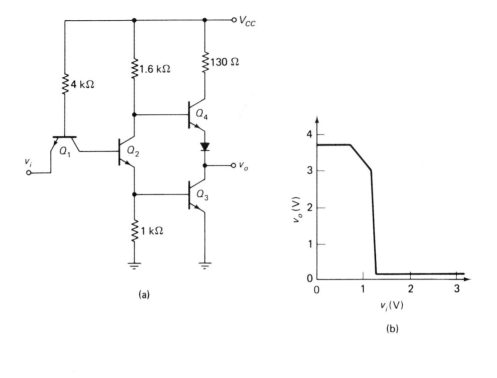

(a)

(b)

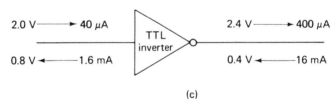

(c)

FIGURE 4.5 (a) Standard TTL inverter where V_{CC} is 5 V. (b) Transfer characteristic of this amplifier when the power-supply voltage is 5 V and the temperature is
25°C. (c) Worst-case TTL gate-loading rule. The gate input can sink a maximum of
40 μA at logic 1 and source a maximum of 1.6 mA at logic 0. The gate output can
source up to 400 μA at logic 1 and sink up to 16 mA at logic 0.

The input impedance of CMOS is very large and the input current is practically zero, so that fan-out of CMOS is very large as long as the output voltage of
the unloaded driving amplifier is above 3 V or below 2 V with a 5-V power supply.
In the case of insufficient fan-out, a buffer amplifier can increase fan-out by raising
the current-handling capability.

Noise.   Noise is the unwanted signal that is superimposed on the wanted signal.
This unwanted signal, if excessive, can make the whole system unreliable. In digital
applications, noise must be eliminated or ignored. There are several sources of

noise. When a switching line is adjacent to an input line, there is coupled noise. When a large amount of current is drawn from the power supply during signal transition, a transient noise voltage appears on the power-supply line.

Noise margin.   Noise margin is the noise voltage that one gate can eliminate. Worst-case TTL noise margins for logic 1 and logic 0 are both 0.4 V, while typical ones are 0.7 V. This means that as long as the noise voltage is less than 0.4 V, a TTL gate has total noise immunity. Because of a more ideal transfer characteristic, the CMOS family has greater noise margins (at least 1 V with a 3-V power supply) than TTL.

EXAMPLE

Verify that worst-case TTL noise margins are both 0.4 V.

Solution

Noise margin for logic $0 = V_{\text{IL}}$ (max) $- V_{\text{OL}}$ (max) $= 0.8$ V $- 0.4$ V $= 0.4$ V

Noise margin for logic $1 = V_{\text{OH}}$ (min) $- V_{\text{IH}}$ (min) $= 2.4$ V $- 2.0$ V $= 0.4$ V

where V_{IL} is the low-level input voltage, V_{OL} the low-level output voltage, V_{OH} the high-level output voltage, and V_{IH} the high-level input voltage.

EXAMPLE

Figure 4.5(a) shows a standard TTL inverter.

1. What is the maximum possible spiking current of this amplifier during signal transition?
2. This inverter package is bypassed by a 0.002-μF capacitor to absorb the spiking current between the power supply and ground lines. Assuming the 5-ns duration of above-maximum spiking current, what is the transient on the power-supply line?

Solution

1. If both Q_3 and Q_4 are turned on, the spiking current will flow from V_{CC} to ground through Q_3 and Q_4. Assuming 0.2 V as the collector-to-emitter saturation voltage and 0.7 V as the forward diode drop, the spiking current is

$$i_s = \frac{5 \text{ V} - 0.7 \text{ V} - 0.4 \text{ V}}{130 \text{ }\Omega} = 30 \text{ mA}$$

2. Current through a capacitor is represented by

$$i_C = C\frac{dv_C}{dt}$$

Constant current for the 5-ns duration makes the preceding equation

$$i_s = C \frac{\Delta V_{CC}}{\Delta t}$$

$$\Delta V_{CC} = i_s \times \frac{\Delta t}{C} = \frac{30 \times 10^{-3} \times 5 \times 10^{-9}}{2 \times 10^{-9}} = 75 \, \text{mV}$$

System bus structure

Figure 4.6 shows a typical system bus structure. Every block shares the bus and only one information transfer between blocks is possible at any given time. Every line in the system bus can represent a bit (binary digit) by being a high voltage (logic 1) or a low voltage (logic 0).

Tristate device. Most digital devices have two states. However a tristate device has one additional state called the high-impedance (hi-Z) state. Figure 4.7 shows a tristate (three-state) inverter and its truth table. If its control line is active, the tristate inverter acts as a normal inverter with two output states. If its control line is at logic 0, the output of the inverter is in the hi-Z state, thereby disconnecting it from the rest of the system. Tristate logic devices make it possible for any line in the bus to be driven by one device selected from many that are connected to the bus. The output of the selected device is in a low-impedance state (logic 1 or 0), while all others are in the high-impedance state. This substantially eliminates the fan-out problem and simplifies system organization.

Address bus. The 16-bit unidirectional address bus is driven by the CPU. Sixteen address lines can address 2^{16} memory locations ($2^{16} = 64 \, k$, where $1 \, k = 1024$). But the memory size of most microcomputer-based instruments does not exceed 8 kbytes. If the CPU wants to read the data stored in RAM, the first step it must take is to put the address on the address bus.

The COSMAC microprocessor has only an 8-bit address bus. The higher 8-bit address byte comes out on this bus first before the lower-bit address byte. Latches must be provided to hold the higher 8-bit address byte to prevent it from being lost.

Data bus. The data bus is an 8-bit bidirectional bus which carries instructions and data. An addressed RAM location may put its contents onto the data bus or accept the contents of the data bus to be written into the addressed location.

Control bus. The control bus consists of several control lines. These lines control all the actions of all the parts of the microcomputer. The names and functions of these lines vary, depending on the microprocessor. Control lines such as WRITE and READ provide for storing and retrieving data in RAM and are used together with the address bus, which specifies the location of interest in the RAM.

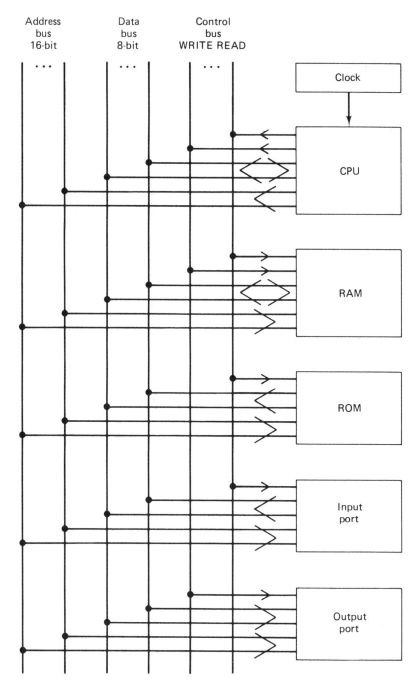

FIGURE 4.6 The microcomputer system bus includes a 16-bit address bus, an 8-bit data bus, and a control bus. Arrows represent the directions of information flow.

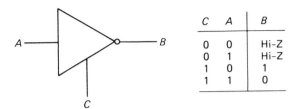

C	A	B
0	0	Hi-Z
0	1	Hi-Z
1	0	1
1	1	0

FIGURE 4.7 Tristate inverter and its truth table.

Clock.   The clock line can be treated as a control line. The clock is essential in every microcomputer to synchronize all actions. Each microprocessor has specific clock requirements of phase, frequency, voltage level, and rise and fall time. Figure 4.8 shows a single-phase and a two-phase clock. In the two-phase clock, the relative timing of the two clock waveforms is specified and the two frequencies are the same. Maximum frequency is limited by the propagation delays through gates and depends on the type of LSI technology. The voltage level identifies the permissible range for high and low clock voltage; maximum rise and fall times are also given.

Clock pulses could be generated by an external clock-driver chip or an on-chip clock circuit. Some microprocessors have extensive clock logic, so the combination of a resistor and a capacitor or a crystal and a resistor may be enough for clock-pulse generation.

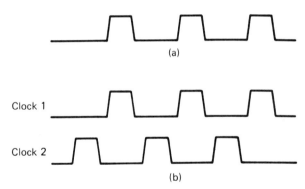

FIGURE 4.8 Microprocessor clocks. (a) Single phase. (b) Two phase.

Multiplexed bus.   Some microprocessors do not have any address bus at all. Instead, the address is multiplexed over the data bus. Control signals and a common clock control the multiplexed bus so that addresses and data are not mixed. This structure makes a simple system, but the speed is lower than a system with a separate address bus.

EXAMPLE

What are the system bus timing relationships for the memory read and write operations in the Z80 microprocessor, one of our model microprocessors?

Solution

Figure 4.9 shows read and write timing for the Z80. For the memory-read operation, the CPU puts the address on the address bus. Then the CPU makes the read control line ($\overline{RD}$) active. (The bar over RD means that it is a negated signal: it is active when it is low.) The $\overline{MREQ}$ control line becomes active (low) whenever the address bus is stable. After some delay, the selected memory location puts its contents on the data bus. Throughout the memory-read operation, the write control line ($\overline{WR}$) is inactive (high). For the memory-write operation, the CPU outputs data to be stored on the data bus. The selected memory location stores the data when $\overline{WR}$ line becomes active (low).

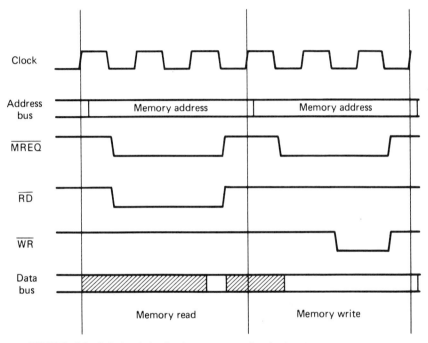

FIGURE 4.9 Relative timing for the memory read and write of the Z80. In the cross-hatched areas, data bus signals are not valid and should not be used.

Processor initialization

When the power switch is turned on, the contents of the program counter, instruction register, accumulator, stack pointer, and status flags are indeterminate. Both hardware and software must initialize the microprocessor at power startup to make sure that it is in a known state.

Figure 4.10(a) shows a simple initialization circuit using one resistor and one capacitor. Figure 4.10(b) and (c) shows power-supply and capacitor voltage waveforms. After power startup, capacitor C charges from 0 V up to the power-supply voltage. When the capacitor voltage v_2 is less than the threshold voltage v_t, $\overline{RESET}$ is at logic 0 and active. The contents of the internal registers are set to zero and the

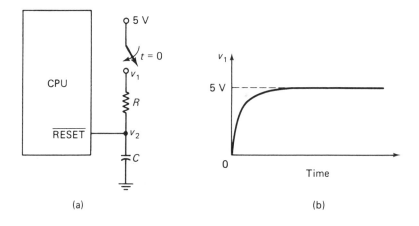

(a)   (b)

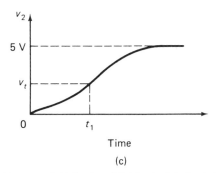

(c)

FIGURE 4.10 Processor initialization. (a) Simple RC circuit for initialization. (b) Voltage waveform of the power supply after the switch is closed at $t = 0$. (c) Voltage waveform of the $\overline{RESET}$ pin of the CPU.

processor tristate lines are driven into the high-impedance state. When v_2 exceeds the threshold voltage, $\overline{RESET}$ is at logic 1 and the CPU goes to a RUN mode.

EXAMPLE

Design an initialization circuit for the COSMAC microprocessor.

Solution

The COSMAC uses two lines, $\overline{CLEAR}$ and $\overline{WAIT}$, to initialize the processor. If $\overline{CLEAR} = 0$ and $\overline{WAIT} = 1$, the CPU is in the RESET state. If $\overline{CLEAR} = 1$ and $\overline{WAIT} = 1$, the CPU is in the RUN state. The CPU should be in the RESET state after power startup. Then the RUN state should follow. We can accomplish initialization by simply connecting v_1 and v_2 from the circuit shown in Fig. 4.10 to $\overline{WAIT}$ and $\overline{CLEAR}$, respectively.

Flags

There are several ways for an external device to signal the microcomputer. One method is to use a flag bit connected to the CPU. A flag may appear on an external flag input pin or a data-bus line. In operation, the CPU repeatedly executes a sequence of instructions until it senses with software that the flag has been set. In a program loop, the CPU scans the flag at regular intervals. Software coordinates every interaction between the CPU and the device connected to the flag. Therefore, software is complex. On the other hand, the hardware is simple. The flag approach is a good solution for detecting a slow and infrequent signal. Unless the flag checking is frequent enough, however, the microprocessor may miss a fast-changing signal. Furthermore, CPU time is used somewhat inefficiently with a regular flag-checking routine.

The COSMAC microprocessor is superb in its flag-handling capability. It has four independent flag input pins, so it can execute four different actions, depending upon the result of the flag-checking software.

Interrupt

A device can ask the microcomputer for immediate service by activating the interrupt line to the CPU. The interrupt approach is useful for a fast response, and the CPU is utilized efficiently compared with the flag approach.

Interrupt request. Most microprocessors have at least one interrupt request line. An external device can request an interrupt at any time through this line. There are two types of interrupts—maskable and nonmaskable. The CPU can ignore a maskable interrupt when it cannot respond to it. The interrupt enable flip-flop (IEF) controlled by enable and disable instructions establishes whether the CPU can respond to an interrupt or not. A nonmaskable interrupt must be serviced regardless of the status of the interrupt enable flip-flop. The CPU cannot ignore it. The power-failure interrupt is one example of a nonmaskable interrupt. If a power failure is imminent, the CPU must respond to it immediately by saving all register contents and status flags into a memory, such as RAM, with battery backup. If the CPU could not respond to a power-failure interrupt, the program could not continue when power was restored.

Interrupt service. If a device requests an interrupt when the interrupt enable flip-flop is set or an interrupt is nonmaskable, the CPU services the interrupt immediately after completing the current instruction. The CPU outputs an interrupt acknowledge signal to indicate that the interrupt was accepted and to cause the interrupting device to deactivate the interrupt request line. The CPU also clears the IEF to prevent further interrupts from being acknowledged. The CPU saves the program counter contents to preserve the return address after an interrupt is serviced. Then the program counter is loaded with the address of the interrupt service routine. The location of this address is peculiar to each microprocessor; for example, it is register 1 for the COSMAC. The interrupt service routine may also save the contents of the accumulator, status flags, stack pointer, and other scratchpad registers that are to be used in this routine. The CPU services the interrupt under the control of an interrupt service routine. After completing this routine, the CPU restores all registers that were previously saved and continues the process that was interrupted. The CPU also sets the IEF. Figure 4.11 shows these steps.

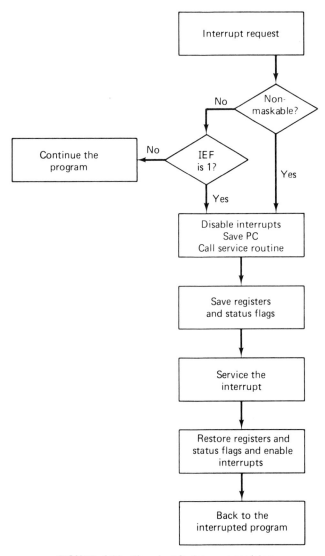

FIGURE 4.11 Flowchart for interrupt servicing.

Types of interrupts. There are three types of interrupts, as shown in Fig. 4.12. Figure 4.12(a) shows the single-level interrupt. The CPU has only one interrupt request line. In case more than one device can request an interrupt, the interrupt request lines from each device are OR gated. There is only one interrupt service routine. If any interrupt is accepted, this service routine is called and determines which device requested an interrupt, so that proper action may be taken.

Figure 4.12(b) shows the multilevel interrupt. The CPU has more than one interrupt request line. If the number of devices is less than or equal to the number of available interrupt lines, the CPU can determine the device automatically; otherwise, OR gating is necessary, as before.

Figure 4.12(c) shows the vectored interrupt. The interrupt controller permits

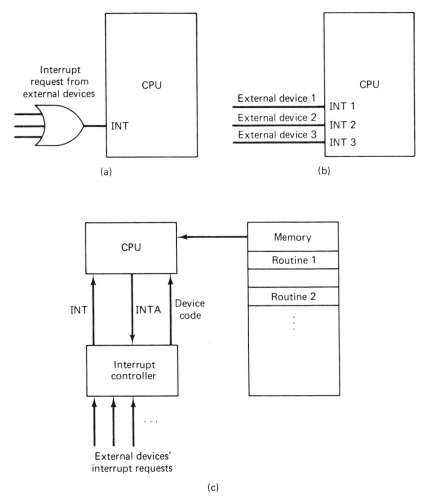

FIGURE 4.12 Types of interrupts. (a) Single-level interrupt. (b) Multilevel interrupt. (c) Vectored interrupt.

several devices to interrupt the CPU. Each device requesting an interrupt has its own service routine at a specific memory location. When the CPU acknowledges an interrupt, the interrupt controller sends it a device code, which identifies the interrupt-requesting device and causes the CPU to load the program counter with the address of a device's service routine. The vectored interrupt provides the fastest response of all but requires more hardware than other techniques.

Interrupt priority. If more than one device requests an interrupt at the same time, to what device should the CPU respond? An interrupt priority may be given to each device to solve this problem. The CPU responds to the highest priority device among the interrupt-requesting devices. Priority determination can be done with either hardware or software. In the hardware method, external devices do the priority determination, and the CPU scans devices one by one from higher to lower priority using the software approach.

One hardware method is to use the priority-interrupt controller. This controller not only handles interrupt priority but can also function as an interrupt controller. The microcomputer usually includes this controller if several external devices are permitted to interrupt it.

Another hardware method to determine priority is daisy chaining, as shown in Fig. 4.13. The nearer the device is to the CPU, the higher is the priority. Device 1 has the highest priority, device 2 has the next highest priority, and so on. Any number of devices can request an interrupt simultaneously. For example, suppose that device 2 and device 3 request an interrupt by lowering $\overline{\text{INT 2}}$ and $\overline{\text{INT 3}}$, respectively. This makes INT change from low to high. If the interrupt is accepted, the CPU lowers $\overline{\text{INTA}}$ to acknowledge an interrupt and to determine the priority in the daisy chaining. Each device senses the DEVIN line. If DEVIN is high, a device is told that its interrupt will be serviced if it is a device that requested an interrupt. In Fig. 4.13 DEVIN 1 is high, but device 1 did not request an interrupt. Therefore, $\overline{\text{INTA}}$ is passed to the next device. DEVIN 2 is high and $\overline{\text{INT 2}}$ is low. $\overline{\text{INTA}}$ is trapped in device 2 and cannot pass any further through the chain because DEVIN 3 becomes low. The interrupt requested by device 3 is ignored because

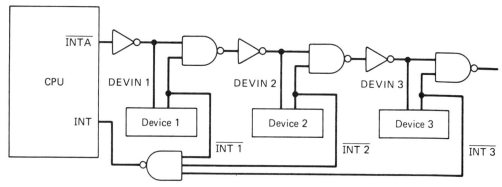

FIGURE 4.13 Priority-interrupt determination using daisy chaining.

device 2 has higher priority. Device 2 sends its identification code to the CPU to let the CPU know that it is the device to be serviced.

Nested interrupt. The priority interrupt controller may also allow the higher-priority devices to interrupt the interrupt service routine being executed for a lower-priority device, but not vice versa. The program counter and other necessary registers should be saved on the stack. This new interrupt service routine could be interrupted again by a higher-priority device's interrupt request, and so on. The COSMAC cannot handle nested interrupts efficiently, because the program counter content is saved in the CPU by register manipulation and register 1 always becomes the program counter for every interrupt request. On the other hand, the stack-oriented architecture of the Z80 facilitates nested interrupts.

Z80 interrupts. The Z80 microprocessor has two interrupt request lines: maskable and nonmaskable. The nonmaskable interrupt causes the program counter to be automatically loaded with hexadecimal address 0066. The maskable interrupt has three different response modes. In mode 0, the interrupting device places an instruction (device code) on the data bus, and the CPU gets the address of the service routine by executing this instruction. In mode 1, the CPU simply jumps to hexadecimal location 0038. In mode 2, the CPU forms the 16-bit memory address and loads the program counter with this address. The higher 8 bits come from the on-chip interrupt vector register, and the interrupting device supplies the lower 8 bits. We must set the interrupt mode and the content of the interrupt vector register by proper programming before any interrupt occurs.

Direct memory access (DMA)

Suppose that fast transfer of data between a device and memory is required in the microcomputer. The flag approach is, of course, a bad choice. Speed is improved substantially with an interrupt approach, but CPU time is still wasted in saving and restoring register contents. Direct memory access (DMA) provides the fastest response, with a higher priority than an interrupt. Using DMA, data transfer occurs directly between RAM and an external device. The DMA operation bypasses the CPU by suppressing the CPU logic, thus speeding up the rate of data transfer.

CPU logic is suppressed for one or more clock cycles and one data byte is transferred at each DMA request. This is called cycle-stealing DMA. Also, CPU logic can be suppressed until a complete block of data is transferred. This is called burst DMA.

DMA controller. The DMA controller coordinates data transfer during either cycle stealing or burst DMA, thus acting as a CPU while the CPU is suspended. Figure 4.14 shows the connections to a DMA controller. The DMA controller has three internal registers: address register, counter register, and status register. The address register holds the first address to be used in the data transfer, the counter register represents the number of memory locations available to the DMA opera-

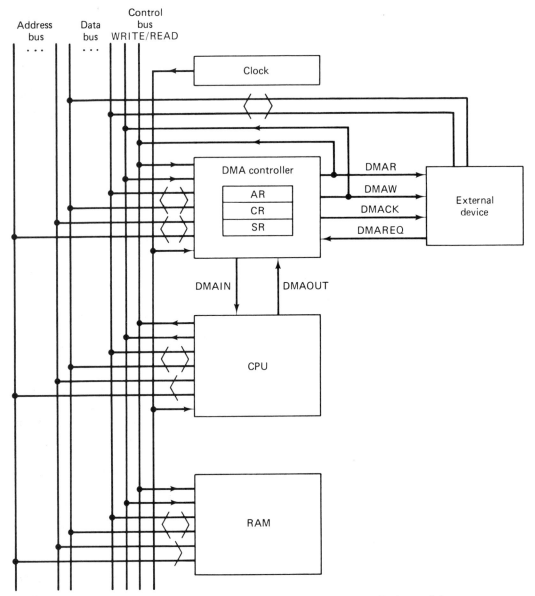

FIGURE 4.14 DMA controller as a part of the microcomputer. Registers of the DMA controller can be addressed under program control. During DMA, the DMA controller takes control over the system bus.

tion, and the status register specifies the mode and direction of DMA. These registers must be initialized by software before DMA starts.

An external device signals a request to the DMA controller when it is ready to transmit or receive data. The DMA controller sets DMAIN to inhibit the internal CPU clock. The CPU disconnects itself from the system bus by driving all connections to the system bus into the high-impedance state. By sending DMA-OUT, the CPU tells the DMA controller that it can now have control over the system bus. DMACK signals an acknowledgment to the external device that requested DMA. Then the DMA controller puts its address register contents on the address bus and issues DMAR or DMAW, depending upon the status register. Data are transferred between the memory and the external device. The address register is incremented and the counter register is decremented to prepare for the next data transfer. READ and WRITE from the CPU to the DMA controller permit the CPU to read and write the three register contents under program control. In the case of cycle-stealing DMA, the DMA operation is completed after 1 byte is transferred. For burst DMA, data transfer continues until the counter register is decremented to zero. Then the DMA controller interrupts the CPU to give control of the system bus back to the CPU. Figure 4.15 shows the flowchart for burst DMA.

Multiple-device DMA. A multiple-device DMA controller can handle many external devices because it has registers dedicated to each device. This DMA controller also contains circuitry to determine the priority when several devices request the DMA at the same time. The DMA controller may have separate DMA acknowledge lines. Otherwise, the external device must have its own select logic.

DMA controller in the CPU. The COSMAC microprocessor is able to do DMA operations without a DMA controller. The COSMAC has 16 internal registers. One of them (register 0) is reserved for holding a DMA address. There are two DMA request lines: $\overline{\text{DMAIN}}$ for sending data to the memory and $\overline{\text{DMAOUT}}$ for receiving data from the memory. Sensing a DMA request, the CPU puts the contents of the DMA address-holding register on the address bus and increments the register contents. The COSMAC does not have a DMA acknowledge output pin, but we can generate that signal externally. In the COSMAC, the CPU floats only the data bus during DMA and drives the address bus and control lines, while the CPU floats the whole system bus with a DMA controller. The COSMAC provides an efficient and minimum-hardware DMA approach.

4.3 MEMORY HARDWARE DESIGN*

All computer systems require some method of storing and retrieving data. In fact, a large portion of the cost of a computer system is for memory. The computer uses memory to hold the data it is going to use, to retain the results of operations or

---

*Section 4.3 written by Kevin R. Colwell.

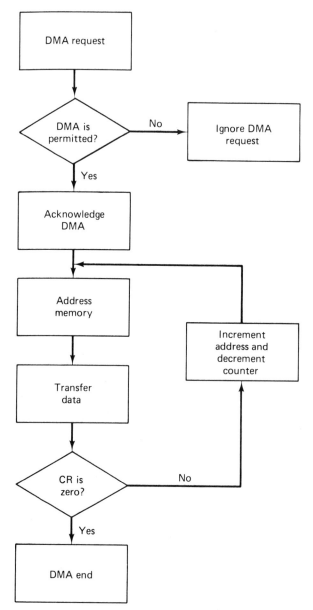

FIGURE 4.15 Flowchart for burst DMA operation.

instructions, and to keep a record of the state of the processor when necessary. Large computers and minicomputers use magnetic core as the storage medium. Although there are some advantages to core memory, it is too expensive and difficult to interface in small systems. Semiconductor memory is the only type used in microcomputers and is rapidly replacing magnetic core in minicomputers.

This section is devoted to semiconductor memory applications in microcomputers. By memory we mean a method of storing information. The fundamental unit of information is 1 bit (binary digit). A bit is either in the logic "0" or the logic "1" state. There are many ways to store a logic state, including a flip-flop or cross-coupled logic gates. A switch that connects a wire to the power supply ($+$V) or to ground (0 V) is a simple logic-state storage device. A capacitor may be charged to a voltage that corresponds to logic one or logic zero. It may require additional circuitry to ensure that the output is not at an intermediate value. Semiconductor memory uses all these techniques for data storage.

For memory to be useful, there must be a way to select or retrieve a particular piece of data and ignore all the others. Each data bit must have a unique address so that we may find it. It is much more convenient to be able to randomly select a piece of data than to have to wait for it to appear in a sequence, as in a serial shift register. For example, it would be simpler to find a given paragraph in this book if you knew the page number and paragraph number than if your only information is that it is the 256th paragraph. It takes longer to count paragraphs than to read page numbers. For this reason most memory is organized so that each bit can be randomly accessed. This gives rise to the name "random-access memory" (RAM). Access time for any location in RAM is independent of the address. A shift register can store and output data bits serially and therefore does not have random access. Such serial memory is usually less convenient to use than RAM.

In some applications it is necessary for the information storage to be permanent. Examples are programs that initiate system operation, programs to perform basic monitoring functions or tables of often used data. For these cases we want the microprocessor to be able to access the stored information but not to modify it. We call this type of memory read-only memory (ROM). ROM is nonvolatile (i.e., loss of power will not change the memory contents).

Thus far we have discussed two types of memory, ROM and RAM. Although both are arranged so that a unit of information can be randomly accessed, RAM is used to indicate memory that can both be read from and written into (read-write memory), whereas ROM refers to memory that can only be read from.

Figure 4.16 shows the semiconductor memory family tree. We have thus far established the three primary branches. Before going into detail about each of these branches, let us compare them.

The smallest unit of information for our purposes is 1 bit. Little information can be stored in 1 bit, so microprocessors are designed to operate on a group of bits: 4, 8 (most commonly), or 16. If a processor operates on groups of 8 bits at a time, it is said to manipulate 8-bit words. It is common to refer to a group of 8 bits

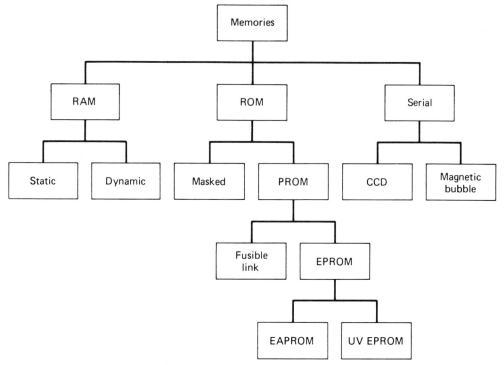

FIGURE 4.16　Semiconductor memory family tree.

as a byte. Therefore, an 8-bit processor has a word size of 1 byte. A 16-bit micro-processor accesses data 16 bits at a time and has a word size of 2 bytes.

Each bit of data in a memory chip (integrated circuit) is stored in a memory cell. There must be some way of selecting one particular cell from all those available. One selection technique uses a decoder. For a 16-bit memory we could use a 1-of-16 decoder with four input or address lines and 16 output lines each connected to a cell. We could then select a given cell by placing the correct address on the inputs, an approach called linear selection (Fig. 4.17). Linear selection is only practical if there are few cells. To make a 1-kbit (1 k = $1024 = 2^{10}$) memory using this approach, we would need a decoder with 1024 output lines. This size of decoder is not practical. Therefore, the cells are usually arranged in a matrix and two decoders used, one to select the column or Y-line, and the other to select the row or X-line. For a 16-bit memory we would use two 1-of-4 decoders with the lower 2 address bits going to the X-line decoder and the upper 2 address bits going to the Y-line decoder. Figure 4.18 shows this technique, which is called coincident selection.

For 8-bit microprocessors the data bus expects 8 bits to be present when a valid address is placed on the address bus. We can supply 8 bits by using one memory chip that outputs 8 bits for each address. Alternatively, we can use eight chips

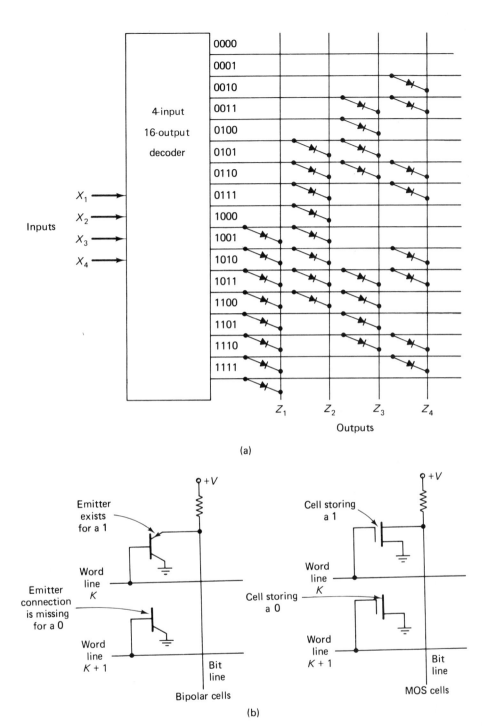

FIGURE 4.17 Read-only memory. (a) Linear selection ROM, address 1000 contains 1100. (b) Bipolar and MOS ROM storage cells. (From Bartee, T. C. 1977. Digital computer fundamentals, 4th ed. New York: McGraw-Hill. Used with permission.)

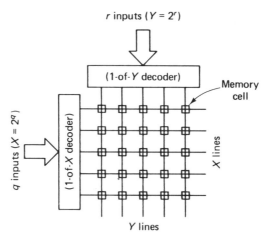

FIGURE 4.18 Coincident selection of memory cells. The number of cells is $N = 2^{q+r}$. Each decoder selects 1-of-$(N)^{1/2}$ lines. If N is large, it is more economical to manufacture two 1-of-$(N)^{1/2}$ decoders than one 1-of-N decoder. (From Hilburn, J. L., and Julich, P. M. 1976. Microcomputers/microprocessors: hardware, software and applications. Reprinted by permission of Prentice-Hall, Inc.)

that each supply 1 bit. We tie the corresponding address inputs of each chip together so that each one sees the same address and contributes 1 bit to the bus. It is, of course, also possible to use two chips that output 4 bits each or any other combination that will supply 1 byte per address.

Memories come in many configurations. For example, the Intel 2141 is a 4 kbit $\times$ 1 chip containing 4096 bits arranged so that each address contains 1 data bit. The minimum number of these chips to form 8-bit words is eight, which would be a 4-kbyte memory. The Intel 2732 is a 4 kbit $\times$ 8 chip with 32,768 bits arranged so that there are 4 k different addresses, each resulting in 8 output bits, or 1 byte. One chip provides a complete 4-kbyte memory system for an 8-bit processor.

Each storage cell in a ROM is usually a single bipolar or field-effect transistor. RAM cells require from three to six transistors and therefore have fewer cells than ROMs per chip. The cells can be implemented in bipolar or MOS technologies. Figure 4.19 compares the different RAM technologies. Bipolar memory can be either TTL (transistor–transistor logic) or ECL (emitter-coupled logic). ECL is used only where cost is secondary to very high speed. Bipolar memories are fast but expensive. MOS cells are slower than bipolar, but cost less, consume less power, and have higher packing densities. They are therefore the usual choice for microcomputer applications.

Read-only memory

There are two classes of read-only memory: masked and programmable. The word ROM usually refers to mask-programmed memory. Mask programming is done by the manufacturer at the time the chip is made. The end user supplies the

Characteristic	PMOS	NMOS		Bipolar	CMOS
		High speed	High density		
Number of bits per chip	4096	4096	16,384	2048	1024
Access time (ns)	300–400	50	150	20	290
Power dissipation (mW/bit)	0.2	0.1	0.02	0.25	0.015 at 1 MHz 0.00050 standby
Average large quantity cost (cents per bit)	0.15	0.5	0.1	0.6	0.7

FIGURE 4.19 Comparison of the various RAM memory technologies. (From Bartee, T. C. 1977. Digital computer fundamentals, 4th ed. New York: McGraw-Hill. Used with permission.)

manufacturer with a listing of the desired contents of the memory (i.e., which switches on Fig. 4.20 are closed). The manufacturer then makes a mask to be used in production of the chips. Once the chip is fabricated, the contents cannot be changed. The initial cost of producing the mask is high, typically several thousand dollars. However, mask-programmed ROM is the least expensive memory available if purchased in large quantities. It is used by companies producing large numbers of identical systems. If a change in the program is necessary, the entire stock of ROM chips is obsolete. For this reason ROM is not used in small volume or prototype systems. ROM chips are currently available in sizes from 256 to 64 kbits.

Programmable read-only memory (PROM) allows the user to program chips individually with a special PROM programmer. There are two types of PROM: fusible link and erasable. Fusible-link PROM chips are manufactured so that all the switches in Fig. 4.20 are closed. Each switch is formed by a fusible link of Nichrome or silicon. Figure 4.21 shows a typical fusible link cell. To program this device the user applies a high-current pulse to the cells that are to be open. This blows the sensitive fuse and opens that cell. Once a fusible link PROM is blown, it is similar to the mask-programmed ROM in that it cannot be changed. PROM is available with up to 16 kbits; 32-kbit PROMs will be available in the near future.

Erasable PROM (EPROM or EROM) allows the user to program a nonvolatile chip but, if necessary, erase the contents and reprogram. Most EPROMs are erased by exposing them to ultraviolet (UV) light. The cells are implemented using a FAMOS (floating-gate avalanche-injection metal oxide semiconductor) technique. A cell is similar to a p-channel FET with the gate floating and surrounded by insulating SiO_2. Whether a FAMOS cell represents a 1 or a 0 depends on the charge on the gate. Increasing the charge on the gate increases the drain-to-source conductance. To program an EPROM, a cell is addressed and a high-voltage pulse is applied to it. The high voltage causes an avalanche injection of electrons into the gate region. Since the gate is surrounded by an insulator, the charge will be trapped

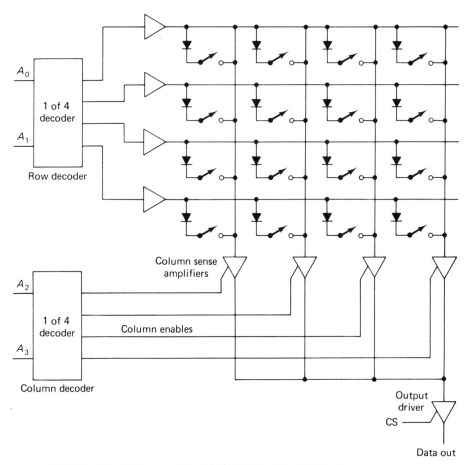

A_0

1 of 4
decoder

A_1

Row decoder

Column sense
amplifiers

A_2

1 of 4
decoder   Column enables

A_3

Column decoder

Output
driver

CS

Data out

FIGURE 4.20 ROM array using coincident selection. The manufacturer closes the appropriate switch during the final steps of fabrication. (Reprinted by permission of Intel Corporation, © 1977, 1978.)

for years. However, exposure of the chip to ultraviolet light causes a photocurrent to flow from the gate to the silicon substrate, and the charge leaks away, thereby erasing the contents of the cell.

EPROMs are very useful for system development and single unit applications. Their price per bit is higher than that for either ROMs or PROMs, but they allow the developer to correct or upgrade software. Once the software has been proven, it can be transferred to PROMs. PROMs are finding an increased usage over ROMs because they are readily available in small or large quantities and can be programmed on an individual basis. Figure 4.22 compares the cost versus size of EPROMs, PROMs, and ROMs.

All ROMs, PROMs, and EPROMs are arranged to store 4 or 8 bits per

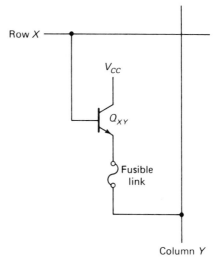

FIGURE 4.21 Typical bipolar fusible-link cell.

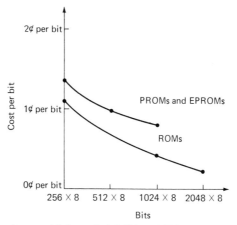

FIGURE 4.22 Cost per bit for typical ROMs, PROMs, and EPROMs (for a lot of 100). (From Peatman, J. B. 1977. Microcomputer-based design. New York: McGraw-Hill. Used with permission.)

address so that it is possible to use a single chip to store a complete program. EPROMs are available with up to 32 kbits (4 kbits $\times$ 8) of storage.

There is another type of EPROM that can be erased electrically. It is usually referred to as an EAPROM (electrically alterable programmable read-only memory) or read mostly memory (RMM). The EAPROM is similar to a RAM but is nonvolatile. EAPROMs use an MNOS (metal nitride oxide semiconductor) cell, and the charge is trapped between two dielectric layers. They are a relatively recent addition to the semiconductor memory family tree. Their high cost and slow access times (1 to 5 μs) have inhibited their use in microcomputer applications.

Interfacing ROMs

As an example of interfacing a ROM to a microprocessor, we will use the 2716 ultraviolet (UV) EPROM. This memory is 16 kbits arranged 2 kbits $\times$ 8. Also produced is a 32-kbit EPROM, the 2732, which has a 4 kbit $\times$ 8 configuration. Figure 4.23(a) shows the 2716 in the read mode. Notice that the chip requires only a single 5-V supply. There are 11 address pins, A0 through A10, to access the 2048 bytes (the 2732 needs 12 address pins for 4096 bytes), eight data outputs, O0 through O7 (these are inputs in programming mode), a chip select $\overline{CS}$ (low to enable outputs, high to put them in a hi-Z mode), and a program pin PGM to provide the programming signal.

We must decide where in memory the 2716 is to reside. Figure 4.24 shows a map of a memory system. The 2716 is to be placed at addresses 8000_{16} through $87FF_{16}$. The chip select $\overline{CS}$ must be low when these addresses are on the bus, to output the data from the referenced byte. We could run the highest address bit, A15, through an inverter (shown in Fig. 4.25) so that an 8_{16} placed in the four high-order address bits makes the chip enable low and selects the EPROM. The data bus then contains the byte selected by the lower 11 address bits. By this point in the discussion, you may have realized that the EPROM will respond to addresses other than 8000_{16} through $87FF_{16}$. In fact, it will be enabled at any address where the most significant address bit is set (i.e., from 8000_{16} through $FFFF_{16}$). By using only the most significant address bit, we have incompletely decoded address 8000_{16}. This incomplete decoding approach is very simple and is often used on small systems where there is only one ROM, one RAM, and one input/output port. However, the memory map in Fig. 4.24 indicates that we have reserved addresses $FF00_{16}$ through $FFFF_{16}$ for stack operations. The incomplete decoding shown in Fig. 4.25 will not work because both the EPROM and the stack RAM will be enabled simultaneously and hence be competing for the data bus. The address decoding must be more complete. Correct decoding may be implemented by connecting the four upper address lines to a 1-of-16 decoder (74154 or 4515) and connecting the decoder outputs to the proper chip enables (Fig. 4.26). A logic circuit using gates can also be designed instead of using a decoder chip.

There is additional chip selection that must be done. The processor can only read from the EPROM, so the EPROM should only be selected when the processor is in the read mode. The $\overline{RD}$ and $\overline{MREQ}$ lines from the processor are used in conjunction with the address lines for chip selection. When the Z80 in Fig. 4.26 executes a read instruction, it places an address on the address bus and subsequently lowers the $\overline{RD}$ and $\overline{MREQ}$ lines. The CPU expects the referenced data byte to be returned on the data bus within a certain time interval. If the EPROM places the correct byte on the data bus within this time limit, the read instruction is executed correctly. Figure 4.23 shows that the manufacturer guarantees that the address-to-output delay will not exceed 450 ns for a 2716 EPROM and that the chip-enable-to-output delay will be less than 120 ns. Both these times are within the limits of operation for a Z80 with a clock frequency of 2 MHz.

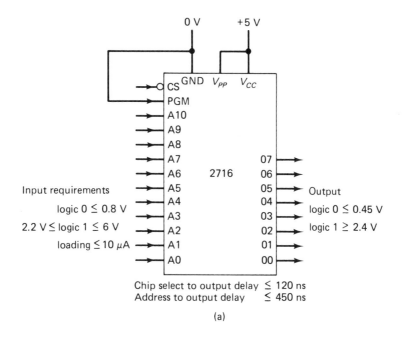

Input requirements

logic 0 ≤ 0.8 V

2.2 V ≤ logic 1 ≤ 6 V

loading ≤ 10 μA

Output

logic 0 ≤ 0.45 V

logic 1 ≥ 2.4 V

Chip select to output delay ≤ 120 ns
Address to output delay ≤ 450 ns

(a)

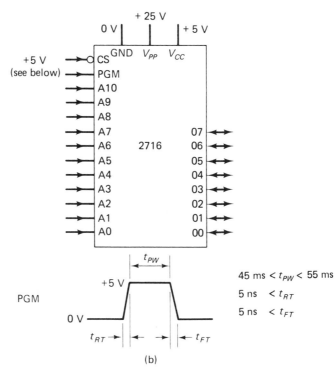

$45\ ms < t_{PW} < 55\ ms$

$5\ ns\ < t_{RT}$

$5\ ns\ < t_{FT}$

(b)

FIGURE 4.23 Intel 2716 EPROM. (a) Read mode characteristics. (b) Programming characteristics.

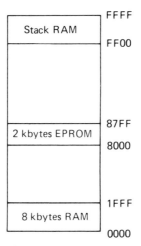

FIGURE 4.24 Memory map.

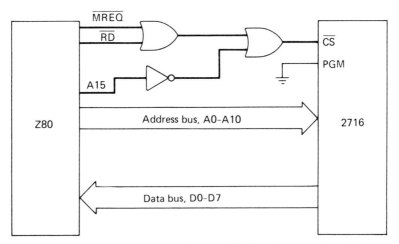

FIGURE 4.25 Interfacing a 2716 EPROM to a Z80. The chip responds to addresses 8000_{16} to $FFFF_{16}$.

To program the 2716 the chip is placed in a special PROM programmer designed to supply the necessary programming pulses. Figure 4.23(b) shows the timing and power requirements for programming. The V_{PP} pin is raised to 25 V and $\overline{CS}$ to 5 V. In this mode the output pins become the inputs. The address and data are placed on the corresponding pins. With the input lines stable, a single 50-ms, 5-V pulse is applied to the program pin. This pulse causes an avalanche injection of electrons into the gate region, where it is trapped. To program the entire 2048 bytes requires about 102 s (2048×50 ms = 102.4 s). The programmed EPROM should be read to verify that programming was successful. If not, it must be erased and other attempts made until the data are correct.

To erase a 2716 or 2732 the chip is removed from the circuit and exposed to

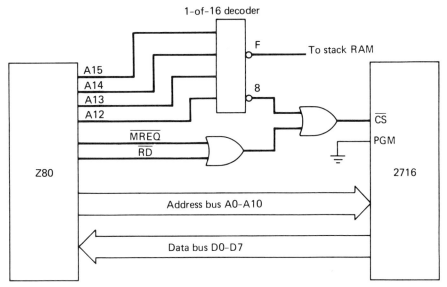

FIGURE 4.26 Interfacing a 2716 EPROM to a Z80. The decoder provides more complete decoding.

ultraviolet light. Because the silicon wafer is covered with a quartz window, the UV light can pass through to the wafer itself. The required exposure time can be calculated by the formula, $T_E = J/I$, where T_E is the exposure time, J the required erasure density (15 W·s/cm² for a 2716), and I the incident power density of the UV light source. For example, if a UV light source has a power density of 5000 μW/cm², $T_E = 15/(5000 \times 10^{-6}) = 3000$ s. The EPROM must be exposed to this light source for 50 min to be erased.

Random-access memory

Semiconductor random-access (read-write) memory is volatile—its contents are lost if the power is removed. There are two types of MOS RAM: static and dynamic. Static RAM cells are flip-flops requiring four to six transistors each (see Fig. 4.27). Static RAM is currently available with 64 bits to 4 kbits per chip; 16-kbit chips will be available soon. RAMs with less than 1 kbit are usually configured to store 8-bit words and are used for system scratchpad storage where 128 bytes or less in one package are required. Larger RAMs have only 1 bit per address, since it is more economical to produce the chips this way. However, a basic memory requires a minimum of eight chips to provide for byte-length storage.

Dynamic RAM cells use stray capacitance as the storage device. Each cell requires a minimum of one transistor, and therefore more cells can be packed on a chip than can be done with static RAM, at a lower cost per bit. Up to 64 kbits are currently available on one chip. Figure 4.28 shows two dynamic RAM cells. The capacitor is usually the gate capacitance of a transistor. The presence of charge on the capacitor indicates one logic state and its absence the other. There is some

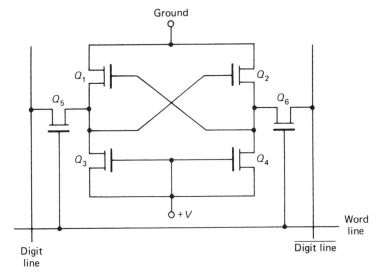

FIGURE 4.27 Six-transistor static memory cell for a linear select memory. Q1 and Q2 serve as resistors. Q3 and Q4 form a flip-flop. Q5 and Q6 serve as switches. (From Bartee, T. C. 1977. Digital computer fundamentals, 4th ed. New York: McGraw-Hill. Used with permission.)

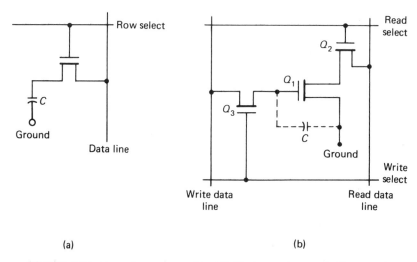

(a)

(b)

FIGURE 4.28 Dynamic memory cells. (a) Single-transistor cell. The capacitor stores information. The transistor serves as a switch. (b) Three-transistor cell. The stray capacitance of Q1 serves as the storage capacitor. (From Bartee, T. C. 1977. Digital computer fundamentals, 4th ed. New York: McGraw-Hill. Used with permission.)

leakage and the capacitor must have its charge refreshed every few milliseconds. Refreshing the cells is accomplished by executing a read or write instruction to the memory chip. The additional circuitry required for refreshing raises the cost of dynamic memory systems above static memory, making dynamic RAM impractical for systems with small amounts of memory. Figure 4.29 compares the cost of implementing static and dynamic RAM. In systems with more than approximately 8 kbytes of RAM, the lower cost, power consumption, and size of dynamic RAM usually outweigh the added cost of refresh circuitry.

Device	Number of memory chips	Power consumption	Power supplies	Relative cost
Intel 2141–4 (static HMOS)	8	0.48 W standby 2.2 W active	5 V	1.00
CDP1821 (static CMOS)	32	1.6 mW standby 0.49 W at 1 MHz	5 V	3.00
MK4027–4 (dynamic)	8	0.2 W standby 3.7 W active	+5 V, −5 V, +12 V	0.35

(a)

Device	Number of memory chips	Power consumption	Power supplies	Relative cost
Intel 2141–4 (static HMOS)	32	1.92 W standby 8.8 W active	5 V	1.00
CDP1821 (static CMOS)	128	6.5 mW standby 1.97 W at 1 MHz	5 V	3.00
MK4027–4 (dynamic)	32	0.86 W standby 14.8 W active	+5 V, −5 V, +12 V	0.35
MK4116–4 (dynamic)	8	0.16 W standby 3.7 W active	+5 V, −5 V, +12 V	0.55

(b)

FIGURE 4.29 Comparison of static and dynamic RAM memories. (a) 4-kbyte. (b) 16-kbyte.

Figure 4.30 is a typical static RAM. This chip has eight data input/output lines, eight address input lines (it is therefore a 256 × 8-bit RAM), two enable lines, and a write control. The WRITE line is used by the processor to tell the memory whether it expects to read data from the RAM or write into it.

To write into this RAM, the correct address is placed on the address pins, the chip enable lowered by the page decoder, the data put on the data bus, and the $\overline{\text{WRITE}}$ line lowered for some minimum amount of time to ensure that the data are transferred correctly. The address and data lines must remain stable while the $\overline{\text{WRITE}}$ line is low. To read data from the memory, the address is placed on the bus. The $\overline{\text{CE}}$ is lowered by the page decoder. The $\overline{\text{READ}}$ line from the CPU is

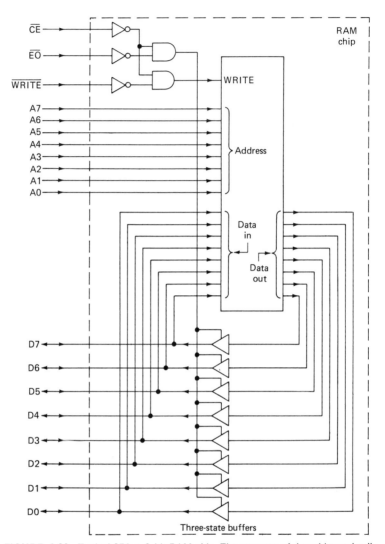

FIGURE 4.30 Typical 256 × 8-bit RAM chip. The contents of the addressed cells are placed on the data bus when the $\overline{CE}$ and $\overline{EO}$ lines are low. The tristate buffers are in the hi-Z state when either $\overline{CE}$ or $\overline{EO}$ is at a logic 1. (From Peatman, J. B. 1977. Microcomputer-based design. New York: McGraw-Hill. Used with permission.)

used to enable the output buffers ($\overline{EO}$). The $\overline{WRITE}$ line remains high for a read instruction. We must be careful when interfacing RAM to a microprocessor that the timing requirements of the CPU are met. For example, a Z80 with a 2-MHz clock frequency expects the RAM to be able to complete a read or write cycle in 750 ns or less. With a 4-MHz clock the RAM must respond within 375 ns. Faster memory is more expensive, so purchasing the fastest chip available is not always a wise decision.

Memory chips often have more than one chip-enable pin, and usually one of these is inverted, allowing for more complete address decoding without external logic. Figure 4.31 shows how several memories can be used together without decoders. The upper 8 bits (high-order byte) form a page address that selects one

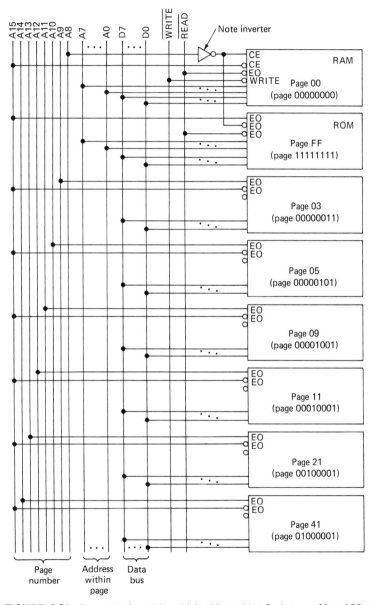

FIGURE 4.31 Page selection with multiple chip enables. Both pages 00 and FF are used and no decoders are necessary. (From Peatman, J. B. 1977. *Microcomputer-based design*. New York: McGraw-Hill. Used with permission.)

chip. Figure 4.32 shows a similar application. When the chips have single select lines, more hardware is required to implement the system.

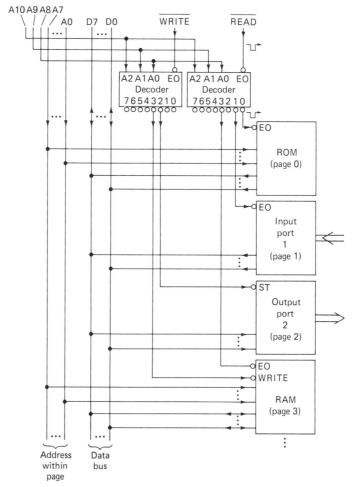

FIGURE 4.32 Page selection with a single chip-enable line. Decoders are required. (From Peatman, J. B. 1977. Microcomputer-based design. New York: McGraw-Hill. Used with permission.)

Interfacing static RAM

The RCA COSMAC has a multiplexed address bus. RCA has elected to use only eight pins (MAO through MA7) for memory address outputs. Addressing a full 64 kbytes requires that the upper 8 bits be output first and latched externally. Then the lower 8 bits are placed on the bus. The upper 8 bits are referred to as the page address and the lower 8 bits as the byte or word address. The COSMAC uses its

TPA line to indicate that the address bus contains a page address. This line is used to clock the high byte into a storage latch. The output of this latch can be used to decode the page addresses. Figure 4.33 shows the connection of CMOS RAM chips to the COSMAC. If more than 1 kbyte of memory is used, the page address must be decoded.

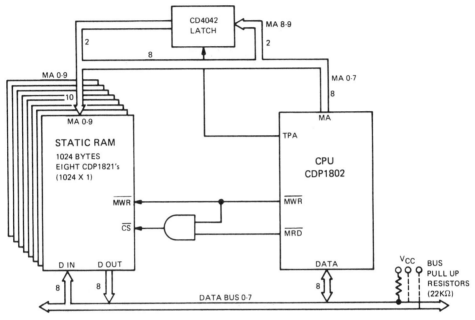

FIGURE 4.33 Interface between the CDP1821 static RAM and the CDP1802 microprocessor in a 1-kbyte RAM system. (Compliments of RCA, 1976.)

CMOS memory requires very little power when not being accessed. The RAM will retain data with a supply voltage as low as 2 V at about 50 μW/chip. This makes CMOS components a logical choice for portable applications or where power failure and subsequent memory loss cannot be tolerated. A small camera battery can maintain a 1-kbyte CMOS RAM for months. Figure 4.34 demonstrates a method of battery backup.

Interfacing dynamic RAM

The Mostek MK4116 RAM contains 16 kbits. The cells are arranged in a 128×128 matrix. The lower seven address lines are used to select the row, and the upper seven, the column. When a read instruction is executed, the cell selected by the row and column decoders has its contents placed on the output pin. At the same time all cells in that row (128 of them) are refreshed. Each of the 128 rows must be refreshed within 2 ms, which means that the chip requires a read or write operation every 15.6 μs. To ensure that the memory is refreshed often enough,

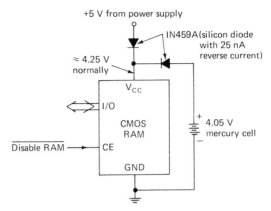

+5 V from power supply

IN459A (silicon diode with 25 nA reverse current)

≈ 4.25 V normally

V_{CC}

I/O

CMOS RAM

+ 4.05 V mercury cell

Disable RAM → CE

GND

FIGURE 4.34 Battery backup for a CMOS RAM. (From Peatman, J. B. 1977. Microcomputer-based design. New York: McGraw-Hill. Used with permission.)

most systems have a separate counter chip that is driven by the system clock. The counter steps through the row addresses and executes a read instruction with the data output disabled. The MK4116 needs a 7-bit counter with a minimum count frequency of 64 kHz. The refresh counter must be disabled and the CPU's address bus connected to the RAM whenever the CPU wishes to read or write to the memory. This requires additional interface circuitry.

The architects of the Zilog Z80 have made it very easy to implement dynamic RAM. The CPU has an internal memory refresh register (the R register) that is placed on the address bus while the current instruction is being decoded. There is no sacrifice in system speed. With the contents of the R register on address lines A0 through A6, the CPU lowers the $\overline{RFSH}$ line for two clock cycles, thus executing a refresh operation. The R register is automatically incremented after each refresh operation. Figure 4.35 shows the timing diagram for a Z80 instruction cycle.

Figure 4.36 shows the basic configuration of a dynamic memory system. During CPU read or write operations the $\overline{MREQ}$ is low, which enables one of the 4-kbit by 8 arrays, depending on the state of A12. If A12 is high, the upper array is selected. During refresh cycles, both $\overline{RFSH}$ and $\overline{MREQ}$ are low and both arrays are enabled.

Serial memory

Serial memories are useful in applications where large amounts of storage are important and speed is not a major consideration. Charge-coupled device memories (CCDs) are shift registers that move clusters of electrons along a channel formed in a silicon chip. The channel consists of a series of closely spaced capacitors. A multiple-phase clock shifts the charge along the channel, where it is periodically refreshed. Texas Instruments is marketing a 65,536-bit CCD in a 16-pin package. The chip is configured so the user can select one of 16 shift registers, each containing 4096 bits. The data are input or output serially at clock rates up to 5 MHz. This results in a maximum latency time (the time required to shift out any

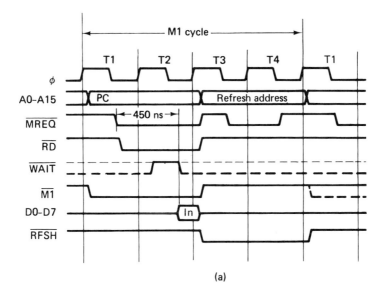

(a)

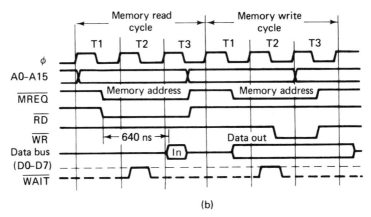

(b)

FIGURE 4.35 The instruction fetch cycle (M1) of the Z80 in (a) is longer than the memory read or write cycle in (b). The extra time is used to refresh dynamic memories. (Reprinted with permission from Electronic Design, Vol. 25, No. 14, July 5, 1977, © Hayden Publishing Co., Inc. 1977.)

given bit) of 819 μs. CCDs have not become popular in microcomputer systems. 1-Mbit CCDs should become available soon.

The newest member of the semiconductor memory family is the magnetic bubble memory, which is a large-capacity nonvolatile device. The first generation has a storage capacity of 92 kbits configured as a set of shift registers where the information is retained in a thin layer of magnetic material by very small cylindrical magnetic domains called bubbles. The bubbles are shifted around by a rotating magnetic field. Magnetic bubble memories are slow. The average access time is

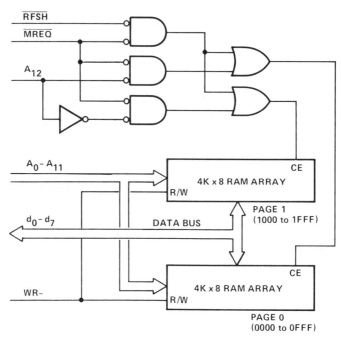

FIGURE 4.36 Interfacing dynamic RAM to the Z80 microprocessor. During a refresh operation A0 through A6 will contain the refresh address. $\overline{RFSH}$ and $\overline{MREQ}$ will go low, enabling both memory arrays. (Compliments of Zilog, Inc., 1977.)

4 ms, which is comparable to floppy-disk storage systems. The technology is still in its infancy, so there is potential for very large capacities at prices near those of present EPROMs.

4.4 INPUT/OUTPUT HARDWARE DESIGN*

The microcomputer, although very powerful for processing data, needs some way of communicating with the surrounding system. Input/output (I/O) hardware provides the needed interface between the computer and the rest of the instrument. I/O hardware is the most flexible area of hardware design in the microcomputer system. Knowledge of the various I/O alternatives often greatly simplifies not only the hardware but also the software as well.

Hardware/software trade-offs

The prime objectives in an overall computer system design are high speed, low cost, high reliability, small program size, and short development time. Because these factors are all directly affected by the I/O hardware design, we must consider

---

*Section 4.4 written by Alan V. Sahakian.

trade-offs between them during the design, and set priorities early to avoid circular conflicts. Consider the following example of such conflicts.

The program size is in part determined by how much processing must be done to data that have been input or are to be output in order to get the data into the proper format. The advantages of hardware processing over software processing are: (1) the program is shorter, and (2) the software development time is shorter. The disadvantages of hardware processing are: (1) it increases hardware cost, and (2) the increased component count decreases reliability.

The speed of a system is primarily a function of the software. If the computer must loop, waiting for input or output devices to become ready to give it data or take data from it, the system slows down. However, if hardware is added that allows the devices to interrupt the computer when they are ready, the time spent on input and output is less and the system speeds up. In many systems the use of interrupt-driven I/O can speed up the computer, often without much increase in the overall hardware complexity.

Subfunctions of input/output hardware

Input/output hardware generally must have the ability to hold data until either the computer or a peripheral device is ready to take the data. This function is called buffering. Without buffering the computer and all its peripheral devices would have to work in perfect synchronism to perform either an input or an output without losing the data to be transferred. The I/O hardware also must often translate data formats between those of the computer and the peripheral device. An example of this data format translation occurs in interfacing systems of different word size. If the computer works with 8-bit words and the peripheral works with 12-bit words, it is the responsibility of the I/O hardware to split the 12-bit word into smaller parts that can be handled by the computer. Two possible formats of 12-bit data are an 8-bit and a 4-bit word or two 6-bit words. Finally, the I/O hardware must often synchronize the data exchange both by signaling the destination device whenever the source device puts new data in its buffer and also by signaling the source device when it is ready to accept new data. Complete synchronization between a microcomputer and an I/O device is called handshaking. Combinations of some or all of these subfunctions are necessary for any input or output.

Parallel input/output hardware

Input or output can be performed one bit at a time (serial) or many bits at a time (parallel). We present parallel I/O first because it is more common.

Input/output control and timing. In parallel I/O the format of the data to be exchanged with the processor is usually the same as that of the data in the processor. In the case of our model processors, the Z80 and the COSMAC, this is an 8-bit parallel word. The function of parallel I/O hardware is then to buffer the data and synchronize the exchange.

The synchronization responsibility of I/O hardware can be met in more than one way. Normally, the processor must be alerted when an input port has a new word of data to be read or when an output port is waiting for one. This can be done by having the processor "poll" each input and output device to see if any are ready to be serviced. In this polling mode each port must have an associated processor-readable bit, signifying its readiness. This bit can either be a bit of a separate input port, or a bit of the input port itself (if the port is handling less than its capacity).

Under all conditions the processor must poll and service each input port more quickly than the device connected to it is loading data into it. If not, data can be overwritten or lost. An example of this possibility is in A/D converter servicing. Consider an A/D converter that generates a new digital value to be input by the processor every 1 ms. We would expect no problems if the processor checks the readiness of this converter every 900 μs and requires less than 100 μs to service it. However, if another device or a combination of devices needs servicing during the cycle, the processor may not poll the A/D converter for more than 1 ms. The converter would overwrite the unread value in the input port with a new value and a data point would be lost. This type of problem is very difficult to find because it may only occur when certain combinations of service routines are performed.

One obvious way of avoiding this problem would be to make certain that the processor checks the converter for readiness more often than every 900 μs. More-frequent checking would, however, tend to slow down the computer. Another approach would be to have the converter's operation initiated by the microprocessor at a time when the microprocessor is sure of its ability to service it. A third (and perhaps the best) way would be for the converter to interrupt the processor when it is ready for service.

An important concept in I/O is that of addressing. I/O ports are similar to memory from the processor's point of view. When the processor performs an input operation from a selected (addressed) input port, it essentially performs a read of this port. Similarly, an output operation is essentially a write. In fact, memory itself can be shared with another device to achieve highly efficient input and output of large amounts of data.

The address of an I/O port must be decoded by hardware just as it must be for memory. To perform this decoding efficiently, we must consider the addressing scheme of the processor as well as the needed number of I/O ports. For example, the Z80 microprocessor addresses an I/O port by sending out an I/O request signal (together with a read signal for an input or a write signal for an output) while also placing the address of the port on its eight low-order address lines. The use of 8 bits of I/O address allows up to 256 input ports (and 256 output ports) to be directly addressed. To address all of these 256 pairs of ports, however, all 8 bits of the address must be decoded. If the number of ports is considerably less than 256, for example 32, then only 5 bits are needed to address these 32 ports. If the 3 bits of address that are not needed are ignored, then any combination of the 8 address bits will select one of the 32 ports, with each port selectable by any of eight possible addresses. This multiple-address decoding characteristic is called redundant addressing because each port is addressable by one intended and seven redundant addresses. Similarly, if only one port is needed, the address need not be decoded.

If the number of ports is equal to or less than the number of I/O address bits of the processor (eight for the Z80 or three for the COSMAC), the address need not be decoded in hardware, but rather each bit of the address can directly select one port. Using this scheme the address decoding hardware is minimal, but so is the number of addressable ports. A problem that can be encountered is that of invalid addresses. If the processor attempts to perform an input operation from an address that has more than 1 bit active (an invalid address), more than one input port will try to place its data on the data bus. This bus conflict results in undefined data and possible damage to the bus drivers of these ports. Bus conflicts are real possibilities when the system software is being developed. They should be carefully avoided. If, on the other hand, the processor attempts to output to an invalid address, all output devices whose address bits are active will simultaneously receive the data on the bus. This can be a useful, simplifying operation in some systems. The possibility of an invalid but harmless address also exists in this scheme: that is when all the bits of the address are inactive. This can be recognized to select an additional port to serve some other useful function.

Input and output ports. Now that we know the functional requirements of a port, we can consider the actual hardware design of typical ports.

Since the functions of input and output ports are so similar, medium- and large-scale integrated circuits are available that will perform either job. An example of such an integrated circuit is the 74S412 multimode buffered latch (see Fig. 4.37). The 74S412 is also commonly available as an 8212 or 3212, depending on the manufacturer. For use with the COSMAC, a pin-for-pin equivalent CMOS version, the CDP1852 is also available. The 74S412 contains eight latching flip-flops (to hold the data), control and selection logic (including a service request flip-flop with an interrupt output), and a set of eight tristate buffers to allow the device to be connected to a common bus. A reset is also provided which clears not only the data-latching flip-flops but the service request flip-flop as well. The 74S412 has two basic modes of operation, which are selected by the mode (MD) input.

When MD is low (logic 0), the 74S412 is in the input mode. In this mode data are loaded into the data latches when the strobe (STB) input goes high (logic 1), and held by the latches when STB is low. When the STB input makes the transition from high to low (a falling edge), the service request flip-flop is activated (a logic 0 is loaded into it), causing the interrupt output to also be active (low). In this mode, the output tristate buffers are controlled by the device select inputs $\overline{DS1}$ and DS2. Both a low on $\overline{DS1}$ and a high on DS2 are required to enable the output buffers. Selecting the device in this way also returns the service request flip-flop to the inactive state. Note that device selection also causes the interrupt line to become active (low). This usually does not cause a conflict because most processors disable their interrupt inputs while in the process of servicing an interrupt.

Figure 4.38 shows the 74S412 configured as an interrupting input port for the Z80. In this configuration the port interrupts the processor whenever a new word of data is loaded into it with the STB line (by the inputting device). The output buffers of the port are enabled when the port is addressed by the processor using its I/O control lines and the eight least significant address bus lines.

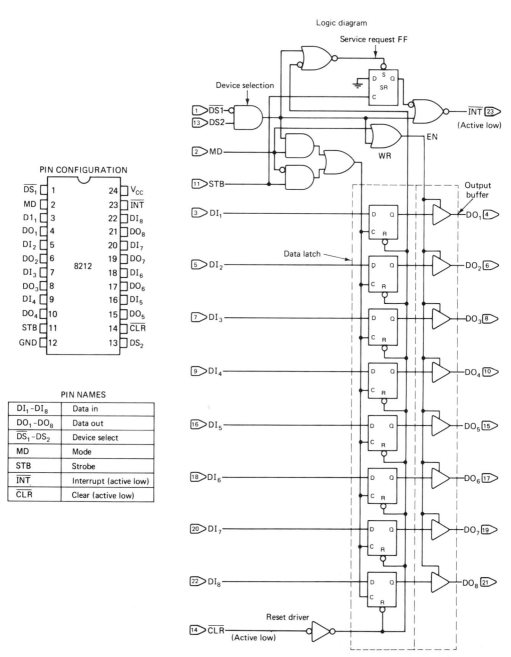

PIN CONFIGURATION

$\overline{DS}_1$	1	24	V_{CC}
MD	2	23	$\overline{INT}$
$D1_1$	3	22	DI_8
DO_1	4	21	DO_8
DI_2	5	20	DI_7
DO_2	6	19	DO_7
DI_3	7	8212	18	DI_6
DO_3	8	17	DO_6
DI_4	9	16	DI_5
DO_4	10	15	DO_5
STB	11	14	$\overline{CLR}$
GND	12	13	DS_2

PIN NAMES

$DI_1 - DI_8$	Data in
$DO_1 - DO_8$	Data out
$\overline{DS}_1 - DS_2$	Device select
MD	Mode
STB	Strobe
$\overline{INT}$	Interrupt (active low)
$\overline{CLR}$	Clear (active low)

FIGURE 4.37 74S412 multimode buffered latch (Intel number 8212). The output buffers are tristate bus drivers. (Reprinted by permission of Intel Corporation, © 1978.)

When its MD input is high, the 74S412 port is in the output mode. In this mode data are loaded into the data latches when the port is selected (using $\overline{DS1}$ and DS2) and held when it is deselected. The service request flip-flop is activated by the falling edge of the STB input. The output tristate buffers are always enabled in this mode.

Figure 4.38 also shows the 74S412 configured as an interrupting output port. This port interrupts the processor whenever the device is ready to accept a word of data, since the STB line is connected to the $\overline{READY}$ line of the output device. The processor outputs to the port by sending the data on the data bus, along with the proper control signals ($\overline{WR}$ and $\overline{IORQ}$) and the port address. These signals drive the device select inputs, which cause the data to be latched into the port.

In the previous two example ports, the device (either input or output) had no way to be sure that the processor had responded to the interrupt. Since the service request flip-flop becomes deactivated when the port is selected by the processor, this signal could be sensed (at the 74S412 $\overline{INT}$ output) by the device as an acknowledgment of the data transfer. This sort of request–acknowledge exchange, referred to as handshaking, is important for reliable operation.

Memory-mapped input/output.   Note from the foregoing discussion that the time involved performing the overhead tasks for an I/O function can be much longer than the actual I/O function itself. When large amounts of data must be transferred through a single port, the time wasted can seriously degrade the system performance.

In memory-mapped I/O the processor addresses the I/O devices just as if they were memory. This concept is similar to direct memory access (see Section 4.2) but differs in that the actual memory hardware is part of the I/O devices rather than part of the computer. The processor can run at full speed, independent of the I/O memory until it needs to access it. Since each location in the I/O memory is just as easily accessed as any other memory location, the software involved in input/output is greatly reduced.

Processors such as the Z80 have capability for memory bit-test and bit-modify, block transfer, and block search. Thus many common I/O tasks can be performed in a single instruction using memory-mapped I/O. It is possible to have the processor execute input data as instructions directly in the I/O section of memory, and very powerful program branching structures can be generated. If the I/O memory can be organized in a careful way such that the relative locations of the individual words in this memory fit the logical structure of the data, more software and time can be saved. This is especially true when dealing with well-structured data such as tables, arrays, and displays.

An example that illustrates the power of memory-mapped I/O is that of the character-oriented video display system shown in Fig. 4.39. In such a display there are a large number of data words (characters) to be output, and these data words are well organized (by row and column location on the screen). The dimensions (number of characters) of the display may be whole powers of 2, for example 16 rows of 64 characters each. These 1024 characters can be directly accessed by their

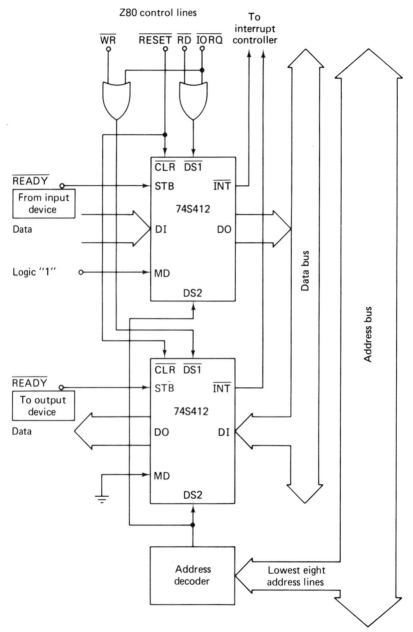

FIGURE 4.38 Interrupting input (top) and output (bottom) ports for the Z80 using the 74S412. The input device loads data into the input port and interrupts the processor using its $\overline{READY}$ line. Similarly, when ready for new data, the output device pulls its $\overline{READY}$ line low.

individual row and column numbers, linked together in a binary series, to produce a 10-bit address. This address corresponds to the actual address of the character stored in the memory. The 63rd character of the topmost row on the screen (character number 111111_2 of row number 0000_2) would be located at address 0000111111_2 in the display memory and could be accessed there by the processor.

Since a typical video monitor (such as a television set) needs to be constantly scanned, the display generator needs to have frequent and regular access to its own memory. Requests from the processor must be interwoven between those of the display generator. The display generator must have the higher priority, since the scanning beam in the video monitor cannot be stopped to wait for the memory, but the processor can (by using its WAIT line). Much of the hardware involved with such a memory-mapped I/O interface deals with this interweaving.

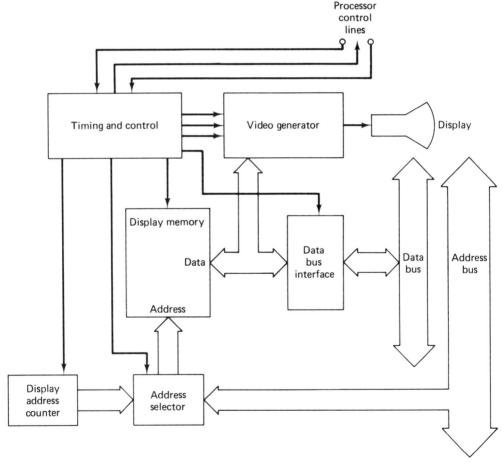

FIGURE 4.39 Memory-mapped video display system. The display memory can be accessed by either the computer or the display itself. The address selector routes the address from either address source to the memory.

The same configuration can be used to interface to a nonfade display (Section 1.2). In this case the memory stores a set of digitized values that represent the display waveform. Each successive location in the memory maps a successive value on the screen. In this way, only a single vertical value on the screen can be stored at any horizontal location (i.e., the waveform must be single-valued). The values are continually displayed by the video generator, using a D/A converter to drive the vertical deflection plates of the cathode-ray tube. The horizontal plates of the cathode-ray tube are driven by a D/A converter fed by the value of the display address counter. Requests for memory access from the processor are again interwoven between those from the display so that the memory (and thus the display on the screen) can be read or modified at any location by the processor.

General-purpose interface bus.   In situations requiring parallel data communication between separate instruments, standard electrical and mechanical specifications are needed. Such a standard was developed by the Hewlett-Packard Company and later adopted in modified form by the Institute of Electrical and Electronics Engineers as IEEE Standard 488–1978. Referred to as the general-purpose interface bus (GPIB), it provides for up to 15 instruments to be interconnected on a single bus with a maximum of 2 m of cable per instrument (or 20 m total, whichever is less). The standard utilizes handshaking data exchange for reliability and versatility and is 8-bit byte-oriented, making it ideal for microcomputer use. The maximum data transfer rate is 250 kbytes/s.

For such a large number of instruments to coexist on the same bus, it is necessary for one instrument to oversee the rest. This instrument is called the bus controller. Along with other duties, the controller enables and disables the other instruments on the bus as "talkers" (data transmitters) and "listeners" (data receivers). This approach allows great flexibility, since the arrangement of the instruments on the bus can be changed at any time under software or hardware control. In fact, the role of bus controller can be reassigned by an overall system controller so that a set of instruments can be totally reconfigured automatically. Although a high degree of control is possible with this bus standard, simple devices can be set up to ignore many of the control signals so that the hardware need not be complex.

The standard bus signal levels can be implemented with common TTL and two resistors, as shown in Fig. 4.40. The driver is an open-collector gate (a gate that can sink, but not source current). The use of open-collector gates driving the bus lines yields a wired-OR configuration in which all drivers on a given line must be high for the line to be high. The receivers should be Schmitt-trigger gates (gates with hysteresis) such as the 7414, to provide good noise immunity.

Figure 4.41 shows the GPIB signal lines DI01 to DI08 are the eight bidirectional data lines over which passes the information to be exchanged. These lines are also used by the controller to issue commands. DAV, NRFD, and NDAC are the three handshaking lines. Three lines are needed instead of two, since the handshaking operation is more complex, taking place between a talker and any number

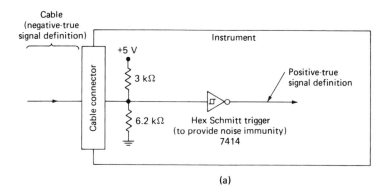

(a)

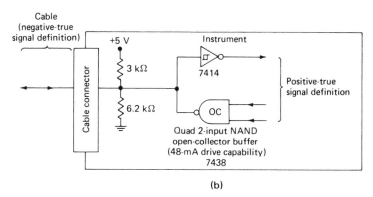

(b)

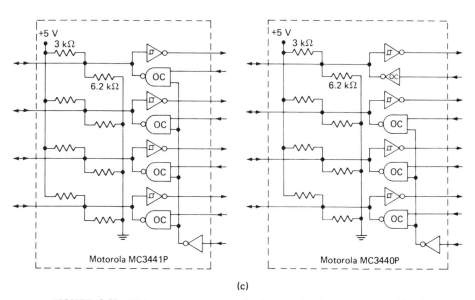

(c)

FIGURE 4.40 GPIB-recommended termination for (a) instruments capable of listening only and for (b) instruments capable of talking as well. (c) Two devices capable of meeting the GPIB standard. (From Peatman, J. B. 1977. Microcomputer-based design. New York: McGraw-Hill. Used with permission.)

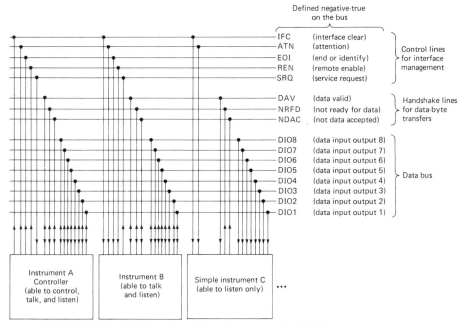

FIGURE 4.41 GPIB signal lines. (From Peatman, J. B. 1977. Microcomputer-based design. New York: McGraw-Hill. Used with permission.)

of listeners. EOI, IFC, ATN, and REN are lines used by the controller to manage the bus. SRQ is an interrupt line to the controller which can be used by any instrument to request the use of the bus.

For good noise immunity there are independent ground lines for the most important control lines. These ground lines are used in a twisted-pair configuration with their corresponding control lines. A common signal ground is provided for all other lines, as is a separate shield for the whole cable, which further improves noise immunity.

Serial input/output hardware

In the previous discussion, I/O data have always been transferred in parallel. That is, all of the bits in a word were sent at once, each on its own wire. It is also possible to send data serially, 1 bit at a time. The main advantage of the serial approach is that only one wire, or more generally only one bit path, is needed. If information is to be transferred over a distance, the use of a serial format can greatly simplify the interconnecting data pathways. However, the conversion to and from the computer's parallel word format requires additional hardware and/or software, so once again we must consider the trade-offs.

Since only one bit path connects the serial source and destination, the data must be time-multiplexed onto it. Along with these data there must also be information about their timing. Specifically, the beginning and end of a word of known length must usually be identified.

Figure 4.42 shows the most common arrangement of this serial information. In this arrangement each bit is allotted a time t_b (called the bit time). The start of a data word is signified by a low on the bit path (also called a space) lasting one bit time. After the start bit is sent, the actual 8-bit data word is sent bit by bit, with the least significant bit first. To finish the transmission of the word, a high (or mark) is sent for either one or two bit times. The number of these "stop" bits sent depends on the speed of transmission, with two commonly being sent at 110 baud and one at 300 baud (the two most common speeds). The transmitter and receiver must both be set to very nearly the same t_b.

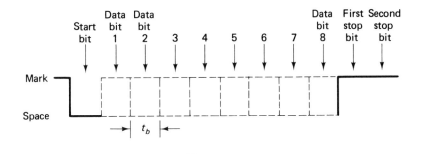

FIGURE 4.42 Serial data format. A mark is a logic 1 and a space a logic 0. t_b is the bit time. The second stop bit is transmitted only at low speeds. The next data word may follow immediately or after any time. In the interim between transmissions, the line remains at mark.

To communicate over telephone lines, tones can be used to represent mark and space. These tones are generated and received by an interface called a modem. If the communication is to take place in only one direction at a time (half-duplex), only one pair of tones is needed. If the communication is to be in both directions simultaneously (full duplex), two different pairs of tones are needed. A specific pair of tones is always assigned to be generated by the originating (calling) modem, and the other pair by the answering modem. In the speed range 0 to 600 baud, the following convention is often used (Hilburn and Julich, 1976):

	Originating modem (Hz)	*Answering modem* (Hz)
Transmitted mark	1270	2225
Transmitted space	1070	2025

Hardware flags. Some microprocessors are equipped with special pins, the state of which can be tested by the processor (as input) or set by the processor (as output). These pins are called hardware flags and can be used for the simplest I/O operation or, with appropriate software, for serial I/O.

A processor that has such hardware flags is the COSMAC. In the COSMAC there are four input pins (called external flags 1 through 4) that can be tested by the processor, and one output pin (called Q) that can be set, reset, or tested by the processor. These pins are ideal for sensing the states of switches, lighting a light, or sounding an alarm. In addition, these pins can be used in conjunction with parallel I/O hardware to establish a simple means of handshaking. If the processor is equipped with a program to sequentially input or output data on these pins, a simple serial interface can be built.

An important consideration here is reliability. Since hardware failures can be reduced by minimizing the hardware, relatively small systems, which must be reliable, can often use these hardware flags to great advantage. Once the software to perform the I/O using the hardware flags is developed, it will always work. Future changes in the protocol of the I/O operations are also easy to effect, by reprogramming the read-only memory, which contains the I/O routines.

Universal asynchronous receiver/transmitter (UART).   The processor's time may be too valuable to be wasted performing the timing and other overhead functions for serial I/O, or the system software development time and/or cost may be very important. Then the job can be performed by a hardware device called a universal asynchronous receiver/transmitter (UART). Figure 4.43 lists some of the many different UARTs that are available.

Two of these UARTs (the MC6850 and the 8251) are especially suited to bus-structured systems such as the microprocessor. Originally designed for use with the

Device	Manufacturer	Comments
S 1883	American Microsystems	Independent receive and transmit
AY–5–1012	General Instruments	
2536	Signetics	
COM 2502	Standard Microsystems	
TMS 6012	Texas Instruments	
TR 1602	Western Digital	
MC 6850	Motorola	Bus-oriented and programmable
8251	Intel	

FIGURE 4.43 Some available UARTs. The first five listed are pin-compatible with each other. The last two are specifically designed for microcomputer use and only require +5 V for supply.

8080 microprocessor, the 8251 UART shown in Fig. 4.44 is especially attractive for use with the Z80 as well. The 8251 is, in fact, a universal synchronous/asynchronous receiver/transmitter or USART. In the synchronous mode the 8251 utilizes one or two special synchronizing characters at the beginning of a continuous stream of serial data words to lock in the receiver. Once locked in, the data are self-synchronizing, and start and stop bits are not transmitted with each character.

The 8251 has an 8-bit bidirectional bus which allows it to receive data from and return data to the processor. In addition, the processor can read the status of the 8251 through this bus, as well as program its mode. Since it requires only $+5$ V (at typically 45 mA) to operate, it is dc-compatible with the Z80.

Teletype interfacing.   One of the most popular I/O devices for any computer system is the Teletype Model 33. This electromechanical device comes in many versions, from printer only to printer with keyboard, papertape punch, and reader. The Teletype uses the serial asynchronous data transmission format shown in Fig. 4.42, but it operates with current rather than voltage levels. A logic 1 or mark consists of 20 mA, and a logic 0 or space is 0 mA. Figure 4.45 shows typical interface circuits for the Teletype.

The keyboard of a Teletype is essentially a quickly opening and closing set of electrical contacts, and the printer, being coupled through an electromagnet, appears to be an inductor. In the slow moving bulky electromechanical environment of the Teletype itself, the electrical noise and contact bounce of the keyboard is inconsequential, but to the high-speed computer it can be totally confusing. To lower the noise susceptibility of the interface circuit, a low-pass filter drives a Schmitt trigger. If the values of R_1 and C are chosen so that the noise is safely less than the hysteresis band of the Schmitt trigger, the noise will be eliminated from the output. R_2 serves to deliver the 20 mA that the keyboard contacts need to establish a good connection.

The inductive load of the printer also presents a problem to the computer. Since (by Lenz's rule) changes in the current flowing through an inductor are opposed by a back electromotive force (inductive kickback), there can be large voltage spikes associated with switching transitions. The diode D helps to damp out the kickback due to the high-to-low current transition; and the resistor, together with the low "on" resistance of the driver, helps to damp out kickback due to low-to-high transitions. The printer circuit should be carefully decoupled from the system's power supply to prevent electrical noise from reaching other circuitry. In systems where 60-Hz interference or static noise due to the Teletype's motor is a problem, optically coupled drivers or reed relays can be used to electrically isolate the Teletype.

RS-232C interface.   Just as the general-purpose interface bus provides a standard of interconnection for parallel devices, the Electronics Industries Association (EIA) RS-232 provides a mechanical and electrical standard of interconnection for serial devices. Originally proposed for connection between data terminals and data sets (telephone interfaces, which are also called modems), the RS-232 is presently

PIN CONFIGURATION

BLOCK DIAGRAM

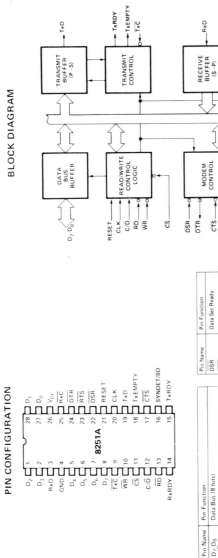

8251A

D₂	1	28	D₁
D₃	2	27	D₀
RxD	3	26	V_CC
GND	4	25	RxC̄
D₄	5	24	DTR̄
D₅	6	23	RTS̄
D₆	7	22	DSR̄
D₇	8	21	RESET
TxC̄	9	20	CLK
WR̄	10	19	TxD
CS̄	11	18	TxEMPTY
C/D̄	12	17	CTS̄
RD̄	13	16	SYNDET/BD
RxRDY	14	15	TxRDY

Pin Name	Pin Function
D₇–D₀	Data Bus (8 bits)
C/D̄	Control or Data is to be Written or Read
RD̄	Read Data Command
WR̄	Write Data or Control Command
CS̄	Chip Select
CLK	Clock Pulse (TTL)
RESET	Reset
TxC̄	Transmitter Clock
RxC̄	Receiver Clock
RxD	Receiver Data
RxRDY	Receiver Ready (has character for CPU)
TxRDY	Transmitter Ready (ready for char. from CPU)

Pin Name	Pin Function
DSR̄	Data Set Ready
DTR̄	Data Terminal Ready
SYNDET/BD	Sync Detect/ Break Detect
RTS̄	Request to Send Data
CTS̄	Clear to Send Data
TxEMPTY	Transmitter Empty
V_CC	+5 Volt Supply
GND	Ground

FIGURE 4.44 Intel 8251 USART. This microprocessor-oriented device can run at any baud rate from dc to 9.6 kbaud (asynchronously) or dc to 56 kbaud (synchronously). The transmit and receive clocks can be 1, 16, or 64 times the baud rate. (Reprinted by permission of Intel Corporation, © 1978.)

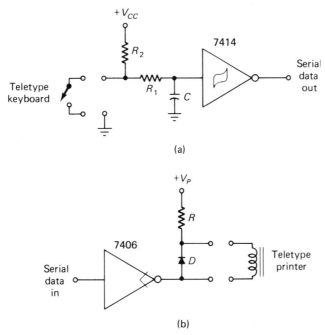

FIGURE 4.45 Typical Teletype interface circuits. (a) Keyboard interface. (b) Printer interface. The 7406 is an open-collector gate which is capable of sinking up to 30 mA. R is selected to deliver 20 mA to the printer with V_P less than 30 V maximum.

used for many other serial applications as well. In the following discussion we will be concerned only with the most recent version of the standard, RS-232C.

RS-232C calls for both specific electrical signals and specific connector and pin-out (Fig. 4.46). The signals are bipolar; that is, a logic 0 is any voltage between $+5$ and $+15$ V, and a logic 1 is any voltage between -5 and -15 V. Because of the wide margin of acceptance of logic levels (10 V), the standard is very tolerant of logic voltage variations between pieces of equipment. The voltage range of -3 to $+3$ V is a transition region where signal voltages may not correspond to specific logic levels. This region should be avoided except during switching transitions. The regions from $+3$ to $+5$ V and -3 to -5 V are settling regions where the logic values should be defined but are out of specification. The slew rate (rate of change of voltage) on any signal lead must be limited to a maximum of 30 V/μs. This requirement ensures that capacitive signal coupling between adjacent wires in cables will be low. The slew-rate limitation also allows the receiver to be set up to ignore fast pulses, which are characteristic of noise.

The connector is a 25-pin D type. Pin 1 is a protective ground which serves to connect the chassis of the various pieces of equipment together in order to bleed off static charges and other electrical noise without affecting any of the signal lines. Pin 2 carries the serial data transmitted from the data terminal to the data set, and pin 3 carries serial data to the data terminal from the data set. Note that a logic 1 on pins 2 or 3 indicates a mark, and logic 0 a space. All the remaining signal pins

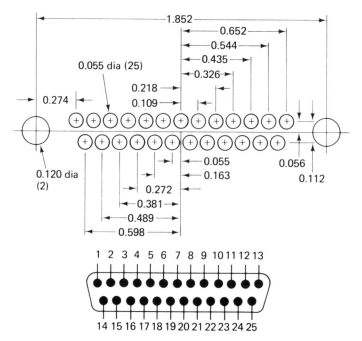

RS-232 pin assignments

Pin	Name	Function
1	FG	Frame ground (not switched)
2	TD	Transmit data
3	RD	Receive data
4	TRS	Request to send
5	CTS	Clear to send
6	DSR	Data set ready
7	SG	Signal ground
8	DCD	Data carrier detect
9		Positive dc test voltage
10		Negative dc test voltage
11		Unassigned
12	(S)DCD	Secondary data carrier detect
13	(S)CTS	Secondary clear to send
14	(S)TD	Secondary transmit data
15	TC	Transmit clock
16	(S)RD	Secondary receive data
17	RC	Receive clock
18		Receiver dibit clock
19	(S)RTS	Secondary request to send
20	DTR	Data terminal ready
21	SQ	Signal quality detect
22	RI	Ring indicator
23		Data rate select
24	ETC	External transmit clock
25		Busy

FIGURE 4.46 RS-232 serial connection standard for a terminal. Typical part numbers for the connectors are DB-25P (plug) and DB-25S (socket), both by Cinch. [From Liming, G. 1976. Data paths. Byte 1 (6) : 32–40. Used with permission.]

are negative logic, however, with a true condition being represented by a logic 0 and false by logic 1. In other words, a -5-V to -15-V signal on pins 2 or 3 would be taken as a true (or mark), but on any other pin it would be taken as a false. Pins 4 and 5 are the handshaking lines for use, if needed, between the data terminal and the data set. Pin 6 signifies the general readiness of the telephone connection to the data set, and pin 20 signifies that the data terminal is on-line and ready to communicate with the data set. Pin 22 signifies the reception by the data set of a "ring" on the telephone line (for automatic answering), and pin 8 signifies the reception of a carrier (data-carrying signal) on the telephone line. Most of the remaining pins are concerned with operation at very high speeds or are unassigned (for future expansion). Because RS-232 was originally intended to serve a specific purpose (connecting data terminals and modems), many of the pin definitions are ambiguous in other applications.

The signal levels called for by the RS-232C standard can either be generated and received by discrete circuitry (Pickles, 1977) or by integrated circuit devices designed especially for this purpose. Two such devices are the MC1488 quad RS-232C driver and MC1489 quad RS-232C receiver (manufactured by Motorola).

The MC1488 requires a power supply of approximately ± 12 V and has two AND-gate inputs on three of its four drivers, thus allowing possible simplification of the circuitry with which it is used. The fourth driver has only one input. To meet the slew-rate limitations of RS-232C, the MC1488 needs to have at least 330 pF of capacitive loading on each driver output. Often the cable to which it is connected has this much stray capacitance, so that no external components are needed.

The MC1489 receiver has voltage thresholds that are presettable using an external resistor for each receiver. The time response can be preset using an external capacitor for each receiver. If neither of these two features is required, the MC1489 needs no external components to operate. It requires only a single power supply of approximately $+5$ V.

Mass-storage hardware

When it is necessary to save programs and data for a period of time, external mass-storage hardware, which usually employs a magnetic medium, is often used. Since most solid-state memory is volatile (i.e., the data stored in it are lost when power is removed), semipermanent records of data must usually be made using some sort of mass-storage device. There are three forms of mass storage commonly used with microcomputers. These are the audio cassette, the digital cassette, and the floppy disk. Paper tape was once popular but is now being replaced by magnetic media.

Audio cassette. The audio cassette is the simplest form of mass storage in common use today. It is especially suited to inexpensive or quickly developed applications. The data are stored serially on a home-entertainment-type audio cassette recorder. One tone represents a logic 1 (mark) and another tone represents a logic 0 (space). Variations also exist that record data as the presence or absence of a tone (Sahakian, 1977). The serial data are most often stored asynchronously and in the same format as that used for data communication over telephone lines.

Because of the many tone-encoding methods and options that are possible and the need for compatibility, a standard (called the Kansas City standard) was established (Peschke and Peschke, 1976). The basics of the standard are as follows. The data rate is 300 baud. The data are recorded using a frequency-shifted tone with a mark consisting of eight cycles of a 2400-Hz tone and a space consisting of four cycles of a 1200-Hz tone. A recorded character consists of a space as a start bit, followed by 8 data bits, followed by two or more marks as stop bits. This is the same as the serial format shown in Fig. 4.42. The data bits are organized with the least significant bit first and the most significant bit last. The start bit is always immediately followed by the least significant data bit, regardless of the number of significant data bits, and all unused bits must be marks.

In the Kansas City standard, the data can be organized as arbitrary-length blocks of the characters defined above. Each block must be preceded by at least 5 s of mark tone, and the first block must start no sooner than 30 s after the end of the clear leader of the cassette (to provide for splicing and wrinkles in the tape). Since the frequencies of the mark tone (2400 Hz) and space tone (1200 Hz) are harmonically related, and the transition between them always occurs after an integral number of cycles, the recorded signal can also be used to derive the bit-clocking information for the UART or other serial data receiver. For example, UARTS often require a clock frequency of 16 times the bit rate (4800 Hz for 300 baud). This clock can be generated from the recorded waveform on the tape by synthesizing a 4800-Hz signal, which is always a harmonic of the tone recorded on the tape. In this way the data are self-clocking and tape-speed variations of up to $\pm 30\%$ can be tolerated. The tape-recorder audio bandwidth required by the standard is 3 kHz, and the error rate has been estimated at roughly 1 per 10^7 characters for 200 passes (Peschke and Peschke, 1976).

The main disadvantage of the audio cassette as mass storage is its slowness, both in getting to the block of data that is to be read and in reading the data once there. The drive motor of the audio-cassette recorder can be started and stopped by the processor through an output port (or hardware flag) driving an appropriate switching circuit, but the tape can only be made to move forward and a manual search for a certain section of the tape can take minutes. Audio-cassette mass storage is best suited to applications in which there is a human operator overseeing the recorder or when there are large amounts of sequential data that can be recorded or read in one continuous operation. Long-term recording of low-density physiological data is an ideal application.

Digital cassette.   The digital cassette is a better choice than the audio cassette for applications requiring high reliability, a high recorded data density, high speed of recording and playback, and automated tape searching.

The primary difference between the digital and audio cassette is that the digital cassette uses tape-oxide-saturation recording and the audio cassette uses linear tape recording. In other words, the digital cassette stores a bit of data by magnetizing the tape oxide either fully in one direction or the other at a given location on the tape. The audio cassette must record a magnetic representation of a number of cycles of a given audio tone to store the same bit of data. Tape saturation recording results in a much greater density of data on the tape, but the tape must be of higher quality and therefore costs more. Since the data density is so high—typically 800 bits/in. (bpi)—a very small defect in the tape can cause the loss of data.

Digital cassette drives are usually capable of bidirectional motion. A search for a particular block of data is therefore possible regardless of its location on the tape. A stepping motor is often used to advance the tape past the recording head. If the cassette is used incrementally, that is, one character or bit at a time, approximately 50,000 to 100,000 8-bit characters can be stored per cassette. If the cassette is used in a continuous fashion, up to 700,000 characters can be stored. The difference is due to the stopping and starting distances necessary for each bit or word in the incremental mode.

Data are usually organized as blocks or records of two to several thousand characters, and files of two to several hundred records. Gaps of 1 to 2 cm separate the records. If the record size is small and the number of records is large, this inter-record gap can accumulate and waste a significant portion of a typical 300-ft (14.2-m) cassette.

Floppy disk.   Digital cassettes are faster than audio cassettes but are still too slow for many computer operations. For high-speed mass storage, the floppy disk is rapidly becoming indispensible.

A "floppy" is simply a thin circular disk of flexible plastic which is coated with a magnetic oxide layer like that used on recording tape. This disk is permanently housed (but free to spin) in a square, flexible protective envelope that has windows to expose certain regions of the disk. The disk (and envelope) has a hole in its center, which allows it to be spun when in use.

Data are stored on the magnetic surface of the disk in concentric rings called tracks. A track is divided into a number of circular arcs called sectors, each of which contains a number of words of data (stored serially). As with the digital cassette, the data are recorded by oxide saturation.

The floppy-disk drive usually has a slot into which the floppy is slid. Once the floppy is fully in the drive, a latching door is generally closed over the slot to seal out dust and other contaminants. Closing the door also engages a spinning hub into the center hole of the disk and it begins to turn. A common speed of rotation is 360 r/min (6 r/s). A movable magnetic head is suspended over a narrow rectangular window in the envelope, which extends over most of the radius of the disk. To get to any track, the head must move radially over the window to the proper radius. This motion is usually accomplished by a stepping motor, which drives a screw and follower or a reel and metal band.

Once at the desired track, the search begins for the desired sector on the track. When the sector is found, the head is pressed against the moving surface of the disk. Data can then be read or written. When the head is not being used to read, write, or search for data, it is lifted back off the surface of the disk to prevent wear. In many disk drives the disk stops spinning, to reduce wear, if there have been no recent requests for access.

Some disks have optically sensed sectors which are located by holes near the edge of the disk. These are called hard-sectored disks because the sectors cannot be moved or changed in size. Other disks have only one such hole and the sectoring is done relative to this by information magnetically recorded on the disk. These are called soft-sectored disks because the sectors can be moved or changed in size under software control.

The standard floppy disk is $7\frac{3}{4}$ in. in diameter and is housed in an 8-by 8-in. plastic envelope. There are 77 tracks, each 0.012 in. wide and spaced approximately 0.02 in. apart. A total of 250,000 to 375,000 8-bit bytes (depending on the specific recording format used) can be stored on a standard floppy disk. Each track stores the same number of bytes, therefore the bit density is greatest on the innermost track. "Mini" floppy disks, which have a diameter of $5\frac{1}{4}$ in., are also available. These mini floppy systems are lower in cost than standard floppy systems but have lower data storage abilities.

To move the head to a specific record takes time. This latency can be broken down into two sources, lateral and rotational. Lateral latency is the time it takes for the head to be moved to a given track, typically 6 ms per track traversed. Rotational latency is the time that it takes once at the track before the record of interest is under the head. On the average, this is one-half of the disk's rotation period, or 83 ms. Figure 4.47 summarizes and compares mass-storage devices.

Technique	IBM 2315 Cartridge Disk	IBM 3740 Floppy	Digital Cassette	Audio Cassette	Units
Data Capacity	48.	3.0	6.0	0.84	Million bits (unformatted)
Average or Typical Access Time	.035	.45	20	120*	Seconds (* = manually controlled)
Data Transfer Rate	2500	250	10.	0.3	k bps
Price of Commercial Package: Drive + Power + Controller	$8000	$1500	$1000**	$100	**Note that personal computing digital cassettes can be much cheaper than commercial drives
System Cost per Unit Data Rate	.32	.6	10	33.3	cents per bps
System Cost per Unit Storage	.016	.05	.016	.012	cents per bit stored
Media Cost	$100	$8.	$4.	$4.	(unit quantity prices)
Storage Cost	1.7	2.2	0.55	3.9	cents/kilobyte of media

FIGURE 4.47 Summarized comparison of mass-storage devices. The IBM 2315 cartridge disk is a full-sized computer peripheral included for reference. [From Rampil, I. 1977. A floppy-disk tutorial. Byte 2(12): 24–45. Used with permission.]

Number-processing hardware

When many complex numerical calculations must be performed, problems can arise with both software development time and processing speed. To overcome these problems, special number-processing hardware has become available. This hardware is independent of the computer in that, once given a numerical problem to solve, it can generate the solution while the computer tends to other tasks. Since such numerical problems can take seconds or minutes to solve, number-processing hardware can be essential.

Number crunchers. To perform scientific calculations on decimal numbers, the National Semiconductor Corp. MM57109 number-oriented processor can be used. This processor, or number cruncher as it is called, is functionally similar to a scientific pocket calculator. It operates in post-fix (reverse Polish) notation and handles data in either floating-point or scientific notation. The data can be from one to eight digits long, and typical operations take between 500 μs and 1 s to perform. The number cruncher can handle trigonometric and other transcendental functions as well as simple algebra. Additionally, it can be programmed (needing only an external program counter and program source) to perform virtually any numerical operation. Figure 4.48(a) summarizes the number cruncher's instruction classes.

Figure 4.49 shows the internal structure of the number cruncher. The device is based on a 4-bit word (being convenient for use with binary-coded-decimal numbers). There is an operational stack of four registers (X, Y, Z and T) as well as a memory register (M). I_1 through I_6 specify the instruction to be executed. During a number cruncher input operation, D_1 through D_4 accept data. Output is multiplexed onto DO_1 through DO_4. Input and output data are sequential and can be in any of the two formats shown in Fig. 4.48(b). In both input and output, the digit address (the sequential location of the digit in the number) appears on DA_1 through DA_4. Three flags are available, including two-user-controlled and one for errors. An external clock of between 320 and 400 kHz must be supplied as well as 9 V at (typically) 12 mA.

Figure 4.50 shows a basic interface between the number cruncher and a microcomputer. Two latches are used, one for instructions and one for output data. The HOLD line from the computer suspends the number cruncher's operation until the computer is ready. To use the number cruncher, the computer loads a 6-bit instruction into the hex latch (which serves as an output port for the computer) and brings the HOLD line low. The number cruncher executes the instruction and signifies its readiness for data or another instruction through its RDY (ready) line. Data are returned to the computer through the quad latch (which serves as an input port). The computer can read the number cruncher's status line ($R/\overline{W}$, RDY, and $\overline{BR}$) through the tristate buffers, addressing them as an input port. The flowchart shows the computer software necessary to control the interface.

For higher-speed number processing, a binary number processor, the Advanced Micro Devices AM9511, is also available. The instruction set of this device is very similar to that of the number cruncher but, being a strictly binary device, it

Digit entry:	
0-9	Each digit is entered into the X register mantissa or exponent if in enter-exponent mode.
.	Fixes decimal point of mantissa of number being entered.
EE	Set enter-exponent mode.
CS	Change sign of mantissa or exponent.
PI	$\pi \to$ X register.
EN	Number entry terminated and stack is pushed. $X \to Y \to Z \to T$
Move:	
Roll	Roll stack. $X \to T \to Z \to Y \to X$
POP	Pop stack. $X \leftarrow Y \leftarrow Z \leftarrow T \leftarrow 0$
XEY	Exchange X and Y. $X \longleftrightarrow Y$
XEM	Exchange X with memory. $X \longleftrightarrow M$
MS	Memory store. $X \to M$
MR	Memory recall. $X \leftarrow M$
Math:	
$X \leftarrow Y + X, X \leftarrow Y - X$	Result in X, stack popped.
$X \leftarrow Y \cdot X, X \leftarrow Y + X$	$Y \leftarrow Z \leftarrow T \leftarrow 0$
$X \leftarrow Y^X$	
$M \leftarrow M + X, M \leftarrow M - X$	Result in memory.
$M \leftarrow M \cdot X, M \leftarrow M + X$	
$1/X, \sqrt{X}, X^2, 10^X, e^X, \ln x, \log X$	Result in X, previous X lost, stack unchanged.
SIN(X), COS(X), TAN(X)	Result in X, previous X lost, stack unchanged.
$SIN^{-1}(X), COS^{-1}(X), TAN^{-1}(X)$	
RTD, DTR	Convert X from radians to degrees or vice versa. Previous X lost, stack unchanged.
Branch:	
JMP	Unconditional jump. On call branch instructions, second word of instruction is the branch address, which is loaded into an external program counter by a load pulse from the NCU.
TJC	Test external jump condition, branch if true.
Input/output:	
IN	Multidigit synchronous input from RAM or peripheral into X register.
OUT	Multidigit synchronous output to RAM or peripheral from X register.
AIN	Single digit asynchronous input. Wait for asynchronous data ready ($\overline{ADR}$) to go low, then read data and pulse acknowledge flag F_2.
Mode control:	
SMDC	Set mantissa digit count from one to eight digits.

(a)

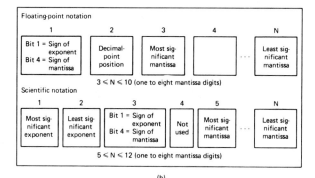

(b)

FIGURE 4.48 Number-cruncher chip. (a) Instructions. (b) Data formats. (Reprinted from Electronics, February 17, 1977; © McGraw-Hill, Inc., 1977, all rights reserved.)

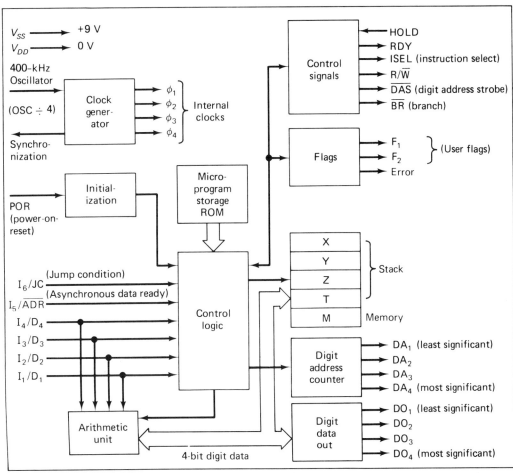

FIGURE 4.49 Internal structure of the number cruncher. (Reprinted from Electronics, February 17, 1977; © McGraw-Hill, Inc., 1977, all rights reserved.)

operates more than 100 times faster. Osborne (1978) compares the MM57109 and AM9511 in microprocessor applications.

Discrete Fourier transform generator. The discrete Fourier transform (DFT) involves much numerical processing (see Section 3.4). However, there is a hardware module that can relieve the computer of this major task. This analog-in/analog-out module is produced by Reticon Corporation and is based on a semiconductor quad-chirped z-transversal filter (the Reticon RC-5601).

The module operates using analog discrete-time techniques to implement the chirped z transform (Rabiner et al., 1969) and generates the power and spectral-density information of a 512-point DFT. Split-electrode weighting techniques (Broderson et al., 1976) are applied to a charge-coupled device (called a transversal filter) to create a discrete analog delay line which also performs an analog sum of its stored values, each weighted by an appropriate factor. This operation is essen-

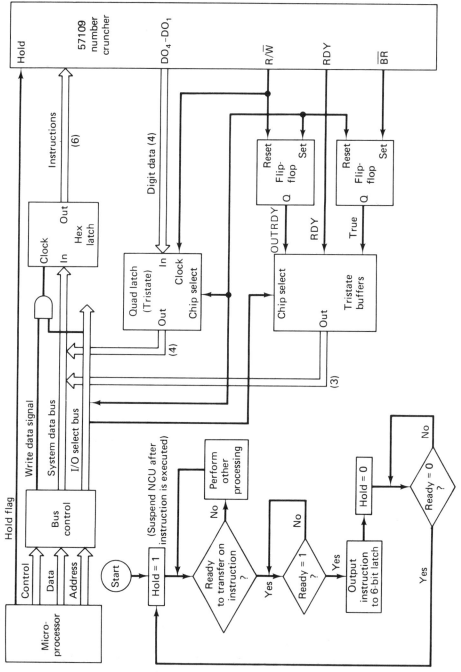

FIGURE 4.50 Basic interface between the number cruncher and a microprocessor. (Reprinted from Electronics, February 17, 1977; © McGraw-Hill, Inc., 1977, all rights reserved.)

tially a convolution and, if performed by the computer, would require a minimum of 2048 multiplications and 2048 additions. The transversal filter is capable of operating at up to a 2-MHz sample rate and of generating the complete DFT, but the module limits the overall performance to a maximum 200-kHz sample rate and to the generation of the power and spectral-density information.

Other input/output hardware

Switches. At first it might seem that a switch could simply be connected from the input of a logic circuit directly to ground or V_{CC}. This is often not the case. Because of mechanical bounce of the switch contacts and other electrical noise, the transitions of the switch are not well defined, but rather accompanied by a short period of fluctuations of resistance. Although these fluctuations are over so quickly that they can generally be ignored, they are poisonous to many high-speed computer circuits. The use of mercury-wetted contacts in switches can lower or eliminate these resistance fluctuations, but these switches are also expensive and must be hermetically sealed. Debouncing of switches can also be done by logic hardware using a single-pole, double-throw switch and a flip-flop made from two cross-coupled gates, as shown in Fig. 4.51(a).

An alternative to this approach is to use a nonretriggerable monostable multivibrator such as the 74121 to produce a fixed-length pulse from a noisy switch closure, as shown in Fig. 4.51(b). The switch is connected to the trigger of the multivibrator so that the output pulse begins at the first transition of the switch and lasts for the period determined by the resistor R_2 and capacitor C. This approach allows the use of a single-pole, single-throw switch and is especially suited to push-button or other momentary switch applications.

Software can sometimes be used to allow the computer to ignore the bouncing

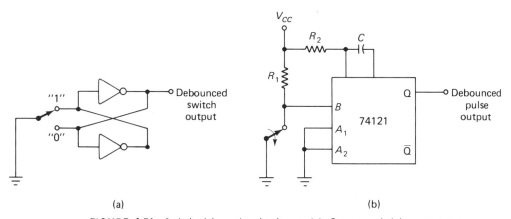

(a) (b)

FIGURE 4.51 Switch debouncing hardware. (a) Cross-coupled inverter gates forming a flip-flop. (b) A monostable multivibrator for momentary switches. R_1 helps ensure that the 74121 input B reaches a logic 1 when the switch is pressed. R_2 and C set the output-pulse duration. In both cases an inverted output is also available.

and noise. Commonly, the first transition of a switch is sensed by the computer, which then waits, ignoring further transitions for a period of perhaps 8 ms, or whatever is necessary for the switch to settle.

Keyboards.   A keyboard is a set of momentary contact switches or keys that are grouped together. There are two basic ways to input switch-closure information from a keyboard. The first and most obvious approach is to allow 1 bit of an input port for each key of a keyboard, as in Fig. 4.52(a). Using this unencoded keyboard, the state of each key is directly readable by the computer.

The second approach—encoded keyboard—uses the fact that often in keyboards, only one key can or should be pressed at a time. This allows the number of input bits to be reduced to roughly the base 2 logarithm of the number of keys. For example, if a keyboard has eight keys, and only one of these keys is to be pressed at a time, it is possible to encode the switch closure information on 3 bits of an input port, as in Fig. 4.52(b). For large keyboards, encoding yields large savings in the number of input port bits needed. If the keyboard is separated from the computer, the number of interconnecting wires can be reduced as well.

Keyboards can also be matrixed to realize a reduction in input bits as well as a reduction in the hardware needed to interface to the keyboard. In a typical matrixed keyboard (Fig. 4.53) the keys are arranged by rows and columns. Each row of the keyboard has a common wire which leads to an input port, and each of the columns has a common wire from an output port. A switch closure connects a row and column wire, establishing a single path from an output bit to an input bit. The computer can then sense which of the switches is closed.

In operation, the computer uses the output port to continually scan the key-

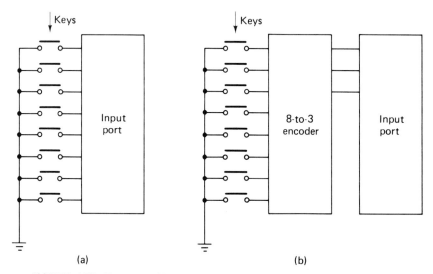

(a)   (b)

FIGURE 4.52 Two ways of inputting from eight-key keyboards. (a) The unencoded approach needs 8 bits of input. (b) If encoded, only 3 bits are needed and the remaining 5 may be used elsewhere.

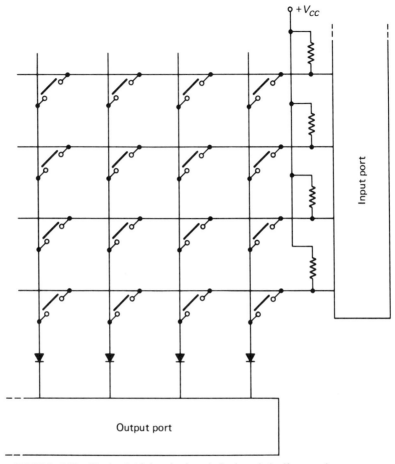

FIGURE 4.53 Matrixed 16-key keyboard. Each switch, if pressed, connects a unique combination of input port pin and output port pin. The diodes guard against short-circuiting of the output port if more than one key is pressed at once.

board columns, pulling each column low, one at a time, in succession. After a column has been pulled low by an output, the computer inputs the logic levels of the rows. Normally, all the rows are high, because they are pulled up by resistors at the input port. If a switch is closed, however, a low in its column will be connected to its row and be inputted by the computer. By knowing which column is low when it inputs the low on a row line, the computer knows which key is pressed.

Matrixing and scanning takes not only extra software to run, but a great deal of time as well. Still, the savings in hardware (especially for a large number of keys or a physically small system) can make it attractive. Virtually all pocket calculator keyboards are matrixed.

Simple displays.   To display a single bit a light-emitting diode (LED) can be used, as shown in Fig. 4.54. The resistor used depends on the LED current and voltage

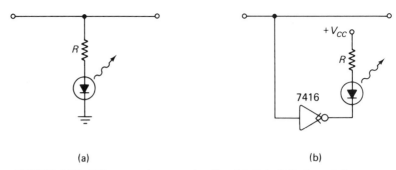

(a)   (b)

FIGURE 4.54 LED connections to a data line. (a) If the LED draws little current, the connection can be direct. (b) For high-current LEDs, an open-collector gate can be used. In both cases, R limits the current through the LED.

specifications. For low-current diodes, a simple connection is adequate. For higher currents, an intervening driver (such as a 7416) is required.

Alarms.   To announce conditions that need immediate attention, sonic alarms are available. One such alarm is the Mini-Bleeptone, manufactured by the Cybersonic Division of the C. A. Briggs Company. This device is a cylinder 24 mm long and 27 mm in diameter. It operates at from 5 to 30 V dc and draws only 3 to 8 mA. The emitted output provides a tone at 800 Hz or, optionally, at 4 kHz, with loudness of 62 to 80 dB, thus making it very hard to ignore. With such a low current requirement, the alarm can be driven directly from a TTL gate output.

Alphanumeric displays.   For applications requiring the display of numbers or alphabetic characters, segment and dot displays can be used. The most common display for numbers is the seven-segment display which we see in almost every digital calculator and watch. Most of these displays have a decimal point as well, either to the left or right of the digit, bringing the total number of controllable elements per digit to eight.

LEDs are often used as the indicating elements. For applications requiring lower power dissipation, liquid-crystal displays are a better choice. Single-package drivers exist for both LED displays (type 7447 integrated circuits) and liquid-crystal displays (RCA CD4055 or CD4056 integrated circuits).

The terminals at one end of each of the indicating elements (segments) in a digit are usually connected together. This allows a reduction in the number of pins on the display package. For LEDs this connection can be either a common anode or a cathode.

For displays requiring many digits, a time-multiplexed matrixing scheme similar to that used in keyboards can simplify the hardware. If, for example, eight digits (each composed of seven segments and a decimal point) are to be displayed, the digits can be flashed by the computer one at a time in rapid succession so that they all appear to be displayed simultaneously. This can be done using the configuration shown in Fig. 4.55.

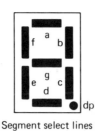

Segment select lines

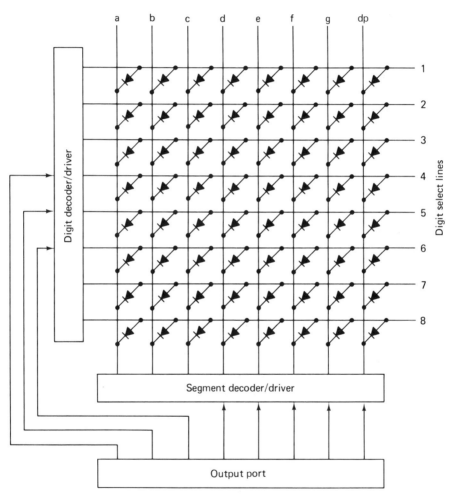

FIGURE 4.55 Matrixed display of eight seven-segment LED digits controlled through one output port. The digit decoder/driver selects and supplies current to one of the eight-digit select lines. The segment decoder/driver sinks current through the appropriate segment lines to display the desired character. (Each horizontal row of LEDs corresponds to one digit.)

If the development time or package count (number of integrated circuit packages) are important factors, single package latch, decoder, driver, and display units are available. One such unit is the Texas Instruments TIL-311 hexadecimal display shown in Fig. 4.56. This device decodes and displays not only the digits 0 through 9 but also the letters A through F. This makes it ideal for hexadecimal applications or for the display of simple messages. Note that the display format does not have seven segments but rather a set of 20 dots. The increased readability of this display is an important feature. Since there is a latch contained in the package, all that is needed to interface this display as an output device is appropriate addressing and control circuitry. The TIL-311 is contained entirely in a red transparent 14-pin dual, in-line package.

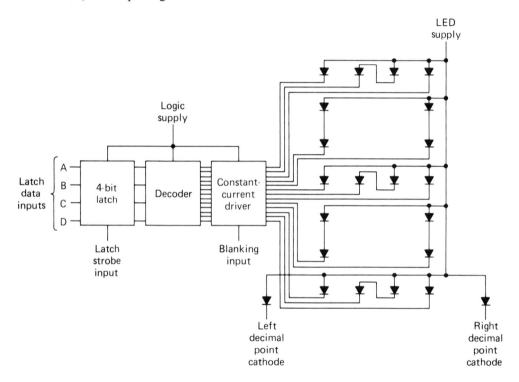

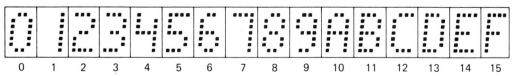

FIGURE 4.56 Texas Instruments TIL-311. This self-contained latch, decoder, driver, and display represents all 16 combinations of 4 bits as their hexadecimal equivalents. (Compliments of Texas Instruments, 1972.)

When the display of any of a full set of alphanumeric characters is needed, dot-matrix displays of typically 5×7 LEDs can serve. The external circuitry used to drive these displays usually incorporates a read-only memory to generate the decoded (5×7 dot) representation of an encoded (often 8-bit) character.

Interfaces. To interface to circuits that are at high voltages, or have different ground potentials, either relay or optically coupled isolators can be used. A typical relay driver is essentially the same as the Teletype printer interface of Fig. 4.45.

The optical isolators shown in Fig. 4.57 are TTL-compatible on the gate side

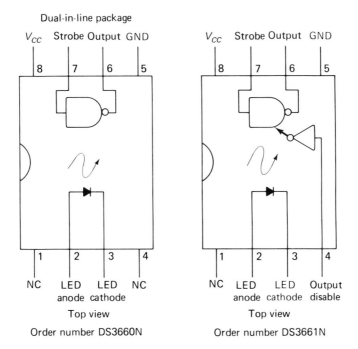

Truth tables (positive logic convention; input "1" when LED is biased on, $I_F > 5$ mA)

DS3660

Input	Strobe	Output
0	1	1
1	1	0
X	0	1

X = don't care

DS3661

Input	Strobe	Disable	Output
0	1	0	1
1	1	0	0
X	0	0	1
X	X	1	Hi-Z

X = don't care

FIGURE 4.57 Optical isolators for digital signals. The DS3660N has an open-collector output, and the DS3661N is tristate. These devices are ideal for communicating between high-speed digital instruments at different ground potentials. (Compliments of National Semiconductor, 1975.)

and require a minimum of 5 mA of current through the diode to cause the gate output to go high. In addition to the isolated input, the type DS3660 has a TTL input and the DS3661 adds a tristate output control. With a propagation delay from the diode to the output of only 70 ns, these isolators can be used to couple high-speed digital circuitry without compromising its performance.

4.5 SOFTWARE DESIGN*

In the previous chapters we illustrated ways in which analog and digital signals are transformed and discussed hardware designs for microcomputers. Hardware designs for microcomputers are so general that the software must specifically define the task. Software refers to the handling of the digital information by the micro-computer hardware. In this section we review some of the basic principles of micro-computer software design and illustrate some of the techniques and tools useful to the software engineer (programmer) to aid in that design.

A systems approach to software design

Our ultimate goals as software engineers are to design and implement reliable soft-ware. Often a complex problem presents too many intricate details to design the entire software package as one complete unit. Figure 4.58 shows that we may break down the overall design goal into a number of smaller blocks. This enables us to concentrate easily on the particular problem in each block without requiring detailed information as to how it fits into the overall design. Later, when we are to

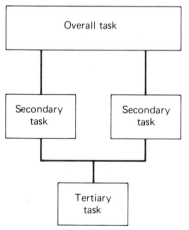

FIGURE 4.58 An overall complex program may be broken down into smaller, easily written modules. Each module is then interfaced to perform the overall program.

*Section 4.5 written by Gary V. Sprenger.

incorporate each block, we may concentrate on the problem of defining block inter-action without reference to the intricate details of each block. In this way each block represents a separate, yet integrated design. In fact, as we build up a library of useful algorithms and programs, our task becomes simply to interface them in different ways for different overall designs. By using this systems approach we gain a better understanding of the software at the level of detail required, without over-whelming ourselves with unimportant or irrelevant details.

Information representation

To effectively translate an algorithm understandable in human terms to the binary language of the microcomputer, we must be familiar with how information is re-presented in microcomputers. Recall that our general microcomputer processes 8 bits of information in a parallel fashion. We can thus uniquely represent 2^8, or 256 states. Each bit added in parallel multiplies the number of unique states by 2, because each bit has only two states. Hence the natural language of the microcom-puter is binary. One of our problems as programmers is to translate information to this binary form.

Binary and hexadecimal number representation. A series of eight ones or zeros to represent information is inherently clumsy for human beings. It would be conve-nient if we could represent our decimal numbers in a binary form directly equivalent in meaning. Since ten distinct digits are used in the decimal system but only two are used in the binary system, we need $2^n = 10$, or 3.32 equivalent binary digits to fully translate the informational content of decimal numbers. In this case the fractional digit presents us with translation problems.

A number system that does have an integer number of binary digits after translation is the hexadecimal or base 16 system. Here $2^4 = 16$, or 4 digits are required to faithfully represent the 16 unique digits of the hexadecimal number sys-tem. Therefore, exact equivalence is accomplished and an 8-bit binary number may be represented by two hexadecimal digits.

$$128_{10} = 1000\ 0000_2 = 80_{16}$$

Figure 4.59 shows some representative examples of the hexadecimal number system and its equivalent representation in the decimal and binary number systems. The case of information translation from hexadecimal to binary representations makes hexadecimal the favorite for use by microcomputer programmers.

Binary-coded-decimal representation. Another shorthand method of representing numbers in microcomputers is the binary coded decimal or BCD code. BCD repre-sentation uses 4 bits to represent the 10 decimal digits 0 through 9. However, extra information not contained in only 10 states is available because four binary digits can represent 16 unique states. To regain exact translational equivalence, six of

Decimal	Hexadecimal	Binary	Binary-coded decimal	
0	0	0000		0000
1	1	0001		0001
2	2	0010		0010
3	3	0011		0011
4	4	0100		0100
5	5	0101		0101
6	6	0110		0110
7	7	0111		0111
8	8	1000		1000
9	9	1001		1001
10	A	1010	0001	0000
11	B	1011	0001	0001
12	C	1100	0001	0010
13	D	1101	0001	0011
14	E	1110	0001	0100
15	F	1111	0001	0101

FIGURE 4.59   Relationships among various number representations.

these states are eliminated and are illegal to use by definition. However, they can still be generated in the microcomputer.

Note also that the absolute range of numbers we may represent is similarly limited.

$$1001\ 1001_2 = 99_{BCD} = 99_{10}$$

Using one 8-bit binary number, we were able to represent uniquely 0 through 255_{10}. Now only numbers from 0 through 99_{10} can be represented in one byte. Rather than a continuous set of integer binary numbers, we must represent each BCD digit as a discrete group of four binary digits. While convenient for human beings to understand, BCD results in important changes in the binary arithmetic of the microcomputer. Nevertheless, BCD codes are widely used partly because of the availability of simple and inexpensive displays that use this code.

Alphanumeric representation—the ASCII code.   In addition to representing numbers in microcomputers, we must also represent the 26 letters of the alphabet, the punctuation marks used in everyday language, and other symbols. Developed by programmers as a standard format of information exchange, the 7-bit American Standard Code for Information Interchange (ASCII) code is easy to implement in microcomputers. A set of 2^7 unique codes is defined. ASCII-encoded decimal numbers present no added problems as compared to BCD numbers. If we remove the three most significant bits in the ASCII code, we have our familiar BCD-coded numbers. Thus any programs written to manipulate BCD numbers can easily be modified to use ASCII-encoded numbers instead. A full listing of the ASCII code characters can be found in Appendix 2.

To use the information we have translated to binary, we must be familiar with the way the microcomputer manipulates and generates information or data. First we shall consider how the microcomputer, via software, can manipulate data without altering its informational content. An important part of this discussion regards how instructions are executed and decisions made by microcomputers. We must also be familiar with how microcomputers can access any distinct piece of information prior to these processes and how we can "teach" the microcomputer to locate the correct piece.

After these basic processes are discussed, we will explore the alteration or generation of information by the microcomputer. Especially important are microcomputer arithmetic and logical capabilities.

Memory pointers, branching, and addressing modes

Information stored in memory may be accessed by microcomputers in many ways. Hence one way to measure the intrinsic power of a microcomputer is to examine the quantity and quality of its addressing modes. Commonly included addressing modes are:

1. Accumulator-implied
2. Stack or scratchpad register
3. Direct
4. Indexed
5. Indirect
6. Doubly indirect
7. Immediate
8. Relative

We will present some of the advantages and disadvantages of these addressing modes along with typical examples of their use.

Memory pointers. Since many of the addressing modes use pointers to memory it is pertinent to review several of the most important kinds of memory pointers. *The single most important memory pointer—the program counter (PC)—is usually a specially dedicated register within the CPU.* This memory pointer has the important function of indicating where in memory the next instruction to be executed is stored. Both instructions and data are stored in memory in the same basic form. Hence for reliable software operation, we must control very carefully how this vital memory pointer is manipulated or changed during the course of our program.

This is not as difficult as it sounds, because most PC manipulations are controlled by hardware. When a microcomputer is turned on (powered-up) or reset by hardware, one particular memory address is forced into the PC. If our program is to run, we *must* store the first *instruction* at this address. Often we must also establish the initial state of the machine—a process called initialization. For example, the RCA COSMAC enables interrupts after a power-up or reset sequence. Initialization must therefore include an instruction to disable or mask interrupt requests until we are ready for them.

After the start address has been forced into the program counter, the contents of this memory address (MA) are fetched via the data bus and placed in a register called the instruction register. The program counter is then incremented by one to point to the next-higher memory address (MA + 1). The instruction is then decoded and, if a multibyte instruction, the remaining bytes are fetched. The PC is incremented after each fetch. The instruction is then executed. This pattern of events occurs for each instruction and is called the instruction cycle. Several typical instruction cycles are illustrated below.

one-byte instruction	fetch–execute
two-byte instruction	fetch–fetch–execute
three-byte instruction	fetch–fetch–fetch–execute

Note that the instruction length is directly proportional to the number of bytes that must be fetched from memory. Since the speed of memory access is the limiting hardware factor, we can speed up program execution by requiring fewer accesses to memory. An added bonus is a conservation of the total memory required for the program. Because memory is the high-cost hardware item in microcomputers, we can keep overall costs down in this manner.

Decision making by branching. The result of incrementing the PC for each instruction is a program that executes in a linear fashion from low memory addresses to high memory addresses. While program execution in this manner is alone quite powerful, it quickly uses the available memory if a particular sequence of instructions is required repetitively. With the inclusion of instructions that modify the program counter, we can break this linear sequence and start a new sequence of instruction execution anywhere in the program.

Those instructions that automatically transfer program execution to another part of the program are called unconditional branches, jumps, or calls. The next one or two bytes following the branch instruction in the program are used by the microcomputer to change the program counter to the address of the new instruction sequence in memory. The alteration of the program counter in this case is done automatically every time unconditional branch instructions are encountered in the program. However, we can make this program branch dependent upon conditions established during the course of program execution through instructions called conditional branches, jumps, or calls.

Conditional branches. Conditional branches are useful to direct program execution in one or two possible directions. Condition codes or flags implemented in hardware are automatically manipulated by instructions in well-defined ways. Conditional branch instructions determine what state one of these condition codes is in at the time the branch instruction is executed and directs program execution accordingly. Condition codes that may be checked in the Z80 are zero, carry, parity, and arithmetic sign. The most frequent use of conditional branches are in program loops. Here a set of instructions is executed repeatedly until the correct condition is established. The branch instruction detects this condition and directs program execution to continue in a linear fashion. This programming technique frees the programmer from repetitive inclusion of this particular sequence of instructions in the program. Determining the number of times to perform the loop requires care. A frequent source of errors is performing the loop one too many or one too few times. As confidence is gained in writing program loops, we may make them dependent upon the particular data to be processed. For example, some processes, such as floating-point arithmetic (described later in this chapter), require that part of a number be left-justified.

$$00110000 \longrightarrow 11000000$$
$$00010111 \longrightarrow 10111000$$

In this case we merely need to know when the most significant bit is high (set to 1). After each shift to the left we can mask out (see bit manipulations) all but the most significant bit and then determine if it is set to terminate the loop.

Stack pointer.   When a branch to another part of the program occurs, we may wish to save the contents of the general-purpose scratchpad registers and program counter. A useful technique to accomplish this is to reserve an area of RAM for temporary storage called a stack. Usually, RAM locations high in memory are chosen and data are saved sequentially in lower addresses by decrementing the stack pointer after each byte is saved. To correctly store and later retrieve data, we must keep track of the location of the next unused storage slot. The stack pointer is a register specially dedicated to this purpose. Originally, the stack pointer must contain the highest address in RAM designated for the stack. After we add or PUSH a byte of data to the location pointed to by the stack pointer, the pointer is decremented and therefore points to the next available location. If we wish to retrieve or POP our stored data back to the CPU registers, we must first increment the stack pointer. Since the last data byte that we PUSH into the stack is the first that we POP out, we call this stack a last-in, first-out (LIFO). Instructions in the Z80 and COSMAC automatically perform these operations on the stack pointer.

Data pointer.   The techniques used for the program counter and stack pointer may also be used effectively to process data. A register can be set aside to contain the address of the first byte of data to be processed. After the data are fetched and processed, the data pointer is incremented or decremented accordingly to point to the next byte of data. The program checks to see if the address of the last byte of data has been processed, and if not, it makes a conditional branch to repeat the processing loop.

Accumulator.   In the discussion thus far we referred to the data as being processed. The general-purpose register where the bulk of this processing occurs is the accumulator—called (A) in the Z80 and (D) in the COSMAC. The instruction sets of all microcomputers with accumulators include a rich variety of accumulator manipulations. Typically, there are instructions that move data to and from the accumulator contents, and shift or rotate the accumulator contents left or right. Since the accumulator of most microcomputers is only 8 bits wide, an extra bit called the carry bit facilitates linkage for multibyte operations. Later we shall see the necessity and usefulness of the carry bit.

To fully appreciate the data-manipulation abilities of microcomputers, we as programmers must become proficient with the addressing modes used. A summary of the addressing mode types is listed below.

Accumulator-implied.   Many instructions included in microcomputer instruction sets imply that the source or destination of the data operand is the accumulator. Typical instructions using accumulator-implied addressing are load, store, rotate, shift, and I/O instructions. Since the source and/or destination of the data operand is implied, the byte length of the instruction is shorter than for other addressing modes.

Scratchpad register.   Similar to accumulator-implied addressing, scratchpad register addressing implies that the source or destination of the data is a particular scratchpad register. Again, short instructions result. An additional advantage of register–register operations is the inherent speed of execution, because memory is not accessed for the data operand.

Direct addressing.   Full direct addressing includes the full 16-bit absolute address of the data operand in the instruction. This necessitates a 3-byte instruction. Present page addressing is a variation in which the upper 8 bits of the address (the most significant byte) are assumed to be the same as the previous instruction—only the lower 8 bits are supplied. In the case of page-zero addressing, the most significant byte of the address is assumed to be zero and the lower 8 bits of the address on page zero are supplied. Both present page and page-zero addressing require only 2-byte instructions.

Indexed addressing.   Indexed addressing makes use of an index register within the CPU that contains the full 16-bit base address of the data operand. The second byte of the instruction contains an offset (e.g., an 8-bit value) to be added to the base address to generate the effective data-operand address. Indexed addressing is useful for processing multibyte data or for complex array manipulations.

Indirect addressing.   A very efficient memory addressing method, indirect addressing can specify any address in memory with a 1-byte instruction. Encoded in the instruction is information that indicates which of the CPU general-purpose register pairs is the 16-bit pointer to memory. Since the pointer must be set up prior to its use, indirect addressing loses its efficiency unless many accesses to memory must be made.

Doubly indirect addressing. Used in the COSMAC as the rule rather than the exception, doubly indirect addressing utilizes a 4-bit register pointer to indicate which CPU register contains the address of the data operand in memory. Many different memory pointers may be indicated uniquely, and thus we may access any one of 16 memory locations with a 1-byte instruction (see Fig. 4.60).

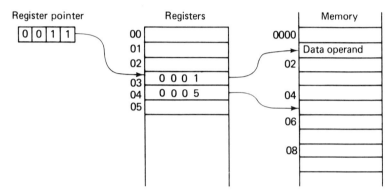

FIGURE 4.60 Doubly indirect addressing. The register pointer contains the address of the general-purpose register to be used as the pointer to the data operand in memory.

Immediate addressing. Unlike the other addressing modes, immediate addressing includes the data operand as part of the instruction necessitating a 2- or 3-byte instruction. Since programs are often stored in read-only memory, the data operand retains the value assigned during program design.

Relative addressing. In relative addressing the second byte of the instruction is interpreted as a signed 2's-complement displacement to be added to the address register to form the effective address. As in immediate addressing, the displacement is a contiguous part of the program and cannot be modified. Relative addressing is used to advantage in branch or jump instructions, where the program counter is modified by the displacement.

Microcomputer data-manipulation basics

Complex signal processing with microcomputers often calls upon our programming skills in mathematics. Chapter 3 presented some of the techniques used, together with algorithms for their execution in microcomputers. While these algorithms are rather trivial programming tasks for the high-level language programmer, we as assembly language programmers are just one step beyond the language of the microcomputer itself. A thorough understanding of the basic arithmetic and logic capabilities of microcomputers is therefore mandatory if we are to implement these algorithms successfully.

Bit manipulation and packing.   Bit manipulation is needed in almost every signal-processing application and in general is required to establish the correct conditions for conditional branches, Any bit may be manipulated by using the logical instructions AND, OR, and XOR (exclusive OR).

For example, we can isolate the fourth bit of a data byte before checking its condition. This is done by selecting the proper bit pattern or mask to AND logically with the data byte.

Bit number	(7) (6) (5) (4) (3) (2) (1) (0)	(7) (6) (5) (4) (3) (2) (1) (0)
Data byte	1 0 1 1 0 1 1 1	0 1 0 0 1 1 0 0
Mask	0 0 0 1 0 0 0 0	0 0 0 1 0 0 0 0
Result after logical AND	0 0 0 1 0 0 0 0	0 0 0 0 0 0 0 0

Notice that we have masked out and lost (reset) all information present in the data byte except bit 4. By choosing the proper mask we can preserve any particular bits of interest.

Data byte	1011 0111	0100 1100
Mask	1111 0000	0000 1111
Result after logical AND	1011 0000	0000 1100

To combine the bit patterns of two data bytes while preserving all information of interest, we can use a logical OR instruction. We continue the previous example:

First data byte	1011 0000	(upper 4 bits preserved)
Second data byte	0000 1100	(lower 4 bits preserved)
Result after logical OR	1011 1100	packed information

In this case the inappropriate information was masked out prior to ORing the two bytes together. The information in the first and second bytes was packed into only one byte by the OR instruction. We can unpack the information using similar techniques.

A method to determine if two bytes are equal uses the XOR instruction. For example, a stack-full condition must be checked before a data byte is PUSHed onto the stack. If we have assigned page 0F of memory to contain the stack (addresses 0FFF-0F00), the stack is full when the stack pointer contains 0EFF. This occurs because the stack pointer is decremented *after* each data byte is stored.

By XORing the most significant byte of the stack pointer with the value of the page assigned for the stack, a nonzero value will result if the stack is full.

Most significant byte, stack pointer	0E	0000 1110	0F	0000 1111
Mask	0F	0000 1111	0F	0000 1111
Result after logical XOR	01	0000 0001		0000 0000
		nonzero— stack full		zero—stack not full

Note that a nonzero value will also result if the stack is empty, but that different bits will be set after the XOR operation. Since the stack pointer is incremented before a data byte is POPed from the stack, the stack pointer will contain 1000 after the last data byte has been removed.

Stack pointer	10	0001 0000
Mask	0F	0000 1111
Result after logical XOR	1F	0001 1111

Combinations of these basic bit manipulations allow the programmer to set, reset, and test any bit(s) required. In addition to the logical instructions, the Z80 has bit set, reset, and test instructions, allowing the programmer direct access to any bit in memory or in the CPU registers without the need for masking.

Microcomputer arithmetic. A look at the instruction sets of our two model microprocessors shows only a small number of arithmetic instructions—ADD, ADC, SUB, SBC, and shift and rotate instructions. Although each instruction is limited, very sophisticated mathematics can be performed using combinations of these instructions together with the bit-manipulation instructions.

A simple addition of two 8-bit bytes can, at most, generate a 9-bit result. The extra bit from the addition is propagated into the carry flag. It is always set if the most significant bits of both numbers to be added are set.

```
                10110111                    10110111
              + 01000111                  + 10000000
 No carry     0 11111110       Carry      1 00110111
```

Furthermore, the value of the sum generated is dependent on the particular number representation used—sign-magnitude, 1's-complement, or 2's-complement (see Chapter 2). To ensure correct mathematical results, different algorithms are required for each of these number representations.

For example, consider the addition of $+5$ and $+2$ in sign-magnitude, 1's-complement, and 2's-complement number representations.

	Sign magnitude	*1's complement*	*2's complement*
$(+5)$	0101	0101	0101
$+ (+2)$	$+ \ 0010$	$+ \ 0010$	$+ \ 0010$
$+7$	0 0111	0 0111	0 0111
	carry	carry	carry

The sums for all number representations are correct. Notice that the results all fall within the range of possible numbers for our 4-bit example.

Consider the addition of $+4$ and -1, however:

	Sign magnitude	*1's complement*	*2's complement*
$(+4)$	0100	0100	0100
$+ (-1)$	$+ \ 1001$	$+ \ 1110$	$+ \ 1111$
$+3$	0 1101 (-5)	1 0010 $(+2)$	1 0011 $(+3)$
	carry	carry	carry

The sign-magnitude result is incorrect. In general, arithmetic problems occur with sign-magnitude numbers if a negative integer is added to a positive one or if integers with like signs are subtracted. Since $X + (- Y)$ is equivalent to $X - Y$, a special subtraction routine is needed. Problems exist because of the two possible zero representations (plus and minus zero).

The 1's-complement result is also incorrect. As in sign magnitude, a direct binary subtraction cannot be performed. We must first determine the signs of the integers and make the appropriate corrections before and after the addition:

		Subtraction		*Addition*	
$(+4)$	0100	minuend (m)		$(+4)$	0100
$- (+1)$	$- \ 0001$	subtrahend (s)		$+ (-1)$	1110
	1110	convert s to			
		1's-complement			
	$+ \ 0100$	add minuend			
1	0010	intermediate result		1	0010
carry	$+ \ \ \ 1$	post-add carry-out		carry $+$	1
	0011	answer			0011

An addition is performed as a simple binary addition and the carry bit is post-added to the intermediate result. To perform a subtraction, the subtrahend is first 1's-complemented, the complement added to the minuend, and the carry-out is again added to the intermediate result.

The carry bit can be ignored in 2's-complement arithmetic since it is included in all negative numbers (hence the synonym 1's complement $+$ 1). All 2's-complement additions generate the correct result if the number range is not exceeded. Most microcomputers include a SUB (subtract) instruction that takes the 2's complement of the subtrahend and then adds it to the minuend. If a carry bit is generated, it is ignored because the correction is included in the 2's-complementation step. The simplicity of 2's-complement arithmetic favors this number representation over the extra program steps required by 1's complement and the difficult problems encountered with sign-magnitude computations. Both the COSMAC and Z80 use 2's-complement arithmetic.

However, we must still deal with the problem of arithmetic overflow. Overflow occurs if the addition of two numbers with like signs results in a sum of different sign. For example, adding the 2's-complement numbers $+7$ and $+1$ generates an overflow condition.

$$
\begin{array}{rl}
(+7) & 0111 \\
+\ (+1) & +\ 0001 \\
\hline
+8 & 1000 \quad (-8) \quad \text{overflow}
\end{array}
$$

Notice that the overflow condition is manifest in the most significant bit of the result. Therefore, a simple test for overflow is to use our bit-manipulation techniques to look at the most significant bit. Overflow is detected in the Z80 by a software-testable overflow flag.

Multiple-precision arithmetic.   The easiest informational unit to manipulate in the microcomputer is the 8-bit byte. However, the range of numbers possible is often too small to accommodate the application. The carry bit serves the purpose of arithmetically linking together 8-bit units into chains of 16, 24, or more bits.

For example, in 2's-complement notation, 16 bits can uniquely represent numbers from 0 through 65,535 ($2^{16} - 1$). The range of positive and negative integers is similarly expanded, to $-32,768$ through $+32,767$. The carry/borrow bit generated as a result of an addition/subtraction of the least significant byte must be used in subsequent addition/subtraction of the more significant bytes.

	Addition		*Subtraction*	
	10001111			01000111
	$+$ 11001000			$-$ 10011000
carry				
1	01010111	01111000		10101111
$+$ 00111000		$-$ 00100001		
$+$ 01000011		$-$	1 borrow	
0 01111100	01010111	01010110		10101111

Add with carry (ADC) and subtract with carry (SBC) are instructions that aid in this process. The carry/borrow bit is automatically included in the addition/subtraction of the next byte. With these two instructions it is possible to link together any arbitrary number of bytes. Note, however, that the carry/borrow bit is *not* to be included in the addition/subtraction of the least significant byte.

Multiplication and division. When two 8-bit bytes are multiplied, a 16-bit result may be generated. Since the majority of microprocessors do not have multiply instructions, we must use double-precision addition to calculate the product.

Multiplication done by hand uses the "sum of partial products" method. The values to be multiplied are treated as absolute values, multiplied, and the sign of the product determined according to the rules of multiplication. For example, $(-212) \times (-125)$ is

$$
\begin{array}{rl}
(-212) & \text{Multiplicand} \\
\times\ (-125) & \text{Multiplier} \\
\hline
1060 \\
424 & \text{Partial products} \\
+\ \ 212 \\
\hline
+\ 26500 & \text{Product}
\end{array}
$$

Another method to do this multiplication is to repeatedly add -212 to itself 125 times and again correct the sign.

Let us use this successive-addition method to multiply $(-2) \times (-2)$ in the microcomputer. We simply add (-2) to itself:

	Sign magnitude	1's complement	2's complement
(-2)	1010	1101	1110
$\times\ (-2)$	$+\ 1010$	$+\ 1101$	$+\ 1110$
$+4$	0100 (4)	1010 (-5)	1100 (-4)
	1	1	1
	Carry Correct	Carry Incorrect	Carry Incorrect
	lost	lost	lost

Notice that in our 4-bit example only sign-magnitude numbers give the correct product. The sign bits have correctly canceled if the carry bit is ignored. The 2's-complement and 1's-complement products are both incorrect.

These results are easy to understand if we keep in mind that 1's- and 2's-complement numbers encode the sign in the representation itself. Thus multiplication cannot be done with simple repetitive additions. We must, instead, extract the sign information in advance and then convert the number to its absolute value. From this point multiplication in the microcomputer proceeds much as by hand.

Figure 4.61 shows one possible method for these conversions. The 2's-complement number is converted to its positive counterpart. The sign is saved and later is used to correct the product calculated.

The multiplication of large numbers by the successive addition method is inherently slow, however. A faster method is the shift-and-add technique. The microcomputer mimics our hand sum of partial products method. For example, if

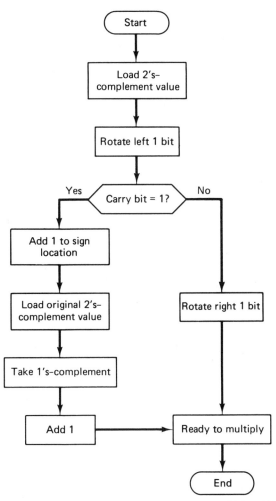

FIGURE 4.61 Absolute value routine for numbers to be multiplied. If MSB of 2's-complement value is set, the value is converted to absolute value (2's complement) and the sign information is added to sign location. The correct sign will be found in the LSB of this location when both numbers are converted. The correct sign of the product may also be found by an exclusive OR performed on the sign bits.

we wish to multiply 8×5 in binary, the process would appear as follows:

$$
\begin{array}{rr}
(8) & 1000 \\
\times\ (5) & \times\ 0101 \\
\hline
& 1000 \\
& 0000 \\
& 1000 \\
& +\ 0000 \\
\hline
(40) & 0\ 0101000
\end{array}
$$

Multiplicand
Multiplier

Partial products

Product

Careful programming allows us to skip the additions of zero values that do not affect the product. As in successive addition, the number representation directly affects the results. Figure 4.62 shows flowcharts for both successive addition and shift-and-add methods. Figure 4.63 shows that our multiplication algorithms will perform division if modified slightly. However, errors due to the finite nature of the division process may appear. Accuracy and rounding errors introduced are passed on to subsequent calculations.

Floating-point arithmetic.   Previously, we have dealt with microcomputer arithmetic on relatively small numbers. A small number may be defined as one that can be represented exactly and used in calculations without introducing significant errors. Integers can be represented exactly and, with the exception of division, used to calculate exact answers.

   If we require the microcomputer to do scientific calculations, often only approximate answers are possible. For example, 2 divided by 3 requires an infinite (nonterminating) series of sixes, $0.6666\ldots$. Depending on the calculation accuracy required, we round off the last digit. In scientific notation we could represent this number as 6.67×10^{-1}.

   Floating point-representation in microcomputers is directly analogous to the scientific notation used in calculators. We express floating-point numbers as powers of 2 rather than 10.

Scientific notation	Floating point
$\pm\ n.nn \times 10^{\pm\mathrm{exponent}}$	$\pm\ 0.nnn \times 2^{\pm\mathrm{exponent}}$

As in scientific notation, floating-point numbers have a sign associated with both the fraction and exponent. We might represent a floating-point number using two successive bytes. The first byte is an exponent giving a power of 2. The second byte is a binary fraction. The fraction and exponent are represented as sign-magnitude numbers; the MSB of each byte is the sign bit. By definition the binary point of the fraction is located just to the right of the sign bit. The most significant bit of the fraction holds a weight of 2^{-1}, the next most significant 2^{-2}, and so on.

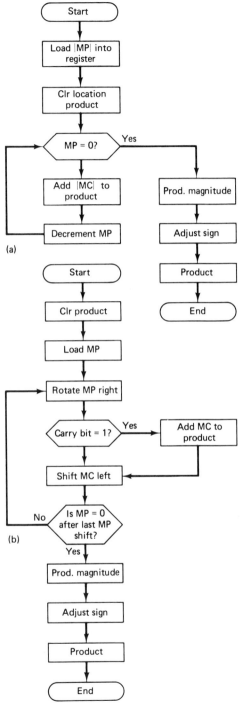

FIGURE 4.62 Multiplication by (a) successive addition and (b) shift-and-add techniques, where MC = multiplicand and MP = multiplier.

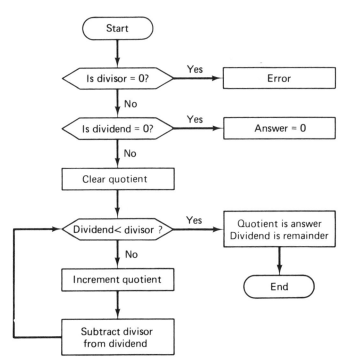

FIGURE 4.63 Method for division by successive subtraction.

By allowing negative exponents, we are able to represent small fractions. The inclusion of the exponent effectively floats the true binary point regardless of how many bits are preserved for the fraction. Therefore, floating-point numbers do not guarantee uniqueness. Since the exponent value floats the binary point, a number of representations for each number are possible.

To guarantee uniqueness, we normalize floating-point numbers. By convention, the fraction for nonzero numbers must be in the range $\frac{1}{2} \leq f < 1$. The normalized floating-point number thus has the most significant bit of the fraction set (= 1). The value for zero is an exception to this rule. In this case the fraction is allowed to be $+0$ (sign-magnitude numbers have a $+0$ and -0).

The algebraic rules for floating-point calculations are similar to those for scientific notation. That is, floating-point numbers cannot be added or subtracted until their exponents are equal. A simplified flowchart for addition of two floating-point numbers is shown in Fig. 4.64. Note that the fraction and the exponent must be manipulated together since each time we add (subtract) one to the exponent we are multiplying (dividing) the fraction by 2. The sum (difference) must be postnormalized and rounded, since the fraction may fall outside our defined range.

Multiplication and division require that we add (subtract) the exponents and multiply (divide) the fractions, respectively. The answer is again postnormalized

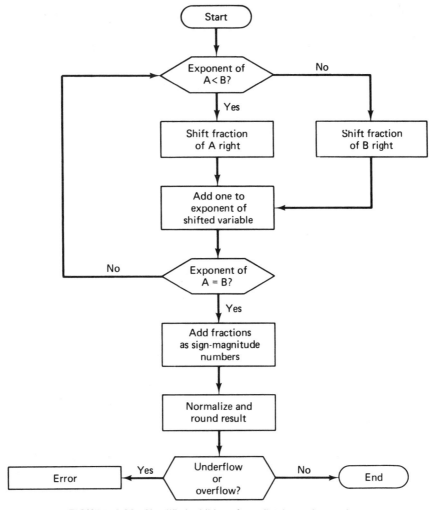

FIGURE 4.64 Simplified addition of two floating-point numbers.

and rounded. After each algebraic operation we must check the result for overflow and underflow.

A fraction length of 1 byte provides a precision of only two decimal digits. In order to obtain more precise numerical representation, we use more bytes to represent the fraction, as in multiple-precision integer arithmetic. A 2-byte fraction provides four decimal-digit representations.

BCD arithmetic. Arithmetic with BCD numbers presents the programmer with a few additional problems. Since each 4-bit group represents one BCD digit but the microcomputer does binary arithmetic on 8 bits, we must adjust the 4-bit codes generated.

For example, we wish to add two BCD numbers, 12 and 28. The binary addition yields an illegal code in the least significant digit.

```
   12        0001    0010
 + 28      + 0010    1000
 ----        ----    ----
   40        0011    1010    Result after addition
             (3)   (Illegal)
```

If we add 6 to the illegal code group and let the carry propagate from bit 3 to bit 4, the correct BCD codes result.

```
     0011    1010
  +          0110
     ----    ----
     0100    0000
     (4)     (0)    BCD
```

We might also wish to add 18 + 18 in BCD. This time a carry from bit 3 to bit 4 results as part of the binary addition.

```
                   Carry
                     1
   (18)        0001    1000
 + (18)      + 0001    1000
 -----         ----    ----
    36         0011    0000
               (3)     (0)    BCD
```

Both 4-bit groups are valid BCD numbers, but the result of the addition is still incorrect. We again need to correct or adjust the results by adding 6.

```
     0011    0000
  +          0110
     ----    ----
     0011    0110
     (3)     (6)    BCD
```

Thus BCD addition must be adjusted if one of two conditions result:

1. A carry-out of a particular BCD digit after addition.
2. Illegal code groups as a result of the addition.

The adjustment must start with the least-significant 4-bit digit, and all carries as a result of our adjustment must be allowed to propagate before adjusting the next digit.

Subtraction of BCD numbers needs similar adjustments, although in this case subtraction of 6 is necessary. For example, if we subtract 9 from 14, the borrow from bit 4 generates an illegal code.

$$
\begin{array}{rl}
(14) & 0001\ 0100 \\
-\ \ (9) & -\ 0000\ 1001 \\
\hline
5 & 0000\ 1011\quad\text{BCD} \\
& \qquad\quad\ (\text{Illegal})
\end{array}
$$

If 6 is then subtracted from the illegal code, the correct BCD result is generated.

$$
\begin{array}{r}
1011 \\
-\ 0110 \\
\hline
0101\ \ (5)\quad\text{BCD}
\end{array}
$$

Some microprocessors facilitate BCD arithmetic by inclusion of a decimal-adjust instruction (DAA). Whenever a binary addition between two bytes is done, two flags are affected—the normal carry flag and an auxiliary or half-carry flag. The half-carry flag is set if a carry from bit 3 to bit 4 has occurred. This flag is then used by the decimal-adjust instruction that follows to make the proper BCD code adjustments. In general, the decimal-adjust instruction works only for addition, because the proper adjustment is different for addition and subtraction. The Z80 includes a decimal-adjust instruction (DAA) that will adjust BCD after both addition and subtraction. A special flag called the subtract flag is set if a subtraction instruction is executed. The decimal-adjust instruction determines the state of this flag and adjusts the code appropriately. The COSMAC does not have a DAA instruction.

Multibyte BCD arithmetic is done the same as binary arithmetic. The only change in the algorithms is the decimal adjustment after each addition or subtraction.

Binary-to-BCD conversion. As human beings we may require the microcomputer to communicate with us in easily understandable form. However, from a software design point of view, binary is the easiest type of information for a microcomputer to manipulate. If our system requires infrequent (in terms of computer time) communication with the human user, it may be simpler to convert the appropriate binary information to BCD just prior to output rather than use BCD numbers throughout the entire program. A subroutine call will convert the numbers only when needed. Throughout the discussion of conversion techniques, we shall assume that only nonnegative numbers are to be converted and that any problems with overflow have been eliminated elsewhere in the design.

The most direct method of binary-to-BCD conversion is the divide-by-10 method. Basically the binary number is divided by 10 (expressed in binary) to yield an integer quotient and remainder. The remainder is directly usable as the least significant BCD digit. The quotient is divided by 10 again and the remainder used as the next more significant digit. This sequence of events proceeds until the quotient after the last division cannot be divided by 10 to yield an integer quotient. The last quotient obtained is thus the most-significant BCD digit.

For example, we wish to convert the binary equivalent of 177_{10}. The conversion to BCD digits would look like this.

$$\textit{BCD digit}$$

$$
\begin{array}{cll}
\quad 17 & & \\
10)\overline{177} & \text{Remainder} & 7\text{—least significant} \\
\quad 1 & & \\
10)\overline{17} & \text{Remainder} & 7 \\
\quad 0 & & \\
10)\overline{\,1\,} & \text{Remainder} & 1\text{—most significant}
\end{array}
$$

We have stripped off the BCD digits from least to most significant. For this example, 18 subtractions are required—17 for the first step and one for the second. However, since the division carried out is done by repeated subtraction of 10, the conversion process is slow for large numbers. The binary equivalent of $32,000_{10}$ would require 3200 subtractions for the least-significant BCD digit alone!

A faster method of conversion is to first determine the largest power of 10 that our binary number can be divided by an integer number of times. This is relatively easy because we know that the maximum number of BCD digits after conversion of an 8-bit number is three. For a single byte number the digit positions carry weights of 10^2, 10^1, and 10^0 from most significant to least significant, respectively. In general, the correct power of 10 to start with can be found by the formula $3N - 1$, where N is the number of bytes in the binary number we wish to convert.

Using the same example, the process would look as follows:

$$
\begin{array}{rll}
& \quad\; 1 & \text{Most-significant BCD digit} \\
10^2 = & 100)\overline{177} & \\
& \quad\; 7 & \\
10^1 = & 10)\overline{77} & \\
& \quad\; 7 & \text{Least-significant BCD digit} \\
10^0 = & 1)\overline{\,7\,} &
\end{array}
$$

Notice that unlike the first method, the BCD digits are stripped off from most significant to least significant and are found in the quotient rather than in the remainder. For this example, the method needs only 15 subtractions in the conversion—1 for the first step, 7 for the second, and 7 for the third. It is easy to improve the algorithm by merely using the remainder after division by 10 as the least-significant BCD digit rather than dividing by 10^0, thus decreasing the number of subtractions to 8 compared to 18 for the first method. Figure 4.65 shows the flowchart for this second conversion method.

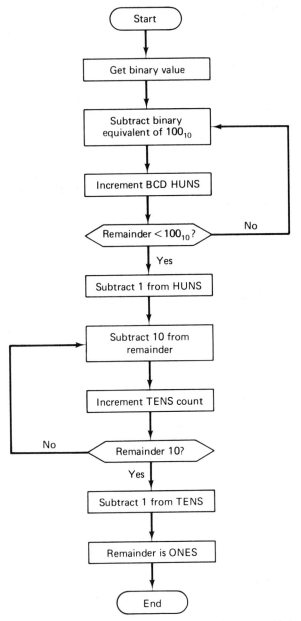

FIGURE 4.65 Method for binary-to-BCD conversion. A more sophisticated program would allow multibyte conversion and leading-zero suppression.

Data structures—stacks, tables, and arrays

The way in which data are input or output from the microcomputer often suggests one data structure that is particularly suited to the task. In this section we shall consider three of the most important data structures and suggest possible uses for each type.

Stacks, register management, and subroutines. A very widely used data structure is the stack. Earlier we saw how the stack pointer is used to move data to and from the last-in, first-out (LIFO) stack. As a temporary storage area the LIFO stack may be used to store intermediate calculation values for example.

The real power of the LIFO stack is in its usefulness in register management and parameter passing to subroutines. Figure 4.66 shows some general considerations and possible sources of error when parameters must be passed to subroutines. In this case the CPU registers are used to pass the required parameters to the subroutine. Unexpected results occur if the subroutine modifies registers containing information to be used later. For example, housekeeping activities within a sub-

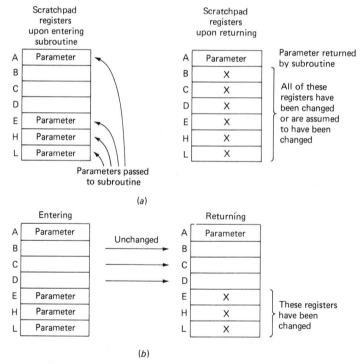

FIGURE 4.66 Subroutine register management using CPU registers for parameter passing. (a) Safe assumption of register usage by a subroutine. (b) Potential source of future trouble. (From Peatman, J. B. 1977. Microcomputer-based design. New York: McGraw-Hill. Used with permission.)

routine long since forgotten may use the same CPU registers as the main program. After the return from the subroutine, the main program will find altered values in these registers.

A safer approach is to store all register contents on the stack before subroutine execution. Figure 4.67(a) shows how the LIFO stack pointer is incremented and decremented to store (PUSH) and retrieve (POP) a parameter. In this way all values can be returned to their proper location after completion of the subroutine. Since we wish to return to the instruction following the subroutine call, the program counter must be saved in this manner as well. At least in the initial design,

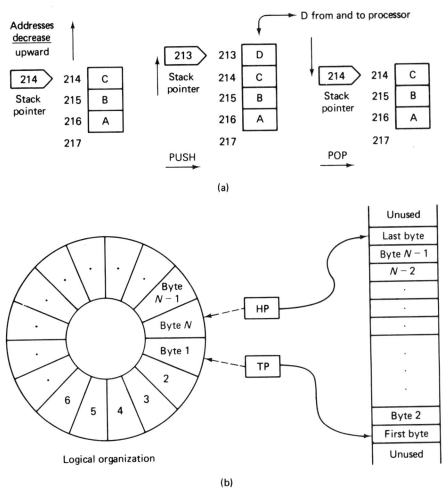

(a)

(b)

FIGURE 4.67 Two types of stack structures. (a) Simple pushdown LIFO stack and use of the stack pointer. (b) Simple FIFO stack in stack-full condition. The tail pointer TP points to first data byte entered on stack. The head pointer HP points to last data byte entered.

this approach increases the efficiency in the development process itself. Since we assume nothing about the CPU registers, the main program and the subroutine can be written independently of each other. The way in which the subroutine is interfaced to the main program takes on a well-defined character. Later in the design we can review the particular workings of each subroutine and eliminate unnecessary instructions.

Interrupt service may also require the use of a LIFO stack. Since interrupts are considered random events, a wise precaution is to save all CPU register contents on the stack. These tasks must be included in the interrupt service routine itself. Just prior to the return from interrupt, the register contents must be restored. Again, the program counter must also be saved.

Figure 4.67(b) shows another type of stack—the first-in, first out (FIFO) stack and illustrates the difference between it and a LIFO. Here we treat the stack as if it were a circular buffer. In this case the last data byte is stored at the bottom rather than at the top of the stack. The first data byte is removed at the top of the stack. To implement the FIFO stack, two pointers are therefore needed—one for the head (top) and one for the bottom (tail) of the stack. Stack-full and stack-empty conditions must be flagged. This is necessary to ensure that the head pointer does not slip past the tail pointer, thus destroying the symmetry of the buffer. Since the real memory used is linear, the link between the high address and low address of the stack must be carefully defined.

Although somewhat more difficult to implement, the FIFO stack can be used to advantage for memory loops or buffering speed differences between the high-speed microcomputer and slower I/O devices. For example, we might wish to collect and update data in a continuous manner. An A/D converter will output a data byte, say 100 times/s. To collect and store the data for a period of 10 s, we need 1000 bytes of memory (assuming that the A/D converter output is 8 bits). Initially, the stack would contain no data. The head and tail pointers point to the first memory location assigned for the stack. Since both pointers contain the same value, a stack-empty condition exists. The first data byte is stored via the head pointer. The head pointer is incremented and a stack-full condition is checked. After 1000 bytes of data are stored in this manner, the stack-full condition is flagged. Now both head and tail pointers are incremented, with each new data byte stored on the stack. Note also that each new data byte is stored in the location of the oldest (or initially the first) data byte.

If we stop the data collection and want to output the data, the tail pointer now points to the oldest data byte on the stack and thus is output first. The tail pointer is incremented and a stack-empty condition is checked. After the 1000 data bytes are outputted, the tail pointer again points to the same location as the head pointer and the stack-empty condition is flagged.

Tables. Another useful data structure is the look-up table. Here data are formatted by the programmer for ease of access to any particular data byte in the table. The address of each data byte is related in a well-defined way to the contents of that address. A commercially available example is the sine/cosine look-up table. The value of sin θ is found by calculating the address via the formula

$$(\theta/90°)128 = \text{address}$$

The contents of that address are retrieved and can be directly used as the calculated sin θ. The routine used to calculate the correct address is called a table-driver routine.

Figure 4.68 shows another possible table-driver routine using indexed addressing. The base address of the table is set up prior to table access. Since we know the input keycodes used (ASCII, for example), we can use this knowledge to format the table. The input keycode is used as an offset and is added to the base address to generate the effective table address.

Arrays. Tables are most often implemented in ROM because of their predetermined data content. We can, however, implement a similar structure for data generated and manipulated by the program itself. A simple array might consist of

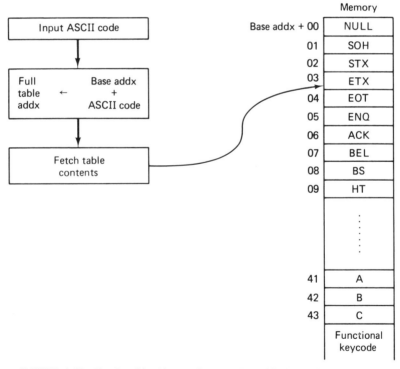

FIGURE 4.68 Simple table-driver and conversion table for ASCII to functional keycode as might appear in a key-parse routine. A complete table can be developed from the ASCII/hex conversion chart in Appendix 2.

two 4-byte numbers we wish to add. If we store the least-significant byte at address 0300, the least-significant byte of the second number could be stored at address 0304 (see Fig. 4.69). A simple method to access both data bytes would be to set up a memory pointer to the least-significant byte of each number and merely increment each pointer as the addition is done.

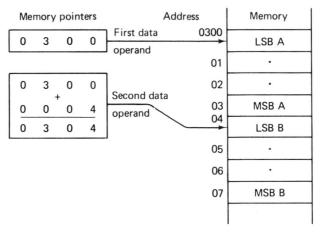

FIGURE 4.69 Method to access two particular data bytes in an array. Two four-byte numbers are accessed—data bytes A by indirect addressing, data bytes B by indexed addressing.

Keyboard parsing—design example

With the design basics presented above, we are now prepared to integrate them into an overall design for user control over microcomputer activities. Basically a multilevel decision-making technique, keyboard parsing allows us to program the microcomputer to accept and intelligently respond to user commands. A great part of this discussion centers on how the machine recognizes a particular character string. Throughout we shall assume that the designer has defined and written each routine needed to execute the user commands.

Suppose that we wish our microcomputer to recognize and execute two commands, formatted as follows for a simple monitor program:

L AAAA DDDD · · · ⟨CR⟩;   Load memory starting at address
                             AAAA with data bytes DD and continue
                             until a carriage return is hit
D AAAA BBBB ⟨CR⟩;   Display memory starting at address
                             AAAA for BBBB bytes; execute command
                             after a carriage return is hit

A full ASCII keyboard has been interfaced to the microcomputer. Routines have been written that automatically input the ASCII character when a key is hit.

From a human factors standpoint we also require that the microcomputer:

1. Accept all address and data information as ASCII coded hex characters 0 through 9 and A through F and convert it to binary.
2. Prompt the user when ready for a command.
3. Prompt the user that a command string error has been made.
4. Ignore space bars unless used to delineate address and data.

If we look carefully at our proposed command strings, we can differentiate six types of keys. Each type is assigned a unique code number called a functional code.

ASCII character	*Type*	*Functional code (FC)*
⟨CR⟩	Terminator	0
A, B, C, E, F, 0–9	Data	1
L	Command	2
D	Command or data	3
Space bar	Delineator	4
All others	Error	5

When a key is hit, a general-purpose input routine will store a copy of the original ASCII code and then use the ASCII code as an index to a conversion table for the functional code number (see Fig. 4.68). Thus every key entered will be converted to its correct functional code.

It is also apparent that the particular sequence in which keys are hit indicates what type of key is to follow. This information is coded in the state or level code defined in Fig. 4.70. By combining the state code with the functional keycode we have a simple means to generate a particular address within another table—the key-parse table. For example, if we are in state 0 and an ASCII L is input, the combination (after input code conversion) is

State	*Functional code*
0	2

By properly coding the contents of the key-parse table we have a method to determine if the proper key type was hit at the correct position in our command string. Overall, with five state codes and six keycodes, we have 5×6, or 30 possible combinations.

However, we still lack the information that allows us to call the proper action routine at the correct place in the key sequence. Seven particular types of action are needed in our example. Each is assigned an action code number, as shown in Fig. 4.70. By combining action codes and state codes in the key-parse table, we can direct the activities of the microcomputer in any manner we choose. The informa-

State code (SC)

0	Initial state — ready for command
1	Input is address information for input to memory
2	Input is address information for output from memory
3	Input is data to store in memory
4	Input indicates number of bytes of memory to output

Action code (AC)

0	Prompt user ready for command (READY)
1	Prompt user entry error (ERROR)
2	Ignore input character (IGNORE)
3	Input used as I/O memory pointer (POINTER)
4	Input used as data — store via memory pointer (INDATA)
5	Input used as number of memory bytes to output (NUMBYTES)
6	Data output routine (OUTPUT)

FIGURE 4.70   State and action codes used in the keyboard parse example.

tion codes in the table are retrieved and each code separated. The action code points to the correct routine to execute. The state code replaces the present state code and becomes the new state code. This allows us to jump from state to state as the key sequence is entered.

The contents of the key-parse table are determined by working through each combination of present state code and functional key code. For example, in state 0 we want an "L" or a "D" to be recognized as valid but the input character itself to be ignored. Hence the correct action code is 2. Since our predetermined command sequence indicates that memory pointer information follows, we need a state change also. For an "L" we want the state to change to 1. Hence the full table entry is 21. For a "D" we want the machine to change to state 2. Here the correct table entry is 22.

In state 0 all other key entries are to be invalid. Since we want the key entry error to be signaled to the user, the proper action code is 1. Because the new state code in the key-parse table automatically replaces the present state code, a 0 must be entered as the new state. This is required to ensure that the user can restart a valid command sequence after any key-entry error. Column 0 of the completed key-parse table in Fig. 4.71 is now filled in. Each column in the table is filled in similarly.

With the heart of the design problem solved, we can now proceed to interface the particular routines that execute the required actions. The action-code table is filled in with the address of the routine appropriate to that code. This allows us to enter the action routines from our general-purpose input and key-parse routine. Since we require that the action routine terminate by returning to the input and key-parse routine, an unconditional branch is added at the end of the action routine in most cases. Figure 4.72 shows the interfaced routines for our design example in general form.

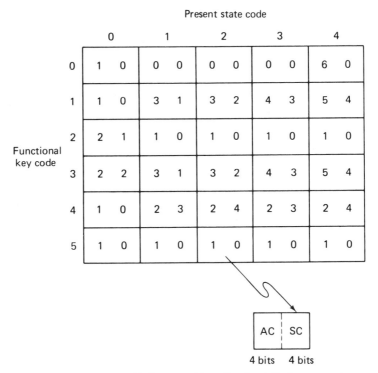

FIGURE 4.71 Key-parse table for recognition of load and display memory instructions. AC, action code; SC, state code. Each table location contains the action code and the new state code for each key entry.

Software development

We may define software development as that process whereby the microcomputer system software objectives are developed into algorithms, implemented by the programmer, and finally translated into the binary language of the microcomputer. Each step of the development process is iterated until the final design objectives are met. In this section we shall explore and evaluate some of the methods and tools used to aid the development process.

Benchmarking. Writing sample programs or benchmarking can yield valuable information concerning suitability and ease of meeting design objectives for a particular microprocessor. We can judge instruction flexibility, program bottlenecks, memory efficiency, and speed. Theoretically, we should evaluate all available microprocessors objectively in this manner before making a choice. Practically, we are often limited in our choices by overriding constraints such as power consumption or speed. Benchmarking is characteristically also application-oriented and thus may favor one microprocessor over another as a result of the application. An objectionable disadvantage to benchmarking is the necessity to be familiar with the detailed

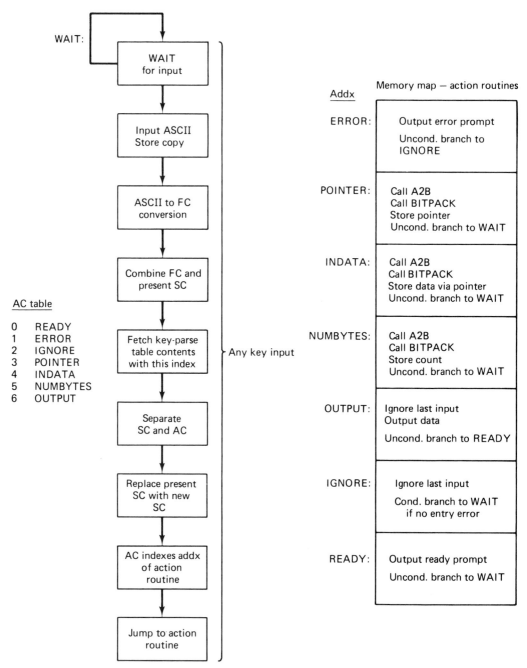

FIGURE 4.72 Interfacing concepts for key-parse design example. The flowchart shown is the general-purpose input and parse routine. The AC table is accessed by this routine to find the proper action routine address. The memory map of the actual action routines shows how they are addressed. Notice that each action routine terminates in unconditional branches which return to the key-input routine (A2B–ASCII-to-binary conversion).

architectures and instruction sets of many microprocessors. In addition, the efficiency and expertise of the software engineer may limit the usefulness of instruction set evaluations by this method.

Hand coding. As programmers we are painfully aware of the fact that programs that look good on paper often fail to run properly in the computer. As human beings we do not naturally speak the binary language of digital computers. Assembly-language mnemonics aid in our translation of algorithms to the particular bit patterns the machine recognizes as instructions.

One method of performing this translation is hand coding. Although tedious and somewhat error-prone, hand coding may be used to advantage if the program is relatively small or a "translator" program is unavailable. Hand coding also facilitates our understanding of hardware–software interactions as well as the subtle nuances of the machine and its instructions.

However, a hand-coded program is extremely difficult to debug. Computer resources are used to aid in debugging. The ease with which programs may be constructed, modified, and coded increases the speed and efficiency of the development of microcomputer software. We shall address several programs supplied as part of a larger computer operating system that are designed for this purpose.

Editors. The editor is a program designed to create and modify symbolic source programs prior to assembly or compiling. User commands allow characters, lines, or groups of lines to be added, deleted, or changed. In this way the editor aids the "cut-and-paste" process of software development. The final product is a source file that can be used by assemblers and compilers.

Assemblers. A program itself, the assembler accepts the mnemonics of an assembly-language source file as data input and generates the linear sequence of machine code (object file) understandable by the microcomputer as instructions or data. Although similar in concept to hand coding, the speed and low error rate of a computer are used to increase the communication efficiency of the programmer and microcomputer. Figure 4.73 shows a flowchart for a typical two-pass assembler.

As part of its translation duties, the assembler must be able to recognize the assembly language that we feed into it. In general, a particular assembler will recognize only one assembly language as valid input. As with any other language, word definitions and semantic rules play an integral role. If we violate those definitions and rules, the assembler will inform us and may point out the area of difficulty. The availability, quantity, and quality of these diagnostics aid considerably in the development of programs for the target microcomputer.

Compilers. Compilers also accept the symbolic source file created via the editor, but in this case the source file is written in a high-level language such as FORTRAN. Algorithm testing and development is facilitated by high-level languages

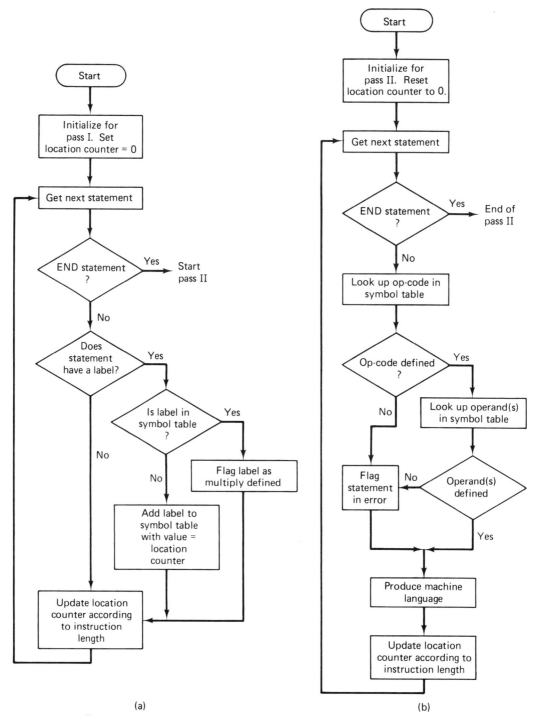

FIGURE 4.73 Simplified two-pass assembler. Notice that the assembler performs the same activities as hand coding but in a slightly different way. (a) Pass I. (b) Pass II. (From Eckhouse, R. H. 1975. Minicomputer systems: organization and programming. Reprinted by permission of Prentice-Hall, Inc.)

because knowledge of the specific machine instructions to perform the task is not needed.

However, an error-free program after assembly or compiling does not ensure that the program will perform as designed. Subtle application or logical errors in the program will not be recognized by the assembler or compiler and often show up unexpectedly later in system development or operation.

Simulators and emulators.   The inherent difficulty of developing software on one machine and running it on another spurred the development of more sophisticated tools for the software engineer. Like an assembler, a simulator is a computer program to aid software development but, in this case, by simulating the software activities of the target microcomputer. Additional diagnostic information is made available to the programmer by halting the simulation under predetermined conditions (breakpoints) such as a simulated memory access or a calculated value. The contents of the microcomputer registers and memory may be reviewed by the programmer at that point in the simulated program. Since the actual target microcomputer is not needed, simulation allows concurrent development of software and hardware independently.

Although this development independence allows great flexibility, it limits the degree to which the software may be developed. Software developed on a simulator depends to a great extent on how accurately the simulator mimics the actual microcomputer. Hence the software will doubtless need further modification when implemented in the real system. Real-time, interrupt, and I/O routines are characteristically difficult to simulate, owing to their intimate hardware interactions.

Specially dedicated microcomputers called emulators ease this problem somewhat as well as providing a degree of hardware–software codevelopment not possible with simulators alone. Software is developed on a microcomputer that often, although not always, uses the same microprocessor as the system under development. Thus the programmer develops a better knowledge of how the target microcomputer is affected by various conditions established through software.

The major advantage of emulators, however, is their ability to perform exactly as the microprocessor in the prototype circuit. A special plug is provided to fit into the prototype board in place of the actual microprocessor chip. The emulator generates all the signals the chip itself does, including control, address, and data. Since the emulator runs at a higher speed than does the microprocessor system under development, real-time, interrupt, and I/O functions are easily and accurately tested in the prototype. Special hardware diagnostic routines may also be available to automatically test the prototype hardware for faults.

We must pay a high price for these advantages, however. Because of their highly dedicated hardware, emulators are expensive. A typical emulator that can emulate several microprocessors may cost $15,000 to $30,000. These disadvantages must be weighed against the predicted product-market and development-time considerations.

4.6 MODEL MICROPROCESSORS*

Because so many microprocessors are available commercially, it is impossible to discuss them all here. We chose the RCA COSMAC and Zilog Z80 because their versatility allows them to meet almost any application needs. For more detailed specification and application literature, refer to information available from the device manufacturers. See Electronic Design (1978) for an extensive summary of microprocessors.

RCA COSMAC

Electrical characteristics. The RCA CDP1802 (COSMAC) is an 8-bit microprocessor which is constructed using silicon-gate complementary symmetry metaloxide-semiconductor logic (COSMOS; often further abbreviated as CMOS). CMOS has the characteristic that, unlike any other logic family, very little power-supply current is drawn in the quiescent state (see RCA, 1978). Significant power is dissipated only when actually switching and is a direct result of parasitic capacitances charging and discharging. Even when operating at its full speed, the COSMAC dissipates only about 40 mW, making it ideal for battery-powered applications. When requirements dictate a lower power drain, the processor can be slowed down or the supply voltages lowered. During periods of inactivity the processor can be "put to sleep" by stopping its clock. Current drain is then negligible and the processor, being dc-stable, retains its state as long as power is applied.

CMOS also makes the COSMAC highly noise-immune. In other words, a signal at any input pin can vary from either V_{CC} (logic 1) or V_{SS} (ground—logic 0) by up to (typically) 45% without losing its logic value.

The COSMAC is available in two versions. The CDP1802 operates from any power-supply voltage within the range 3 to 12 V, and the CDP1802C from 4 to 6 V. The maximum speed of the COSMAC is primarily a function of the processor's supply voltage V_{DD}, with a minimum cycle time for the CDP1802 version of 2.5 μs at 10 V and 5 μs at 5 V. The COSMAC's maximum speed is also in part a function of temperature over its wide operating range of -55 to $+125°C$. The speed must be derated by 0.35%/°C above 25°C.

Two independent supplies can be used if desired, one to the internal processing circuitry (V_{DD}) and one to the processor's interface circuitry (V_{CC}). This allows the processor to be run at full speed with $V_{DD} = 10$ V while interfacing to TTL logic circuits, which operate at $V_{CC} = 5$ V. V_{CC} must always be less than or equal to V_{DD} (including during power-up and power-down) to prevent damage to the processor. Also as with any MOS device, unused inputs must be connected to either V_{CC} or V_{SS} (whichever is appropriate), and no logic input voltages should ever be greater than V_{CC} or less than V_{SS}.

The COSMAC has an internal oscillator which generates the necessary clock

---

*Section 4.6 written by Alan V. Sahakian.

from an external quartz crystal. Optionally, an external clock signal can be applied and the internal oscillator ignored.

Architecture.   Figure 4.74 shows that the COSMAC is organized around an array of sixteen 16-bit scratchpad registers, R(0) through R(F). The contents of each of these R registers is divisible into two 8-bit bytes and can be directed to any of three destinations. The first destination is the set of eight memory address lines, where a 16-bit R register's contents are multiplexed, 8-bits at a time, and made available externally. The second destination can be the 8-bit D register (the accumulator), which holds data for ALU (arithmetic and logic unit) operations. The third destination can be the register itself, through the increment/decrement circuit, which allows the contents of any 16-bit R register to be increased or decreased by one.

Any of these 16-bit R registers can be designated (by the 4-bit P register) as the program counter. Instructions to be fetched from memory are addressed by the

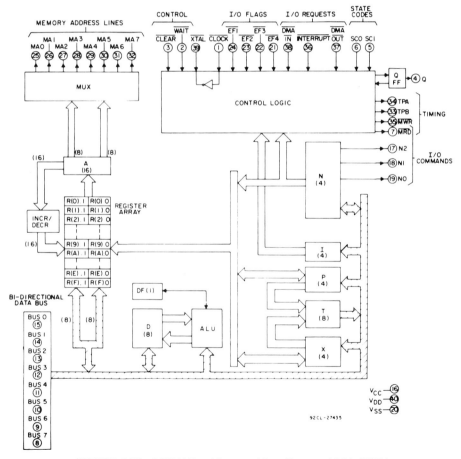

FIGURE 4.74   COSMAC architecture. (Compliments of RCA, 1979.)

processor by placing the program counter's contents on the memory-address bus as above, after which the program counter is incremented. To call a subroutine, the P register is simply changed so that it designates a new 16-bit R register as the program counter. In this way the subroutine address is specified by the initial contents of the new program counter. To return from the subroutine, the contents of the P register are restored to their original value, which redesignates the original program counter. Unfortunately, the COSMAC has no single-word subroutine call instruction, making the foregoing operation a common programming task. Whenever an interrupt occurs, R(1) automatically becomes the program counter, which allows the location of interrupt service routines to be at any address in memory specified by the initial contents of R(1).

Aside from the 4-bit P register, the 4-bit X and N registers can also select any of the 16-bit R registers for other operations. In certain ALU and I/O operations the X register can designate one of these R registers as a memory pointer for data exchanges with memory. The N register can designate which of the 16-bit R registers participates in such operations as load and store. To do this, the N register is always directly loaded with the least significant 4 bits of a fetched instruction. During I/O operations the N register specifies one of the seven possible I/O ports (with its least-significant 3 bits). Additionally, the N register must also help specify other instructions and act as a transfer agent when loading the X or P registers. The 4-bit I register (instruction register) is always loaded with the most-significant 4 bits of a fetched instruction. These bits specify (to the control logic) the type of operation to be performed.

The Q flip-flop is settable, resettable, and testable by the processor. A separate pin on the package is connected directly to the output of this flip-flop, allowing simple single-bit output. Similarly, $\overline{EF1}$ through $\overline{EF4}$ are processor-testable input flags which allow simple input. Together, the Q pin and an $\overline{EF}$ pin can serve (with appropriate software) as a serial interface (Section 4.4).

Direct memory access (DMA) is easily accomplished with the COSMAC. When the processor receives a DMA request on either its $\overline{DMA\ IN}$ or $\overline{DMA\ OUT}$ lines, it finishes its current instruction and places the contents of R(0) on the address bus. External devices can then write into memory (if a $\overline{DMA\ IN}$ was requested) or read out of memory (if a $\overline{DMA\ OUT}$ was requested) at the location pointed to by R(0). R(0) is then automatically incremented and the processor continues with whatever it was doing before the DMA request.

Timing. Figure 4.75(a) shows the timing for the COSMAC. All but three instructions take two eight-clock-pulse machine cycles to execute. During the first machine cycle, the processor fetches an instruction, and during the second (and third if necessary) executes it.

TPA and TPB are two timing pulses generated by the COSMAC every machine cycle. The falling edge of TPA is used to strobe the high-order byte of the 16-bit address on the eight address lines into an external latch. TPB's falling edge marks the start of a new machine cycle.

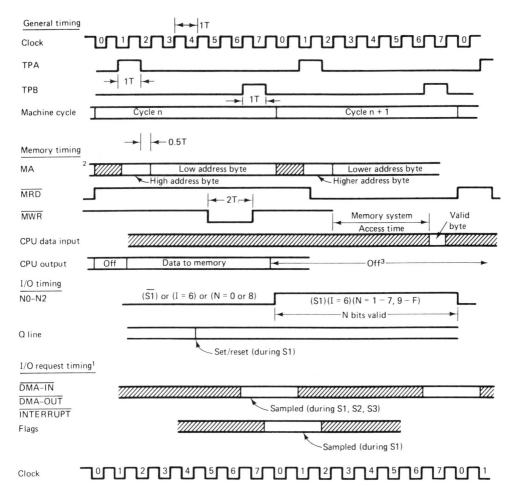

Notes:

[1] User-generated signals
[2] Shading indicates "dont care" internal delay
[3] "Off" indicates high-impedance state

(a)

CLEAR	WAIT	MODE
L	L	Load
L	H	Reset
H	L	Pause
H	H	Run

(b)

State type	State code lines	
	SC1	SC0
S0 (Fetch)	L	L
S1 (Execute)	L	H
S2 (DMA)	H	L
S3 (Interrupt)	H	H

(c)

FIGURE 4.75 COSMAC timing and control. (a) Timing diagram. (b) Mode control inputs and their resulting modes. (c) State types and their corresponding state code outputs. (Compliments of RCA, 1979.)

Control lines. Figure 4.75(b) shows that the $\overline{\text{CLEAR}}$ and $\overline{\text{WAIT}}$ lines to the COSMAC allow control of its mode. When both $\overline{\text{CLEAR}}$ and $\overline{\text{WAIT}}$ are low, the COSMAC enters the load mode. In this mode, the CPU idles, and an input device can load data into memory using the $\overline{\text{DMA IN}}$ line.

When only $\overline{\text{CLEAR}}$ is low, the CPU is reset. A reset forces registers I, N, and Q to zero, and enables interrupts. During the first machine cycle after a reset, the CPU initializes by zeroing registers X, P, and R(0). This allows execution to begin, with R(0) as the program counter, at location 0. The CPU can be automatically reset on "power-up" by connecting $\overline{\text{CLEAR}}$ through a capacitor to V_{ss} and a resistor to V_{cc}. In this way, $\overline{\text{CLEAR}}$ is held low momentarily after power is applied.

The pause mode occurs when the $\overline{\text{WAIT}}$ line only is low. When paused, the CPU suspends all operations but holds its state. This is useful for slowing the CPU down to interface to slow memory or I/O devices. Having both $\overline{\text{CLEAR}}$ and $\overline{\text{WAIT}}$ high allows the processor to run normally.

SC0 and SC1 are the state-code lines from the CPU. Figure 4.75(c) shows how they indicate the type of machine cycle that the CPU is presently executing.

$\overline{\text{MWR}}$ is the write pulse from the CPU to memory. $\overline{\text{MRD}}$, if low, indicates that the CPU is requesting a read from memory. Additionally, during an I/O operation, $\overline{\text{MRD}}$ indicates the direction of data flow (low for output and high for input).

N0, N1, and N2 are lines used to select I/O devices. They remain low except during I/O operations, when they carry the value of the three least-significant bits of the N register.

Instruction set. The highlights of the COSMAC instruction set are covered here. A complete listing of the instructions and their operations is included in Appendix 4.

Data can be transferred between the 8-bit D register (accumulator) and memory using the load and store instructions. Register operations (called get and put) exchange data between the accumulator and the high or low byte of a 16-bit R register.

The COSMAC also has instructions to perform simple logic and arithmetic on 8-bit data. Included are shift, shift with carry, AND, OR, exclusive OR, addition, and subtraction. In these instructions, the accumulator is always one of the operands. The other operand can either follow the instruction itself in memory (immediate mode) or be pointed to by the register specified by the 4-bit X register (memory mode). This register is more simply called R(X).

Two types of jump instructions are included in the COSMAC's repertoire. The first type, the branch, has two variations, long and short. In the long branch, both bytes of the program counter are replaced, allowing a jump to any location in memory. The short branch replaces only the least-significant byte of the program counter, limiting the jump to the bounds of the current 256-byte page of memory. The second type of jump instruction, the skip, advances the program counter by 1 (short) or 2 (long). Both types of jump can be performed conditionally, based on the value of the accumulator, the carry flag, and certain other registers and flags.

Input and output instructions transfer data either from the memory to an output device, or from an input device to the memory and (simultaneously) the accumulator. In both cases, the memory location is pointed to by R(X).

Finally, there are control instructions, to halt (IDLE) the CPU, do nothing (NOP), set and reset the Q flip-flop, exchange data between 4-bit registers, push data onto a memory stack, enable and disable interrupts, and other operations.

Simple system.   Figure 4.76 shows a simple system based on the COSMAC (CDP 1802). Only five integrated circuits are needed to realize this system. Included are 512 bytes of ROM, 32 bytes of RAM, and 8-bit parallel input and output ports. Note that the high-order memory address from the CPU is strobed (by TPA) into a latch contained within the ROM package. The ROM then enables the RAM, when appropriate, thus simplifying the hardware. The I/O ports are each selected by a different N line, also simplifying the hardware.

Zilog Z80

Figure 4.77 shows the Zilog Z80, which is the most powerful 8-bit microprocessor commonly available. Capable of performing 158 instructions, it is well suited to complex control and processing applications.

Electrical characteristics.   The Z80 is an N-channel MOS (NMOS) microprocessor which operates from a single 5-V power supply. All inputs and outputs are TTL-compatible [except the clock input, which requires an external 330-Ω resistor to V_{cc} (+5 V) if driven by common TTL].

The two versions of the Z80, the Z80 and Z80A, are capable, respectively, of operating at a minimum 400-ns and 250-ns clock periods, with maximum power consumptions of 750 mW and 1 W. Like the COSMAC, the Z80 is dc-stable and has no maximum clock period.

Architecture.   Figure 4.77(c) shows that the Z80 has eighteen 8-bit registers, and four 16-bit registers. Of the eighteen 8-bit registers, twelve are general-purpose which are also usable as six 16-bit register pairs. The main and alternate register sets are exchangable, with only one set being in active use at a time. The program can select which set to work with at any time by simply executing an exchange command. This is ideal for interrupt servicing, where it is necessary to maintain an unmodified copy of the preinterrupt registers and where time is important.

The stack pointer register allows a last-in-first-out (LIFO) stack to be located anywhere in memory. Data can be pushed onto or popped off this stack from and to certain CPU registers. This stack allows subroutine nesting to virtually any level, as well as multilevel interrupts and general data storage and retrieval.

Two index registers are provided which can be used to reference tables in memory. These registers each hold a 16-bit base which points to a given address, thus locating the table. An 8-bit displacement from this base is specified by instructions that reference the table. In this way, tables of up to 256 bytes can be located anywhere in memory and can be easily referenced.

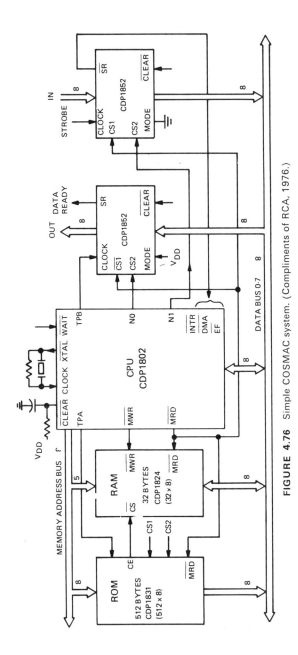

FIGURE 4.76 Simple COSMAC system. (Compliments of RCA, 1976.)

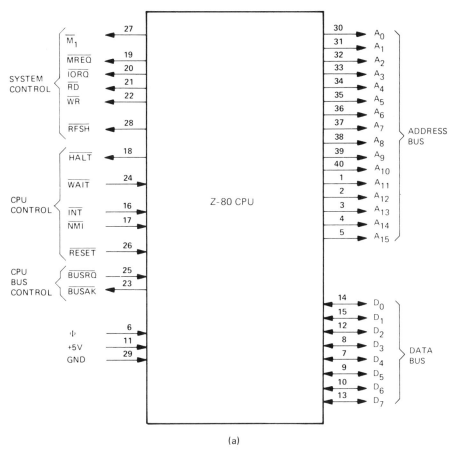

(a)

FIGURE 4.77 Z80 microprocessor. (a) Pin-out. (b) Architecture. (c) Internal register configuration. (Compliments of Zilog, Inc., 1977.)

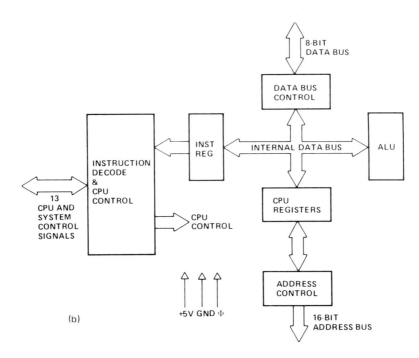

(b)

Z-80 CPU BLOCK DIAGRAM

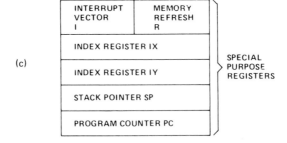

	MAIN REG SET		ALTERNATE REG SET		
	ACCUMULATOR A	FLAGS F	ACCUMULATOR A'	FLAGS F'	GENERAL PURPOSE REGISTERS
	B	C	B'	C'	
	D	E	D'	E'	
	H	L	H'	L'	

(c)

INTERRUPT VECTOR I	MEMORY REFRESH R	SPECIAL PURPOSE REGISTERS
INDEX REGISTER IX		
INDEX REGISTER IY		
STACK POINTER SP		
PROGRAM COUNTER PC		

Z-80 CPU REGISTER CONFIGURATION

FIGURE 4.77 (continued)

The Z80 has three software-selectable modes of response to a maskable interrupt. In mode 0, the Z80 behaves exactly like the Intel 8080 upon receipt of a maskable interrupt, jumping to any one of eight fixed locations on page zero of memory. A restart vector supplied on the data bus by the interrupting device specifies the jump to one of these eight locations. In mode 1, the Z80 always jumps to location 0038_{16}. In mode 2, the most powerful mode, the Z80 can jump to any 16-bit address.

The memory refresh register R enables dynamic memory to be used without external refresh circuitry. The lowest 7 bits of this 8-bit register are automatically incremented after each instruction fetch, with the eighth remaining as programmed by a load register R instruction. While the CPU is decoding and executing an instruction, these 8 bits are placed on the address bus (together with register I) and a refresh command is issued.

The ALU performs 8-bit operations. Some of these are add, subtract, AND, OR, exclusive OR, compare, shift (left or right), rotate, increment, decrement, bit set, bit reset, and bit test.

The instruction decode and CPU control section holds and decodes instructions after they are fetched. It generates all the signals necessary to control the CPU, and external devices as well. In addition, this section responds to external control inputs.

Timing and control. Figure 4.78 shows timing diagrams for the Z80. $\overline{\text{M1}}$ is a CPU output which indicates that an instruction is being fetched. ($\overline{\text{M1}}$ is also used to help acknowledge interrupts). $\overline{\text{RFSH}}$ indicates that the address bus holds the refresh address for dynamic memory. $\overline{\text{RD}}$ and $\overline{\text{WR}}$ are the read and write request signals from the CPU. These indicate the directions of both memory and I/O operations.

$\overline{\text{MREQ}}$ and $\overline{\text{IORQ}}$ indicate that a memory or I/O operation is being requested by the CPU. ($\overline{\text{IORQ}}$ also occurs with $\overline{\text{M1}}$ to acknowledge an interrupt.) $\overline{\text{HALT}}$ indicates that the CPU is halted and must be interrupted or reset to resume operation. Refresh activity continues while the CPU is halted to prevent loss of data in dynamic memories. $\overline{\text{BUSAK}}$ acknowledges an external request for use of the bus. When $\overline{\text{BUSAK}}$ is low, the address and data buses, as well as some of the CPU control outputs, are disabled (put in the high-impedance state). Refresh ceases during this state, so it must be kept short. ϕ is the clock input.

$\overline{\text{WAIT}}$ is an input that allows the CPU to be slowed down to interface with slow memory or I/O. As long as the $\overline{\text{WAIT}}$ line is low, the CPU continues to idle. Refresh also ceases in this state. $\overline{\text{INT}}$ and $\overline{\text{NMI}}$ are the maskable and nonmaskable interrupt inputs. The maskable interrupt can be ignored (disabled) by the CPU until it wants to service it, but the nonmaskable cannot. The nonmaskable interrupt is usually reserved for alarm conditions. $\overline{\text{RESET}}$ clears the program counter, the I and R registers, and disables the maskable interrupt. $\overline{\text{BUSRQ}}$ requests the use of the CPU bus and is acknowledged by $\overline{\text{BUSAK}}$ as above.

Instruction set. The Z80's instruction set is a superset of that of the Intel 8080, one of the most popular microprocessors. This allows programs originally written

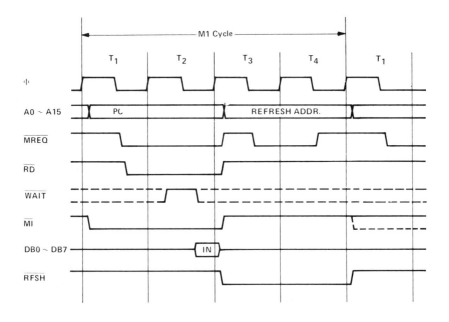

INSTRUCTION OP CODE FETCH

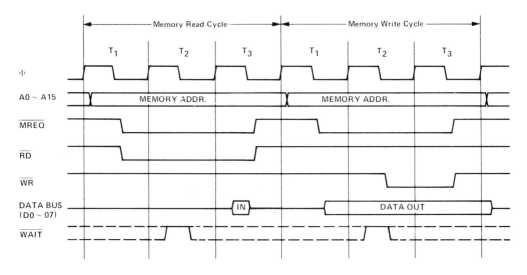

MEMORY READ OR WRITE CYCLES

FIGURE 4.78 Some common Z80 timing cycles. (Compliments of Zilog, Inc., 1977.)

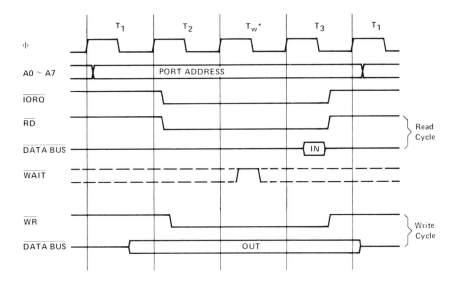

INPUT OR OUTPUT CYCLES

FIGURE 4.78 (continued)

for the 8080 to be used with the Z80. Only a minor incompatibility exists between the two processors. This concerns the Z80's redefinition of one of the 8080 flags. The Z80 instruction set is listed in Appendix 4.

The Z80 incorporates no less than nine addressing modes. These include immediate, immediate extended, modified page zero, relative, extended, indexed, register, implied, register indirect, and bit addressing. Many multioperand instructions allow the mixing of addressing modes.

Data can be stored into memory from a register or loaded into a register from memory. Data can also be transferred and swapped between certain registers. Sixteen-bit words can be handled using register pairs.

The Z80 can search any section of memory for a given data word with its block-search instructions. This content addressability simplifies character-oriented programs. Block transfer instructions are also provided. These copy an entire section of memory into another. The block-oriented instructions save not only programming effort but CPU time as well.

All the common 8-bit arithmetic and logic operations are implemented in the Z80. Sixteen-bit add, subtract, increment, and decrement can be performed using specific register pairs. Data can also be rotated or shifted in the accumulator, any general-purpose register, or any memory location in a single operation. BCD arithmetic is also provided for, including a BCD digit (4-bit) rotate.

Individual bits in registers and memory can be set, reset, or tested in a single operation. This means that a virtually unlimited number of flags are available. Data can be packed into memory bit by bit, which increases memory utilization for odd or variable-length words. Status bits of I/O devices are also easily handled.

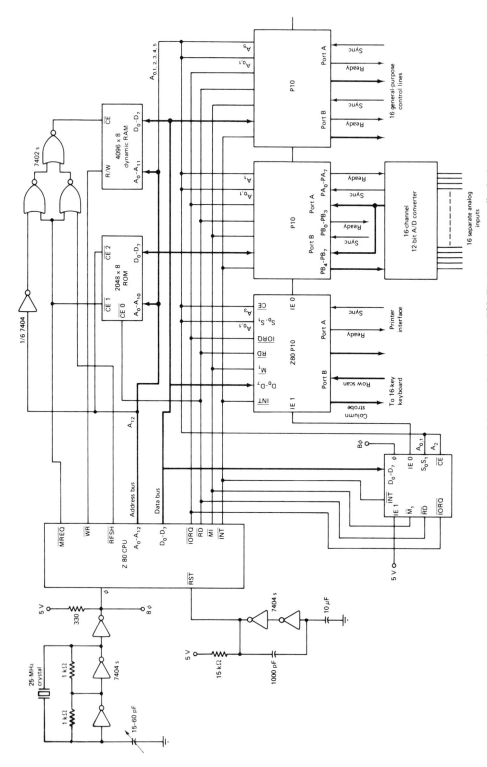

FIGURE 4.79 Simple but very powerful system based on the Z80. The interrupt controller is the circuit below the CPU. (Reprinted with permission from Electronic Design, Vol. 25, No. 14, July 5, 1977. © Hayden Publishing Co., Inc. 1977.)

Single-instruction subroutine call and return are provided. Jump instructions can use either the immediate extended, relative, or register indirect modes. Conditional versions of some of the above are also provided. A particularly useful instruction is DJNZ (decrement B, jump if not zero). It provides a very simple means of implementing indexed loops in programs.

I/O can be carried out with a device specified either immediately or indirectly (through the C register). Block I/O instructions, which transfer up to 256 words between I/O devices and memory, are also included.

Finally, the CPU has certain control instructions that allow enabling and disabling the maskable interrupt, changing between any of the three maskable interrupt modes, and, for the computer that has everything, a "do-nothing" instruction, the NOP.

Simple system. As with the COSMAC, all that is needed to build a simple system around the Z80 is memory (RAM and/or ROM) and I/O. A clock generator is also needed and can be an *RC* or crystal oscillator, depending on the speed and accuracy needed.

Figure 4.79 shows a slightly more substantial system. Here the Z80 is interfaced with 2 kbytes of ROM, 4 kbytes of RAM, six I/O ports [two in each parallel input/output (PIO) package], and an interrupt controller. A "power-up" sensing circuit holds the reset ($\overline{RST}$) low when power is first applied. The crystal oscillator clock runs at a 2.5-MHz rate, which is the maximum for the basic Z80. The variable capacitor allows fine tuning of the crystal to achieve accurate timing.

A 16-channel, 12-bit A/D converter is interfaced to two input ports. Its 12-bit word is split into an 8-bit and a 4-bit word, and each is routed through a separate input port. Handshaking is transacted with the SYNC and READY lines.

A keyboard and printer are interfaced through the first PIO circuit. The keyboard is matrixed to reduce hardware, as discussed earlier in this chapter.

The interrupt hardware configuration is daisy-chained, as discussed in Section 4.2. With this approach, the acknowledge line to all interrupting devices strings them in "series" so that the device closest to the CPU has the highest priority. In this system the highest-priority devices are the keyboard and printer. Daisy chaining requires time for an interrupt acknowledge to be rippled to a low-priority device through all those with higher priorities. In larger systems, where this may be a problem, the CPU can be slowed down by using its $\overline{WAIT}$ line during an interrupt acknowledge.

REFERENCES

BARNA, A., AND PORAT, D. I. 1976. Introduction to microcomputers and microprocessors. New York: Wiley.

BARTEE, T. C. 1977. Digital computer fundamentals, 4th ed. New York: McGraw-Hill.

BRODERSON, R. W., HEWES, R., AND BUSS, D. D. 1976. A 500-stage CCD transversal filter for spectral analysis. IEEE J. Solid-State Circuits SC-11: 75–84.

BURSKY, D. 1979. Microprocessor data manual. Electron. Des. 27(24): 49–112.

ECKHOUSE, R. H. 1975. Minicomputer systems: organization and programming. Englewood Cliffs, NJ: Prentice-Hall.

ELECTRONIC DESIGN. 1978. Microprocessor data manual II. 26(21): 53–217.

HARTENSTEIN, R., AND ZAKS, R. (EDS.). 1975. Microarchitecture of computer systems. Amsterdam: North-Holland.

HILBURN, J. L., AND JULICH, P. M. 1976. Microcomputers/microprocessors: hardware, software and applications. Englewood Cliffs, NJ: Prentice-Hall.

HUSS, D. A. 1977. Magnetic bubble memory. Kilobaud 1977(11): 54–56.

INTEL. 1977, 1978. Intel memory handbook. Santa Clara, CA.

INTEL. 1978. MCS-85 user's manual. Santa Clara, CA.

KLINGMAN, E. E. 1977. Microprocessor system design. Englewood Cliffs, NJ: Prentice-Hall.

LANCASTER, D. 1977. CMOS cookbook. Indianapolis, IN: Sams.

LEWIS, T. G., AND DOERR, J. W. 1976. Minicomputers: structure and programming. Rochelle Park, NJ: Hayden.

LIMING, G. 1976. Data paths. Byte. 1(6): 32–40.

MOSTEK. 1978. Mostek 1978 memory data book and designers guide. Carrollton, TX.

McGLYNN, D. R. 1976. Microprocessors. New York: Wiley.

NATIONAL SEMICONDUCTOR. 1975. Interface integrated circuits. Santa Clara, CA.

OSBORNE, A. 1977. An introduction to microcomputers. Vol. 1, Basic concepts. Berkeley, CA: Osborne and Associates.

OSBORNE, A. 1978a. An introduction to microcomputers. Vol. 2, Some real microprocessors. Berkeley, CA: Osborne and Associates.

OSBORNE, A. 1978b. An introduction to microcomputers Vol. 3, Some real support devices. Berkeley, CA: Osborne and Associates.

PEATMAN, J. B. 1977. Microcomputer-based design. New York: McGraw-Hill.

PESCHKE, M., AND PESCHKE, V. 1976. Byte's audio cassette standards symposium. Byte 1(6): 72–73.

PICKLES, G. 1977. Who's afraid of RS-232? Kilobaud 1977(7): 50–54.

RABINER, L. R., SCHAFER, R. W., AND RADER, C. M. 1969. The chirp z-transform algorithm. IEEE Trans. Audio Electroacoust. AU-17: 86–92.

RAMPIL, I. 1977. A floppy disk tutorial. Byte. 2(12): 24–45.

RCA. 1976. User manual for the CDP1802 COSMAC microprocessor. Somerville, NJ.

RCA. 1979. Preliminary data sheets for the CDP1802D, CDP1802CD. Somerville, NJ.

SAHAKIAN, A. 1977. Computer/cassette interface takes tone from clock. Electronics 50(1): 115.

TEXAS INSTRUMENTS. 1972. Optoelectronics data book. Dallas, TX.

TEXAS INSTRUMENTS. 1975. The microprocessor handbook. Dallas, TX.

TEXAS INSTRUMENTS. 1977. TMS 3064VL 65,536-bit CCD memory data sheet. Dallas, TX.

TOONG, H-M. D. 1977. Microprocessors. Sci. Am. 237(3): 146–161.

UNGERMAN, R., AND PEUTO, B. 1977. Get powerful microprocessor performance by using Z80. With 158 instructions it offers more flexibility than other μPs, plus 8080 code compatibility. Electron. Des. 25(14): 54–63.

WEISSBERGER, A. J. AND TOAL, T. 1977. Tough mathematical tasks are child's play for number cruncher. Electronics. 50(4): 102–107.

WINFIELD, J. 1977. Dynamic memories offer advantages. Electron. Des. 25(14): 66–70.

ZILOG. 1977. Z-80-CPU, Z-80A CPU technical manual. Cupertino, CA.

PROBLEMS

4.1 Low-power Schottky TTL is becoming more popular because of its low power consumption and small propagation delay. Its worst-case loading rule is shown in Fig. P4.1. (a) How many standard TTL gates can a low-power Schottky TTL gate drive? (b) How many low-power Schottky TTL gates can a standard TTL gate drive? (c) What are the noise margins in part (a)?

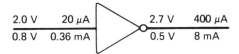

2.0 V	20 μA		2.7 V	400 μA
0.8 V	0.36 mA		0.5 V	8 mA

FIGURE P4.1 Low-power Schottky TTL inverter.

4.2 Fig. P4.2 shows two tristate inverters. (a) What Boolean function does this configuration realize? (b) What will happen if both C_1 and C_2 are active? (c) Realize the Boolean function in part (a) using ordinary (two-state) gates.

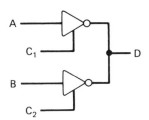

FIGURE P4.2 Tristate inverter circuit.

4.3 If there is small noise voltage on v_2 in Fig. 4.10(c), the CPU will fluctuate between the RESET and RUN state around the threshold voltage. Design a more reliable initialization circuit, using a Schmitt trigger to make sharp transitions.

4.4 The contents of the address register and the counter register of the DMA controller of Fig. 4.14 are 0060_{16} and $00A0_{16}$, respectively and the status register indicates that the burst DMA operation is active. (a) What are the contents of the address register and the counter register at the end of the DMA operation? (b) If each byte transfer takes 1 μs, how long does it take to end the DMA operation?

4.5 An RCA CDP1821SD 1204 × 1-bit RAM will retain data with a power-supply voltage of 4 V at 500 μA maximum. How long can a single 4.05-V mercury camera battery with a 190-mA/h rating maintain a 1 kbit × 8 memory?

4.6 The manufacturer of a microprocessor-controlled instrument must decide whether to store the controlling program, subroutines, and table of constants in a single large PROM or several smaller PROMs. What are the advantages and disadvantages of each method?

4.7 Show how two 256 × 4-bit RAM chips can be connected together to form a 256 × 8-bit memory to be used with the COSMAC. You may assume that no other memory is present in the system.

4.8 Show that it is possible to decode a full 256 pages of memory for the COSMAC using three chips. (*Hint:* An 8-bit latch and two 1-of-16 decoder chips.)

4.9 Draw a block diagram of a circuit to program and verify 2716 EPROMs. For simplicity you may use output ports.

4.10 Draw a flowchart of an algorithm to program an EPROM with the circuit of Problem 4.9.

4.11 The R register of the Z80 CPU allows dynamic memories to be used with a minimum amount of hardware. With 64-kbit dynamic chips on the horizon, very large memory with few chips would seem possible. Why will the Z80 not refresh 64-kbit dynamic memories?

4.12 (a) Design an address decoder (to serve in Fig. 4.38) which compares the incoming address with the state of eight switches (allowing the port address to be changed at will). Use any common gates (including exclusive OR). Assume that the switches are SPDT and that switch bounce is not a problem. (b) Repeat part (a) for SPST switches.

4.13 (a) A Z80 system is to have seven I/O ports. Briefly describe the scheme that you as the I/O designer would use to address these ports. (b) Repeat part (a) for a COSMAC system.

4.14 Two microcomputer systems communicate using the serial data format shown in Fig. 4.42. Estimate how far the relative timing of the receiving system can differ from the transmitting system before data errors occur. (*Hint:* Assume that the receiver begins timing with the falling edge of the incoming start bit, and samples the incoming data at what it anticipates to be the center of each bit time.

4.15 (a) An 800-bpi digital cassette is used with a record size of exactly ten 8-bit characters and interrecord gaps of 2 cm. Estimate the number of characters that can be stored in this way on a 14.2-m cassette. (b) Repeat part (a) with a record size of 1000 characters.

4.16 Estimate the total latency from track 1 to a specific record on track 77 for a typical floppy disk.

4.17 Design an 8-key-to-3-bit keyboard encoder as in Fig. 4.52. Use only NAND and NOT gates and assume bounceless SPST keys switching to ground with pull-up resistors.

4.18 Design a circuit to add on to the encoder of Problem 4.17 which senses when any key is pressed.

4.19 (a) In the matrixed keyboard of Fig. 4.53, can the computer be made to correctly recognize the simultaneous closure of any two keys? Explain. (b) How about three keys?

4.20 Show the software needed to use the matrixed keyboard of Fig. 4.53. Only be concerned with single-key closures and assume that switch bounce is not a problem. Use any suitable descriptive flowchart convention and return a 4-bit number identifying the key pressed.

4.21 In the debounced switch of Fig. 4.51(b), the values of R_2 and C set the output pulse width. The nonretriggerable monostable multivibrator ignores its input during the output pulse. What happens if the pulse width is set too short? Too long?

4.22 Design an interface between an 8-bit output port and an X-ray machine that has a different ground potential (you need only show "a bit" of circuitry). Use the DS3661 optical isolator (Fig. 4.57) and assume that the LED is driven with 5 mA and has a forward drop of 1.75 V.

4.23 In the matrixed seven-segment display of Fig. 4.55, it is possible to use two output ports (one for digits and one for segments) and work with unencoded data. In this way each digit is selectable by one bit of the digit port and each segment in that digit (including the decimal point) is selectable by one bit of the segment port. Comment on the advantages and drawbacks of this scheme.

4.24 Design a circuit that generates the COSMAC mode control inputs [Fig. 4.75(b)] from a set of three noisy SPDT switches. One switch should generate the LOAD code, one the RESET code, one the PAUSE code, and when all switches are inactive the RUN code should be generated.

4.25 Design a circuit to decode and indicate (on a set of four LEDs) the state code of a COSMAC [Fig. 4.75(c)].

4.26 A COSMAC (CDP1802C version) operates at room temperature with $V_{DD} = 5$ V. How long does it take to execute an ADD instruction (two machine cycles) at the maximum speed? What clock frequency does this correspond to?

4.27 A COSMAC (CDP1802D version) operates at 3.2 MHz in a simple battery-powered application. The processor idles in a "time-killing" loop for 95% of the time. (a) Estimate the lifetime of a 150 mA/h (5 V) battery driving only the processor (see RCA, 1979). (b) Repeat part (a) if the clock is turned off when the processor is not needed.

4.28 Show a scheme to input from an eight-key keyboard using the hardware flags of the COSMAC.

4.29 A Z80 system has 8 kbytes of EPROM and 16 kbytes of dynamic RAM (using CPU refresh). A floppy-disk drive is interfaced to the system in such a way that whenever the CPU makes a request for data from the disk, the drive pulls the CPU's $\overline{\text{WAIT}}$ line low until it finds the data. Often, when the drive is accessed, the system "crashes." Why?

4.30 For a Z80A running at maximum speed, use Fig. 4.78 to determine (roughly) how much time an output port address decoder has before it must settle.

4.31 The Z80 samples its $\overline{\text{WAIT}}$ line upon the falling clock edge of T_2 (and every falling clock edge while it is in a WAIT state). Notice in Fig. 4.78 that a WAIT state (identified as T_w^*) is automatically inserted by the CPU regardless of the $\overline{\text{WAIT}}$ line. Why is this feature needed?

4.32 Our microcomputer has no subtract instruction. How can we implement a subtraction on 2's-complement numbers?

4.33 Our microcomputer has no rotate right (ROR) instruction. Flowchart a possible method to rotate a number right one place and load the LSB into the MSB.

4.34 Why is indexed or indirect addressing useful for input/output in memory-mapped I/O systems?

4.35 We wish to implement a nested subroutine structure with a COSMAC microcomputer, but the COSMAC stores the PC in a temporary register T after each subroutine. Write a program to save the PC after each subroutine call.

4.36 How do the various addressing modes increase the (a) efficiency of memory utilization, and (b) flexibility of programming options?

4.37 In Fig. 4.61 we illustrated one possible way to do a 2's-complementation of a number. An easier way exists, however. After considering the instruction sets of the Z80 and the COSMAC, can you find it?

4.38 Why is correction by adding or subtracting 6 necessary for BCD arithmetic?

4.39 An overflow has occurred after an addition. Can the overflow be corrected? If so, make a flowchart showing the method. If not, how can we circumvent the problem?

4.40 We wish to round off the product obtained after multiplying two 8-bit numbers. Suggest a way in which this can be done.

4.41 A digital pH meter has been interfaced to the microcomputer. The range of values after A/D conversion is 0.00 to 2.55. A reference electrode output is available at input port 1 (in a pH 7.000 solution). The unknown electrode output is available at input port 2. Describe a way in which we can calibrate the instrument and use a standard curve (in computer form) to find the unknown pH.

4.42 In the key-parse design example in the text: (a) How is a data "D" differentiated from the command "D"? (b) Can the design be modified easily if we wish to reformat our commands? (c) Suggest a possible addressing scheme to locate the correct action routine. Is there a method that is particularly suited?

4.43 A number of errors can occur in floating-point arithmetic. Specify two major sources and explain why they can be troublesome.

4.44 A digital filter is needed to smooth our collected data points. We decide to use one with the format $[1/4][2x_{-1} + 4x_0 + 2x_{+1}]$. Suggest two ways we can implement the filter. Is one way simpler (in terms of programming difficulty) than the other?

5

Applications
in Existence

This chapter brings to one place information on a large number of medical applications of microcomputers. Because little information is available in journals, we extensively searched conference proceedings for recent applications. We gathered up-to-date information by mailing a questionnaire to each source.

Although the medical applications of microcomputers will expand greatly in the future, we hope this information will give you ideas for possible applications. It should suggest how to select a microcomputer, the memory size required, the software effort required, and interfacing techniques.

5.1 GENERAL SIGNAL PROCESSORS*

Signal averaging

Many biopotential signals have very small amplitudes and large noise components. If the noise has frequency components that are higher or lower than those of the desired signal bandwidth, we can use conventional filtering techniques [Fig. 5.1(a)].

*Section 5.1 written by Kevin R. Colwell.

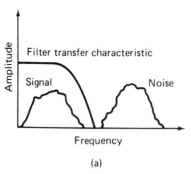
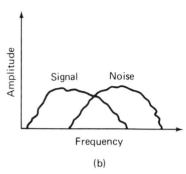

(a)   (b)

FIGURE 5.1 Amplitude spectra of signals mixed with noise. (a) A conventional filter can be used to reject noise if the noise spectrum is not in the signal band. (b) Filtering is ineffective when the spectra overlap. [From Ellis, R. C., Jr. 1976. Signal averaging and medical applications. Medical Electronics, Pittsburgh, Pa. 15216. 7(2) : 41–43. Used with permission.]

However, filtering will not work if signal frequency components and noise components overlap [Fig. 5.1(b)]. In this case we may use signal averaging to improve the signal-to-noise ratio (SNR).

Averaging sums the signal and the random noise. The noise sums more slowly than the signal, and we achieve a net gain in SNR. Multiple-exposure photography and variable-persistence oscilloscopes have been used to average signals for years. Digital logic has made this process more convenient and precise. Averagers require a synchronization between the sweep and the desired signal. For signal averaging to be successful, the signal must be repetitive (not necessarily periodic) and the noise and signal uncorrelated.

The input waveform, $f(t)$, has a signal portion, $S(t)$, and a noise portion, $N(t)$. Then $f(t) = S(t) + N(t)$. Let $f(t)$ be sampled every T seconds. The value of any sample point ($i = 1, 2, \ldots, n$) is the sum of the noise component and the signal component.

$$f(iT) = S(iT) + N(iT)$$

Each sample point corresponds to a memory location. The value stored in memory location i after m repetitions is

$$\sum_{k=1}^{m} f(iT) = \sum_{k=1}^{m} S(iT) + \sum_{k=1}^{m} N(iT) \qquad \text{for } i = 1, 2, \ldots, n)$$

The signal component for sample point i is the same at each repetition if the signal is stable. Then $\sum_{k=1}^{m} S(iT) = mS(iT)$. We assume that the signal and noise are uncorrelated, that the noise has a mean of zero, and is random. After many repetitions, $N(iT)$ has an rms value of σ_n. Then for any sample point on any repetition, the SNR $= S(iT)/\sigma_n$. The rms value of the noise after m repetitions for any sample point is $\sqrt{m}\, \sigma_n$. The signal-to-noise ratio after m repetitions is then

$$SNR_m = \frac{mS(iT)}{\sqrt{m}\ \sigma_n} = \sqrt{m}\ SNR$$

The averaging improves the SNR by a factor of $m^{1/2}$ (Moore, 1970).

Signal averaging is a kind of digital filtering process. The Fourier transform (Section 3.4) of the transfer function of an averager is composed of a series of discrete frequency components. Each of these has the same spectral characteristics and amplitudes (Fig. 5.2). This represents a comb filter. The width of each tooth decreases as the number of sweep repetitions increases. The desired signal also has a frequency spectrum composed of discrete frequency components, while noise has a continuous distribution. The comb filter passes the discrete frequency components and rejects all the other frequencies. The signal averager, therefore, passes the signal while rejecting the noise.

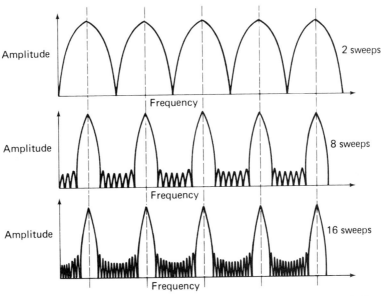

FIGURE 5.2 A Fourier transform of a signal averager shows that it is a comb filter. [From Ellis, R. C., Jr. 1976. Signal averaging and medical applications. Medical Electronics, Pittsburgh, Pa. 15216. 7(2) : 41–43. Used with permission.]

Figure 5.3 shows the block diagram of a typical averager. To average a signal such as the cortical response to an auditory stimulus (a clicking sound or a tone), we input the EEG (Section 1.5). The stimulus provides the synchronization necessary to trigger the sweep. It is important that the trigger-pulse-to-response latency be very stable; otherwise, the averaged signal will be smeared. When the averager receives the trigger pulse, it samples the waveform at the selected rate, digitizes the signal, and sums the numerical value with the contents of a memory location corresponding to that sample interval. The process continues, stepping through the memory addresses until all "addresses" have been sampled. The sweep is terminated

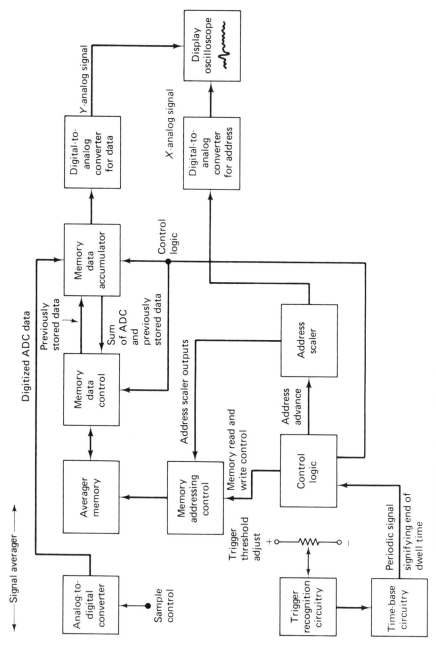

FIGURE 5.3 Block diagram of signal averager. [From Ellis, R. C., Jr. 1976. Signal averaging and medical applications. Medical Electronics, Pittsburgh, Pa. 15216. 7(2) : 41–43. Used with permission.]

at this point. A new sweep begins with the next trigger pulse and the cycle repeats until the desired number of sweeps have been averaged. The interval between samples is used to convert the sums stored in memory back to analog values so that they can be displayed on a CRT. Figure 5.4 shows the improvement in SNR versus number of sweeps.

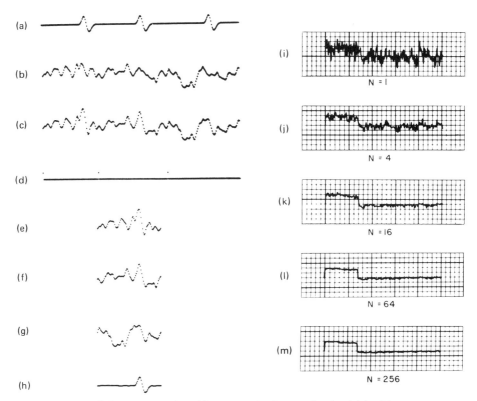

FIGURE 5.4 Demonstration of how averaging improved a signal (a) with respect to noise (b). (c) is the signal and noise. (d) shows the synchronization signal. (e), (f), and (g) are averaged to give the signal (h). (i), (j), (k), (l), and (m) illustrate the improvement in SNR as a function of sweep repetitions. [From Cox, J. R., Jr. 1965. Special purpose digital computers in biology. In R. W. Stacy and B. D. Waxman (eds.), Computers in biomedical research, Vol. 2. New York: Academic Press. Used with permission.]

The equations above represent the ideal case for Gaussian-distributed noise. This assumption is not always valid. The noise distribution may be related to the signal and misleading results can occur. If the noise has low-frequency components, there is a possibility that a correlation may exist between the noise samples in adjacent stimulus periods. Cox (1965) shows how to calculate the loss in SNR from this type of correlation. This problem can be minimized by randomizing the period between stimuli.

A problem may occur if the repeating signal itself is used to initiate the sweep, as for example when the R wave is used as a trigger to average the ECG. In this case triggering occurs when the signal plus noise crosses a threshold. Noise causes jittering in the time of occurrence of the synchronization pulse and consequently produces a blurring of the averaged signal.

Since signal averaging involves sampling an analog signal and converting it to a digital form, the process must adhere to the sampling theorem (Section 2.1). Problems related to the frequency-folding effect (Ross, 1957) can be reduced by filtering the signal before averaging.

Signal averaging uses an infrequent repetition of the stimulus to enhance the SNR. Therefore, rare phenomena that might be observed in a single sweep may be lost in the averaging process.

Commercial signal averagers are available in two types, computer-controlled systems and instruments employing conventional logic control. Most can average signals in both the time and frequency domains. Computer-controlled systems provide more versatile data-acquisition instruments, but at a higher cost.

Digital oscilloscopes

The advent of digital storage oscilloscopes brings a new dimension to data acquisition and analysis. Digital oscilloscopes combine the features of conventional oscilloscopes, x-y-t plotters, and A/D and D/A converters. They permit human judgment to enter the analysis process at an early stage. A digital oscilloscope can be controlled by conventional logic circuits, but microprocessors are now being used to produce more flexible instruments.

A plug-in with knobs similar to a conventional oscilloscope provides for amplifying or attenuating an analog signal to a level appropriate for the internal A/D converter. The A/D converter samples the input wave at a selected rate and stores it in sequential RAM memory addresses until the memory is filled. These data represent one sweep. Between samples, the contents of the memory are read out to a D/A converter. The restored analog signal is amplified and applied to the deflection plates of a CRT. In y-t operation the value stored in any address represents the y value or amplitude and the address itself the x value.

A sweep is started by a trigger circuit similar to that of conventional oscilloscope. The oscilloscope can then continue in one of several different modes. With the address counter initialized to the bottom of memory, each location is filled until the top of memory is reached. The counter then resets to zero and the process repeats with the next trigger. The memory is arranged as a circular buffer producing a display similar to a triggered analog oscilloscope. The memory can be filled once and the contents held indefinitely, disabling further conversions. This is analogous to the single sweep function on conventional oscilloscopes, except that the data are held in memory. The CRT can be refreshed continuously, resulting in a nonfade display.

With a circular memory the trigger can start storing data at any address. It need not correspond to the left side of the screen. For example, consider the case where the trigger point is set in the middle of the screen and a complete sweep requires time T. If the trigger event occurs at $t = 0$ and the current sweep is terminated when the highest address is reached (corresponding to $T/2$), the right half of the display will contain events following the trigger (0 to $T/2$), and the left half will show events preceding the trigger ($-T/2$ to 0). The portion of the signal preceding the trigger occurs at times $t < 0$ or in negative time. This is a very useful feature which allows the operator to see events that preceded or caused the triggering event.

Digital processing can manipulate data stored in digital form. The trace can be raised or lowered on the screen by adding a constant value to each memory location. It can be expanded (magnified) by multiplying the contents of each location (for vertical expansion) or the address counter (horizontal expansion) by the magnification factor. Also, the contents of each location can be output in digital form to a storage device or to a computer for processing. After processing, digital data can be returned to the oscilloscope memory and displayed.

The normal display process can be slowed down and used to plot the waveform on an analog recorder. A fast waveform can be digitized and then the contents of each address sent to the D/A converters at a rate slow enough for x-y plotters. Since the waveform can be moved or expanded, the operator can scale the trace as necessary before outputting it in analog or digital form for storage or further processing.

Digital oscilloscopes do not have time bases like conventional oscilloscopes. The operator selects a sample rate that must be fast enough to satisfy Shannon's law and eliminate the possibility of aliasing (Chapter 2). Since there are a discrete number of data words, selecting a sample rate too fast will exhaust the memory before the signal has terminated.

The resolution of an oscilloscope depends upon the length of the word (number of bits in the A/D converter) and the sampling rate. The larger the word size, the more accurate (Fig. 2.3) but slower the conversion. A compromise must be reached between speed and accuracy. Currently, 12-bit conversions can be performed at 500-ns intervals and 6-bit conversions at 2-ns intervals.

There are two types of commercially available digital oscilloscopes that use microprocessors for control. One type is the processing oscilloscope, which provides a programming capability to do generalized signal processing, including differentiation, integration, and other programmable signal processes. The other type is the nonprocessing oscilloscope, which provides only button and knob manipulation of the captured signals (Electronics Test, 1979).

Processing oscilloscopes.   An example of a processing oscilloscope is the Norland NI 2001A. It is the first marketed device to combine the features of a digital oscilloscope and the computational power of a microprocessor. It is intended to fill the gap between general instrumentation and expensive minicomputer-based automatic data systems. Figure 5.5 shows a block diagram of the oscilloscope. The Intel 8080A microprocessor is used with a large amount of software in ROM (24 kbytes).

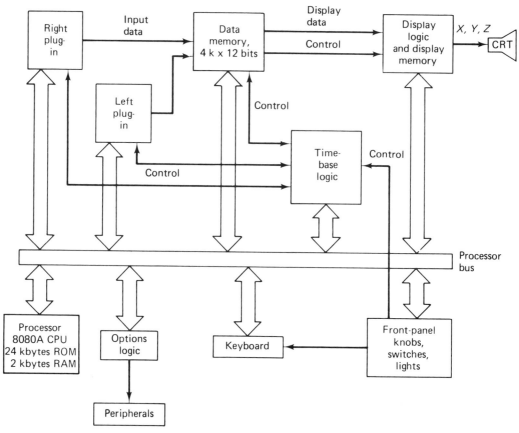

FIGURE 5.5 Block diagram of Norland Instruments NI 2001A digital oscilloscope. (Compliments of Norland Instruments, 1976.)

The signal is digitized in the left and right plug-ins with 8 or 10 bits of resolution. The maximum sampling rate is 1 MHz. The data are stored in a 4 k × 12-bit RAM memory array. The memory can be divided into two arrays of 2 kwords each or four arrays of 1 kwords each. This allows up to four signals to be read in simultaneously. Each array can be presented as a y-t display, or any array can be plotted against any other for an x-y display. Once the signal is in memory, the user can display the numerical value and time of any sample point by placing a movable cursor on that point. The scope in this mode functions as a digital voltmeter. The signal amplitude can be expanded up to 2^6 times and reduced 2^{-2} times.

The operator can program the microprocessor to perform many numerical computations on the data. Figure 5.6 shows the control keyboard of the instrument. It is possible to add, subtract, multiply, or divide an array (the data for one sweep) by a constant, thus scaling the waveform to any desired size. The numerical readout may then be scaled to any desired units, such as amperes or watts. The processor can also do mathematical operations on arrays. For example, if it records two

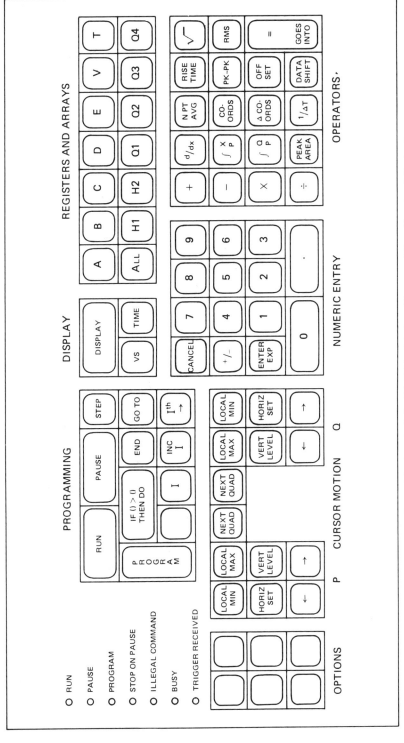

FIGURE 5.6 Control keyboard of the NI 2001 digital oscilloscope. (Compliments of Norland Instruments, 1976.)

signals in separate arrays, one representing the time-varying voltage to a device and the other the current through it, the processor can multiply the two arrays together point by point and display the product waveform representing the power consumed.

Norland has implemented many of the commonly used arithmetic functions in firmware. By pressing the appropriate operator button, the processor can compute the square root, derivative, rise time, integral, or peak value of a recorded signal. In the example above, it computed the power by multiplying the current and voltage signals. The operator can position the cursors to contain an integral number of periods, and with a single key can compute the true rms power and display it on the screen. These are only a few of 19 operations available.

The programming language is simple and has been designed to minimize the number of key strokes necessary to manipulate arrays of data. The program to multiply two waveforms and display the result is as follows:

$$Q1*Q2 \Longrightarrow Q3$$

$$DPLY \ Q3 \ vs \ T$$

The program reads "multiply array Q1 times array Q2 (1024 words) and put the result into Q3 (1024 words); display Q3 versus time."

The scope has seven floating-point registers to hold numerical results such as the peak value or the frequency. Conditional branching is possible, and the program can generate both digital and analog output signals for feedback control of experiments. Some of the signal computations are slow. For example, several seconds may be required to compute the integral of a trace.

The NI 2001A has added frequency-domain calculations. It can perform the Fourier transform, inverse Fourier transform, autocorrelation, cross correlation, convolution, cross spectra, coherent output power, and convolution spectra.

A plug-in is available that performs true signal averaging where the digitized signal is summed and divided by the number of repetitions. Throughput is 200,000 samples/s for 8-bit resolution and 60,000 samples/s for 12-bit resolution. It can average up to 999,999 repetitions. The Norland 3001 is an updated version that uses an 8085-based 1-MHz mainframe.

Nonprocessing oscilloscopes. An example of a nonprocessing oscilloscope is the Nicolet 2090 general-purpose digital oscilloscope. It costs less than half the price of the Norland but is not programmable. Nevertheless, it is a very versatile instrument for data collection. The oscilloscope can accommodate three plug-ins. The input can be sampled at intervals from 500 ns to 200 s. Eight-bit and 12-bit A/D converters are used to give an amplitude resolution of up to 0.025%. The oscilloscope has 4096 13-bit words. Sweep durations of from 512 μs to 9.5 days are possible (up to 76 days if a built-in floppy disk is used). The memory can be divided into two or four quadrants of 2048 or 1024 words, respectively. This allows up to four traces to be retained at one time in the main-frame. A trace can be expanded up to 64 times, inverted or moved vertically. The only mathematical operation possible between quadrants is the subtraction of one trace from another.

The 2090 has one vertical and one horizontal cursor. The screen numerically displays the value of the data point at the intersection of the vertical cursor and the waveform. The screen displays both the voltage and the time after trigger. The operator can move the cursors to any position on the signal to provide the coordinates of that point. The operator can set the oscilloscope so that the trigger point corresponds to the vertical cursor's position, thus permitting pretrigger information to be displayed.

The storage controls establish one of three modes of operation. *Live* mode corresponds to a conventional triggered scope. A trigger event initiates a sweep that terminates when the quadrant is filled. The next sweep begins automatically with the next trigger event. The *Hold Last* button allows the sweep in progress (or the next sweep if the scope is waiting for a trigger) to be completed but disables further events from triggering a sweep. This holds the current contents of the memory until the scope is returned to the *Live* mode. The *Hold Next* mode finishes the current sweep and then places the oscilloscope in the *Hold Last* mode. The next sweep will be retained. These three modes, together with cursor triggering, makes the 2090 very versatile at capturing single events.

The oscilloscope can be equipped with an optional floppy-disk drive that fits within the oscilloscope case. The disk holds 32 kwords and is divided into eight tracks of 4096 words. The oscilloscope can be set to store one long sweep of 32 kwords (only for sweep speeds of 500 μs/point or slower) or autocycle, where consecutive waveforms are stored on the disk until it is full. To read the disk back into memory the user selects a track and executes a recall.

The user can output the contents of the memory in both digital and analog form. The data are output through a parallel I/O port for further processing. The memory can then be reloaded by a handshaking process and the processed waveform displayed. Slow analog outputs are provided for use with *x-y* recorders. Figure 5.7 shows a block diagram of the oscilloscope. The processor has a bit-slice architecture based on the Advanced Micro Devices 2900 family of chips. Bit slicing involves having several microprocessor chips controlled by a common program counter, program ROM, and clock. Each microprocessor chip manipulates 4 bits of the word. In this way, variable-length words are possible. The 2090 uses three chips, each handling 4 bits, for a word length of 12 bits. There are other benefits to bit slicing. Because each chip handles only 4 bits, the number of transistors per chip is reduced. This allows higher-speed but less-dense technologies (TTL for the AMD 2900) to be used. Also, the manufacturer can microprogram the controlling ROM to implement any desired set of instructions. Bit slicing is not practical for all microprocessor applications because the hardware and development costs are much higher than for single-chip microprocessors.

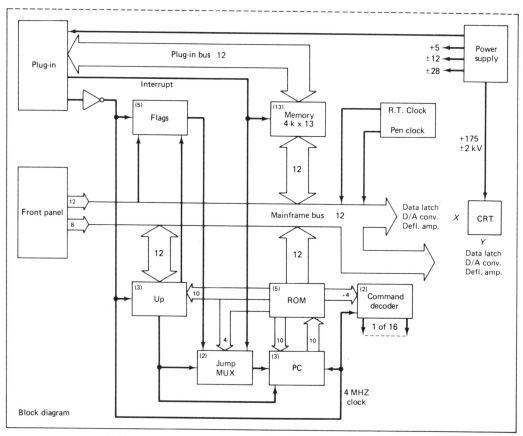

FIGURE 5.7 Block diagram of the Nicolet 2090 digital oscilloscope. (Compliments of Nicolet Instrument Corp., Oscilloscope Division, 1978.)

General laboratory instruments

In addition to the commercial systems just described, there have been several microcomputer-based instruments developed for use in general medical laboratories.

Histogram averager. Schoenfeld et al. (1977) describe several microcomputer-based instruments developed for biologists by their engineering support group. One instrument is a histogram averager used to monitor the activity of multifibered nerves or muscles. The histograms are plots of the number of responses occurring in successive selectable time intervals following a stimulus. There are 341 time bins and repeated histograms can be averaged. Figure 5.8 shows the basic hardware. The microcomputer includes a Motorola 6800 microprocessor, 1 kbyte of primary RAM, with an additional 128-byte scratchpad RAM. The software is stored in a

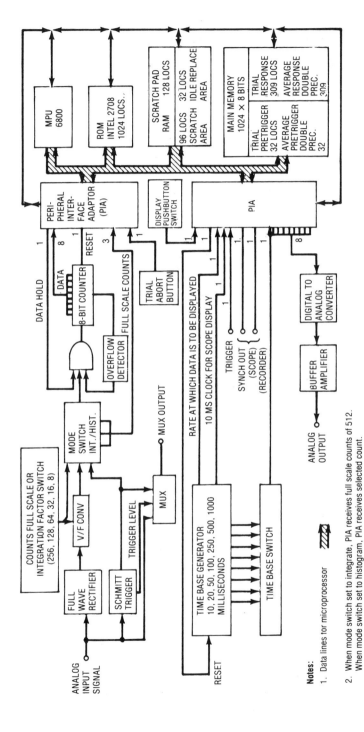

FIGURE 5.8 Histogram averager. [From Schoenfeld, R. L., et al., 1977. The microprocessor in the biological laboratory. Computer 10(5): 56–67.]

Notes:

1. Data lines for microprocessor

2. When mode switch set to integrate, PIA receives full scale counts of 512.
   When mode switch set to histogram, PIA receives selected count.

1-kbyte EPROM. Input and output are handled with two parallel I/O chips (PIAs). The data are displayed on an oscilloscope, and hard copy is available.

Signal averaging is a difficult application for most microcomputers because their speeds are too slow to do the necessary data manipulation in real time. The sampling rate must therefore be limited. Burkowski and Trenholm, (1978) developed a powerful physiological data averager based on the LSI-11 microprocessor. The hardware is basically a minicomputer and beyond the limits of this text.

Flight recorder.   Jolda and Wansek (1978) utilized an 8080 to build a prototype of an in-flight physiological data acquisition system. It acquires data on heart rate, acceleration, and breathing flows and pressures. The proposed version will incorporate a bubble memory to replace the present tape recorder. A ground-based computer will use FORTRAN programming to reformat the data and plot results.

Biomedical computer module.   A biomedical computer module (BMC) developed at the V.A. Hospital in San Diego, California, is a stand-alone microcomputer system for physiological signal processing (Fleming et al., 1976). It is physically designed to exactly replace a plug-in analog processing module such as an ECG amplifier in a Hewlett-Packard multichannel strip-chart recorder. The BMC accepts an analog input signal, processes it with a program stored in UV EPROMs, and outputs the resultant signal to the recorder. If several signals each require different processing, a number of these BMC modules can be plugged into a single Hewlett-Packard recorder mainframe. The BMC was designed for use in a hospital environment, so its designers took special care to ensure patient safety.

In operation, the microcomputer (1) notifies the operator if patient leads fall off or are improperly grounded, (2) switches patient leads to use the ones with the highest SNR, and (3) checks the program flow to make sure it is executing properly. Additional safety features are an isolated amplifier, diode networks to hold current below 10 μA, and inductor protection to keep high-frequency diathermy current from exceeding 6 mA.

The BMC contains an 8080A microprocessor, 8 kbytes of EPROM, and 256 bytes of CMOS RAM with battery backup. It also includes a power-fail circuit, which gives the microprocessor a 20-ms advance warning so that it can execute a power shutdown subroutine to preserve important data in the battery-backed-up RAM.

The front panel consists of the operator controls and displays including a keypad and seven-segment LED displays. A real-time clock composed of CMOS digital logic runs from the battery backup to allow timing intervals from 8 μs to 97 days. The analog input board contains optically isolated inputs that safely permit up to a 2500-V difference between the patient and the digital supply voltage and a 5000-V difference between the patient and the supply ground. The leads go through a switching matrix to permit the microprocessor to check impedances (to detect leads that are shorting or have fallen off) and then through a differential amplifier with CMRR exceeding 120 dB to reject 60-Hz and other common-mode-voltage interference present in the leads.

Upon power-up the BMC has an initialization software procedure that (1) checks all the boards for correct operation, (2) calibrates boards whose characteristics might vary, (3) checks to see if memory has been stored and maintained correctly, and (4) applies a calibrated signal to the strip-chart recorder.

The last two bytes of memory in both PROM and RAM are reserved for a cyclic redundancy check (CRC) sum and a checksum character. After initialization, the memories are read and the checksums are compared to the last two bytes. If any dropped bits are detected, the microcomputer notifies the operator of such an error. If an error occurs in the RAM sum, this implies that the last shutdown probably caused the mistake and the test must be repeated from the beginning.

A technique called watchdog threading permits checking the program flow to assure that there are no errors in program execution. At the end of each software subunit, the program takes several bytes from specific locations in RAM, encodes them using a polynomial correction code, and then puts the encoded bytes back into RAM. At the end of a major segment of code, the bytes are read and compared to a reference value. If the values are equal, the watchdog timer gets reset. This timer provides a means of detecting when the program goes awry (from power-supply noise or other processor glitches) and executes improperly. When this happens, the timer overflows and the entire program resets and starts over.

The program subunit that handles the data from the A/D converter constantly checks for 60-Hz interference. Interference indicates that the patient leads are not properly attached or that some other ac coupling is occurring, and the microcomputer notifies the operator with an audible alarm and visual display.

The program checks the input leads by switching the crosspoint matrix and selects the ones with the largest SNR. It also checks for dc offset voltage and supplies a negative voltage through a D/A converter to center the signal around 0 V. This allows the signal to be monitored through the full scale of the A/D converter. The amplitude of the signal can also be adjusted to make use of the full dynamic range.

The analog outputs to the strip-chart recorders have gain and offset calibrated by the operator during the initialization procedures. The scaling factors for these two variables are stored in RAM, so that recalibration is not necessary should the power fail.

The BMC can do any signal processing that can be programmed for the 8080A processor. Since the program is stored in EPROMs, changing the function of the device is simply a matter of replacing the EPROMs with others having a different program.

An example of an existing BMC program is a Fourier transform algorithm. With this program, the BMC accepts an input physiological signal, computes the transform in real time, and produces an output result on a strip-chart channel which plots frequency across the width of the paper, time along the longitudinal axis of the paper, and amplitude as the darkness (controlled by modulating the current in the thermal stylus). If the Fourier transforms of simultaneous signals are desired, two BMCs with identical programs are used.

This approach shows how microprocessors can provide redundant and reliable operations in the implementation of complex algorithms to process physiological signals.

5.2 ECG ACQUISITION AND TRANSMISSION*

Large time-shared computers at regional sites are doing a substantial number of computer interpretations of electrocardiograms. These computers normally receive the ECGs over the voice-grade telephone network from remote hospitals. We discuss here instrumentation for acquiring, preprocessing, and transmitting ECG signals.

ECG acquisition carts

Microcomputer-based ECG carts which can be rolled to the bedside of a patient (1) capture multichannel ECG signals, usually the standard 12-lead ECG; (2) preprocess the data in different ways; (3) display the ECGs locally, usually on a strip-chart recorder; and (4) transmit them over the voice-grade telephone system to a remote computer. Figure 5.9 summarizes the general features of these carts. The ROM stores the program that defines the instrument's operating characteristics. The RAM saves discrete-time ECG signals. The A/D converter samples three ECG leads simultaneously because this is the number that can be transmitted simultaneously over the voice-grade telephone network using frequency modulation.

In normal operation the microprocessor sequences the lead selector to send four groups of three leads to the multiplexer, each group for 2.5 s. The microprocessor reconstructs the analog signals from the captured discrete-time ECGs by outputting to a three-channel multiplexed D/A converter. The D/A converter drives an FM modem that produces modulated audio signals in the telephone frequency band. Simultaneously, the D/A outputs to a three-channel strip-chart recorder, and the microprocessor turns the recorder on.

Most telephone transmission of ECGs is done with FM techniques. Figure 5.9 shows in dashed lines an optional digital telephone-transmission link using a UART and a digital modem. This approach transmits the signals in their discrete form as a serial bit stream. Although this is an inherently less noisy approach than FM, the baud rate using the voice-grade telephone network is too low to achieve real-time transmission of three simultaneous channels. Therefore, digital transmission is not currently used extensively.

The operator of the ECG cart enters patient information and other data through a keyboard or thumbwheel switches. The processor sends these data and other information, such as the identification number of the cart, as a preamble before transmitting the ECGs. An alphanumeric display gives the operator feedback, such as error codes and parameters derived from the ECG. These ECG carts

*Section 5.2 written by Hossein Baharestani and Yongmin Kim.

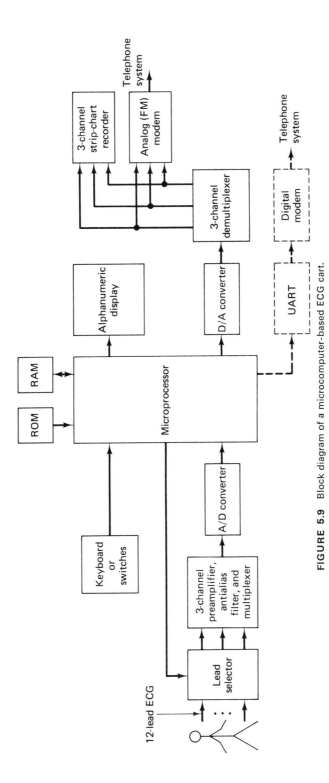

FIGURE 5.9 Block diagram of a microcomputer-based ECG cart.

facilitate capture of high-quality signals that are noise- and artifact-free and reduce operator procedural errors. Furthermore, by preprocessing the ECG signal to eliminate such problems, they simplify the analysis algorithms of the central computer by guaranteeing reliable data.

Microcomputer augmented cardiograph.   Marquette Electronics (1978) offers a commercial three-channel electrocardiogram cart, called the Microcomputer Augmented Cardiograph (MAC-1), that makes extensive use of microcomputer capability. Its microprocessor is a Motorola 6800 that uses 2 kbytes of UV EPROM for program storage.

When the instrument is first turned on, it goes through a dynamic memory check and provides a single beep if the memory test succeeds. If problems exist, it beeps a number of times. It has an LED display to provide messages to the operator.

Except for an analog antialiasing filter which is part of the ECG preamplifier, the MAC-1 does all its signal processing with digital filters. These filters are programs stored in its EPROM memory.

During recording three digital filters improve signal quality.

1. It has a complex digital filter that minimizes baseline drift without the distortion that usually accompanies simple filters [see Fig. 5.10(a)].
2. With another filter, it observes maxima and minima and automatically centers the trace, as shown in Fig. 5.10(b). If a gain change is required, it notifies the operator through its LED display.
3. It measures the constant value of 60-Hz interference and, with an adaptive digital filter, subtracts the 60-Hz signal out, without distorting the ECG, thus producing the interference-free signal shown in Fig. 5.10(c).

Additional features of the MAC-1 are a sampling rate of 500 samples/s, a heart-rate meter with LED readout of an eight-beat average, elapsed-time meter, and three-channel FM telephone transmission. Also, it senses arrhythmias and automatically records a 5.4-s or 10.8-s rhythm strip. The MAC-1 is also useful for continuous-rhythm recording of three ECG leads during exercise—a task that normally requires specialized ECG instrumentation. This is possible because the digital filter eliminates the usual baseline-drift problems associated with recording exercise ECGs.

In the self-test mode, it cues the paper to run out at 5, 25, 50, and 100 mm/s and records step and sine-wave responses of several amplitudes through each amplifier. It adds ± 200 mV of offset voltage in all leads and checks for proper operation. It checks patient cable continuity. It requires that Leads I and V_5 be of the same polarity or notifies the operator if the leads are reversed.

Purchase of an additional 16-kbyte RAM permits R-wave synchronized averaging of surface His bundle potentials for research applications.

Office ECG terminal.   Comp-U-Med (1977) offers a commercial office ECG terminal that incorporates a microprocessor. Cue lights direct the operator to enter

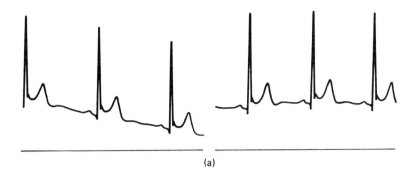

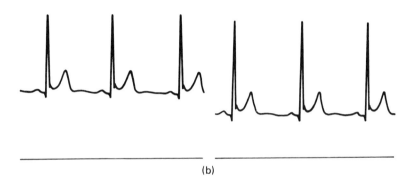

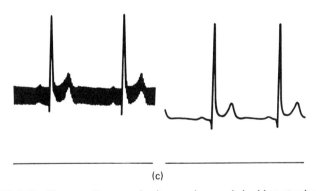

FIGURE 5.10 Electrocardiograms simultaneously recorded with a standard ECG machine (left traces) and the Microcomputer-Augmented Cardiograph (MAC-1) (right traces). (a) Lead V_5 with baseline drift. (b) Lead V_5 with amplitude saturation. (c) Lead II with excessive 60-Hz interference. (Compliments of Marquette Electronics, 1978.)

specific patient data into the pressure-sensitive keyboard. These include age, height, weight, blood pressure, medications, and I.D. An alphanumeric LED display verifies the patient data. The terminal automatically dials a remote computer center, which receives and analyzes the standard 12-lead ECG. In less than 30 s, the terminal's thermal printer and strip-chart recorder provide an ECG analysis and interpretation for the patient's medical record.

ECG data checking and compression

Several research systems using the microcomputer to check and compress ECG signals have been implemented, but they are not yet available commercially. We can easily transmit at most 1200 bits/s (baud) through the voice-grade telephone line, while at least 7500 baud is necessary for real-time ECG transmission of three channels simultaneously (i.e., 250 samples/s/channel, 10 bits/sample). But we know that ECG signals change their amplitude significantly only during a small percentage of the total ECG cycle. If we discard portions of the signal that are clinically unimportant, the signal can be compressed without any severe loss of information.

Bertrand et al. (1975) developed a data-compression device using an Intel 8008. The compression algorithm is based on the difference in amplitude between successive signal sample points. Whenever the difference exceeds a preset threshold value, the microprocessor saves the differential amplitude and the elapsed time since the last saved data. These data are transmitted by modem to the central computer. Such data compression solves the problem of limited baud rate of the telephone channel by reducing the amount of data that are sent. Also, this approach decreases the required ECG data-storage space required by the computer. Since this algorithm is based on the differences between successive data points that exceed a prespecified level, it is called delta coding with threshold. We discuss other coding algorithms for ECG data compression in Chapter 6.

ECG transmission

Only medium-size and large computers are used for diagnostic interpretation of the 12-lead ECG, because of the requisite complex algorithms, large amounts of digital data, and required processing speed. On the other hand, microcomputers are useful for acquiring, preprocessing, and transmitting ECG signals. Large hospitals can afford to install and maintain expensive ECG interpretation computing facilities, but small hospitals and rural clinics cannot generally afford their own facilities for this purpose.

One approach to providing such resources is hardwire connections between clinics and remote central facilities which are cost-shared by many users. However, the wiring cost increases as the distance increases. Therefore, a simple and reliable transmission system is important for ECG analysis. There are two basic techniques available for transmitting signals: telephone and radiotelemetry.

Telephone transmission. ECG signals are transmitted either using the voice-grade dial-up telephone network or by using a specially designed dataphone. We may select either digital or analog transmission. For digital transmission, three ECG leads at a time are amplified and filtered. After A/D conversion, these digital signals are transmitted over the telephone line by a digital modulator-demodulator (modem). Multiplexing permits several signals to be transmitted at the same time. The synchronized digital ECG signals are transmitted serially with individual identification codes. If each signal is transmitted for 3 s, it takes 12 s to transmit the complete 12-lead ECG. At the central computer, another modem translates the multiplexed signal into three digital signals; these signals are stored by the computer, where subsequent ECG analysis takes place, or by the digital tape recorder when the computer is busy or inoperative.

Analog transmission differs from digital transmission in that (1) data are transmitted over the telephone system in analog form using FM modems, (2) an A/D converter is interfaced to the central computer, and (3) an analog tape recorder is required. Although the analog method is used extensively, it has poor resolution and high sensitivity to noise. The digital method overcomes these difficulties but is more expensive.

Radiotelemetry. Wireless transmission by radiotelemetry gives maximum mobility for the patient. This method is used for transmitting ECGs from ambulatory patients in the intensive-care unit and from patients undergoing exercise ECG testing.

Because of its excellent electrical isolation, radiotelemetry is sometimes employed to reduce the possibility of electrical shock. Time- or frequency-division multiplexing provides for transmission of more than one signal on one carrier frequency.

5.3 PHYSIOLOGICAL MONITORING*

Intensive-care-unit (ICU) monitoring systems continuously monitor critically ill patients. They give a warning (visual or audible) to hospital personnel if any of the patients' vital body systems fail to perform properly, as measured against a predetermined set of criteria. Some of these vital body systems include the circulatory and respiratory systems, acid–base and metabolic control systems, and the central nervous system. An ICU monitoring system must provide enough measurable or computable quantities to permit a complete assessment of the vital body systems by comparing these quantities with the criteria predetermined by the physician. Only a small number of quantities need to be measured because the rest of the critical values may be computed from the measured ones. This means that the primary goal

---

*Section 5.3 written by Gregory S. Furno.

of ICU instrumentation is computation of critical patient parameters from acquired physiological data.

There is now a trend to distribute some of the computing into the patient bedside units. A microcomputer at the bedside can do data acquisition, display, reduction, and transmission to a central ICU computer. The bedside microcomputer thus acts as a preprocessor for a larger computer. We examine monitoring systems that use microprocessors in this section.

Cardiac monitoring

Electronics for Medicine (1979) uses a Z80 microcomputer in its ECG amplifier plug-in. It uses a special electrode that has two active elements in one housing. If skin motion causes a difference in potential between the two active elements, the microcomputer identifies the artifact, suspends QRS processing, and causes the rate meter to hold the last good data. The microcomputer's algorithm recognizes artifact from muscle noise and similarly prevents false-positive alarms. A digital filter permits QRS detection in the presence of moderate artifact. The microcomputer also automatically resets the baseline, adjusts triggering sensitivity, and provides troubleshooting diagnostics.

Intensive care unit monitoring

A microprocessor-based bedside patient monitor utilizes an Intel 8080 microprocessor with 1 kbyte of RAM, 4 kbytes of ROM, and a real-time digital clock (Moritz and Murdock, 1975). Currently, the instrument monitors heart rate, systolic, diastolic, and mean blood pressures, central venous pressure, pulmonary arterial pressure, and left arterial pressure. Any channel may be displayed along with the clock time either on command, or sequentially. The monitor may be connected to a minicomputer to provide mass data storage and to perform complex data manipulations.

The Unibed patient monitoring system replaces an entire range of traditional monitoring devices with a single, general-purpose unit (Deutsch et al., 1977). It recognizes the nature of the signal source and performs the appropriate processing step. All of the usual switches, knobs, dials, and meters have been replaced by a touch-sensitive character board and display. Firmware modules, microprocessor programs in ROMs, perform the physiological signal analysis, information display, and user interaction. Prototype clinical testing and evaluation are under way at the Dijhzigt Academic Hospital, Rotterdam, The Netherlands.

Commercial patient monitors

Figure 5.11 shows the major components of the General Electric Patient Data System. The bedside stations contain up to four plug-in modules which process the incoming data. The bedside station may function as a stand-alone unit, or it may communicate with a central or nurse's station containing an analog and alphanu-

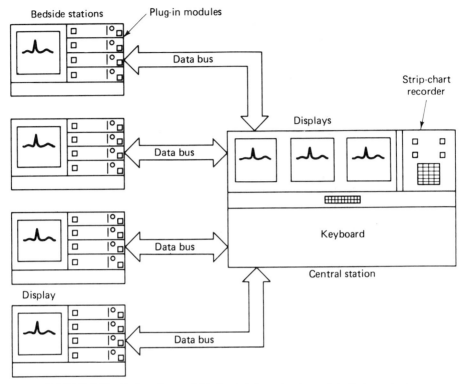

FIGURE 5.11 Each patient variable feeds into a plug-in module that may incorporate a microcomputer. This distributed processing in the bedside stations lightens the workload of the minicomputer in the central station.

meric CRT display and a special strip-chart recorder that prints parameter information directly for the patient's chart. Both stations incorporate microprocessors.

In an alternative system, more complex bedside stations communicate with a central station, which in turn communicates with a minicomputer station. The minicomputer station, consisting of a PDP-11, 28 kwords of memory, a disk controller, and a 1.2-Mword DEC pack cartridge disk, can serve up to three central stations, which in turn can each serve a maximum of 12 bedside stations. Any bedside or central station can access all of the computer functions, which include a simple patient admission and discharge routine, 32-h data storage, manual data entry, rapid data retrieval, trend plots, hard-copy report, cardiac output determinations, and dysrhythmia analysis. Microprocessor circuits in each bedside and central station organize, format, and transmit data over the various buses in ASCII code. Plug-in modules for the bedside stations are available to monitor the ECG; arterial, pulmonary artery, and venous blood pressure; thermal dilution cardiac output; respiration; temperature; and the EEG.

In the Spacelabs Alpha System plug-in circuit modules, or "cardules," accept input data from the patient, perform data processing, and communicate with other cardules over a common bus, referred to as simply a databus. The system uses two types of cardules called source and slave cardules. Source cardules, designed for bedside use, connect to the patient and process the incoming data, be it ECG, blood pressure, or temperature, depending upon the type of cardule. Slave cardules, used in larger systems where remote monitoring and control are desired (such as a nurse's station), communicate with designated bedside source cardules over the databus, providing a duplicate display and some control over the source cardule from remote locations. The cardules are housed in display terminal cabinets, which contain CRT displays for the presentation of data from either source or slave cardules. Strip-chart recorders may also be connected to the databus, controlled by the various cardules (both source and slave). Cardules are available that can process ECG, pressure, temperature, and respiration data, as well as perform trend analysis and selective monitoring of only those channels that exceed alarm limits. The Alpha system uses various microprocessors, including the Intel 4004 and the Rockwell PPS 8. This system required 20 worker-months of effort to develop the hardware, and 14 worker-months to develop the software. A combination of hand coding in machine code and in-circuit emulators was used to develop the software. Use of a microprocessor in this system allows for a redundancy and parallel processing capability for vital information, a higher benefit-to-cost ratio, and ease of service.

A microcomputer-based ICU system is available that uses the hospital's existing instrument front ends (Midwest Analog and Digital, 1978). The system acquires up to eight parameters on each of eight patients. It displays four nonfade traces in four different colors and shows alphanumeric patient data. It provides trend plots, alarms, and arrhythmia rates. A cursor feature provides opportunity for waveform examination; time intervals within ECGs and pressure traces; specific values of pressures or trends; and mean, maximum, and minimum values of pressures within selected intervals.

Arrhythmia analyzer

Jenkins et al. (1978) used an Intel 8085 to develop a bedside arrhythmia analyzer. It uses a swallowable pill-electrode for recording sharp atrial A waves from the esophagus and records a standard surface lead II on a second channel. Use of a 500-Hz clock permits accurate resolution of four intervals: AA, AR, RR, and QRS width. The program operates between clock pulses and classifies a number of arrhythmias.

Hemodynamic monitoring

Another instrument monitors hemodynamic variables derived from arterial blood-pressure measurements (Donati et al., 1978). It has greater pattern recognition and storage capabilities than does an analog monitor and is less expensive than a dedicated minicomputer-based system. For each of two patients, it can acquire an electrocardiogram and arterial and left atrial blood pressures. It can recognize the beginning of each cardiac cycle, eliminate aberrant beats, identify the dicrotic notch, and compute 10 hemodynamic parameters on a minute-to-minute basis. It can print results every minute and can store in memory 4 h of results for each patient. The monitoring proceeds according to this fixed cycle.

For $T = 0$ to 15 s, the instrument (1) acquires signals from patient A; (2) defines the beginning of each cardiac cycle based on timing criteria derived from recognition of the QRS complex; (3) eliminates all but four cardiac cycles, rejecting those showing the largest deviation from the mean systolic pressure; and (4) recognizes the dicrotic notch.

For $T = 15$ to 30 s, the instrument (1) computes the systolic pressure, diastolic pressure, mean pressure, endocardial viability ratio, heart rate, peripheral resistance, stroke volume, stroke work, stroke power, and cardiac output; (2) performs averaging over the retained cardiac cycles; and (3) prints the results and the time of day.

For $T = 30$ to 45 s, the instrument performs the procedure of the first 15 s for patient B, and for $T = 45$ to 60 s, it computes and prints results for patient B.

A 30-character/s printing terminal and an x-y cathode-ray tube are the peripherals. The system uses a prioritized interrupt structure and a simple, 10-command monitor to allow the user to interactively define parameters, inquire about system status, request printouts and trend displays, and control calibration procedures. A prototype is presently undergoing clinical evaluation.

Respiratory monitoring

The Chemetron Corp. has developed the RICS II microprocessor-based respiratory intensive-care system (Chemetron, 1977). It sequentially monitors up to 16 critical patients and continuously monitors one patient.

The system displays the following parameters in graphic form for trend analysis or in tabular form for the patient history (see Fig. 5.12):

1. F_1O_2—fractional inspired oxygen concentration.
2. P_EO_2—expired oxygen concentration.
3. F_1CO_2—fractional inspired carbon dioxide concentration.
4. P_ECO_2—expired carbon dioxide concentration.
5. Respiratory rate.
6. Expiration/inspiration ratio.

Respired gases from up to 16 patients are sequentially drawn into the Medspect medical mass spectrometer for analysis. The RICS II microcomputer contains 8 kbytes of RAM and 12 kbytes of program stored in EPROM. The microcomputer is dedicated to the acquisition, storage, analysis, and display of the raw data acquired by the Medspect.

In one mode, the RICS II sequentially monitors up to 16 patients selected

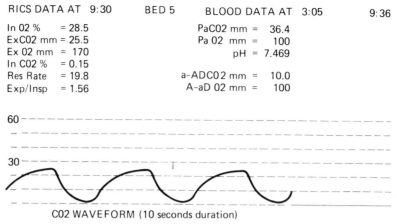

RICS DATA AT 9:30   BED 5   BLOOD DATA AT 3:05   9:36

In 02 %   = 28.5   PaCO2 mm =   36.4
ExCO2 mm = 25.5   Pa 02 mm =   100
Ex 02 mm = 170   pH = 7.469
In CO2 %   = 0.15
Res Rate   = 19.8   a-ADCO2 mm =   10.0
Exp/Insp   = 1.56   A-aD 02 mm =   100

CO2 WAVEFORM (10 seconds duration)

FIGURE 5.12 Example of patient status format, showing parameters obtained during most recent ward scan. The CO_2 waveform displayed is from a stored record of 10 s duration of the waveform at that time. (Compliments of Chemetron, 1977.)

from a maximum of 28 beds. Up to 24 h of data are stored in the microcomputer if the ward scan is performed every hour or up to 12 h of data are stored in the microcomputer if scanned every half-hour. Other features of RICS II are high and low alarms of F_IO_2 and P_ECO_2. Whenever F_IO_2 and P_ECO_2 are beyond the preset limits, the alarm light on the diagnostic panel indicates an alarm condition and the ward display indicates the specific patient.

In another mode, the RICS II is used for continuous, uninterrupted single-patient monitoring. It displays patient respiratory data, including the breath-by-breath real-time CO_2 waveform. All the six parameters measured are updated every 2 min and displayed on the console.

The RICS II system provides information to help wean the patient from the ventilator systematically and safely. This information displays (1) trends in the alveolar–arterial O_2 and arterial–alveolar CO_2 gradients; (2) changes in alveolar CO_2 concentrations that may indicate changing respiratory status; (3) actual and expected inspired O_2 concentrations, thereby detecting potentially hazardous errors in gas mixing; and (4) regulator function. This information reduces the dangers of over- and underoxygenation.

Obstetrical monitoring

DeHart and Barclay (1978) use a Cromemco Z80 microcomputer system to monitor uterine pressure. The system has keyboard display, mini-floppy disk, and 24 kbytes of memory. The system samples uterine pressure every 2 s and computes and displays for each contraction: (1) maximum pressure, (2) maximum time derivative of pressure, (3) the velocity of muscular contraction, and (4) the flow per unit force (which represents the effectiveness with which the uterus is expelling the fetus). The system is programmed primarily in BASIC and has its own operating system, which provides assembly, listing, loading, editing, and testing capabilities. It provides for reading or writing to memory, calls to assembly subroutines, access to disk data files, chaining from one program to another stored on the disk, and access to all input/output devices.

Figure 5.13 shows a microprocessor-based data acquisition and preprocessing system used to monitor obstetrical patients (Lin et al., 1977). The system continuously monitors the fetal heart rate (FHR), intrauterine pressure (IUP), cervical dilation, and fetal descent, and it determines the fetal trajectory during labor and delivery. The system preprocesses fetal descent signals obtained from ultrasonic transducers and converts the raw data to the "station" measurements routinely used by clinicians. Preprocessing also helps reject random noise, and performs some preliminary data compression to put the data in more traditional clinical terms. A PDP-11/45 program which uses pattern recognition to extract and recognize uterine contractions from intrauterine pressure data will be adapted for use in the microprocessor preprocessing unit. A multichannel oscillograph provides real-time display of selected raw signals or preprocessed data, and an *x-y* plotter plots trends

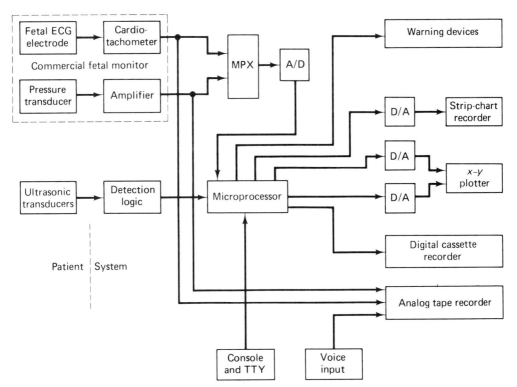

FIGURE 5.13 Obstetrical data-acquisition and preprocessing system. (From Feng, C. H., et al., 1976. A microprocessor-based data acquisition and preprocessing system for obstetrical patient monitoring. Proc. Annu. Conf. Eng. Med. Biol. 18:189. Used with permission.)

of the cervical dilation or fetal descent data during labor. An analog tape recorder provides secondary backup for the analog data and also provides a voice channel for recording clinical information for future study. A digital cassette recorder retains preprocessed data in quantitative engineering terms for detailed off-line analysis.

The microprocessor controls the timing and sequence of data acquisition and data transfer among the various I/O devices. It also performs calibration, identification of acquired data, monitoring of the status of peripheral I/O devices, and outputting of error messages in case of any hardware failure. The microcomputer may be programmed to perform data reduction, analysis, and presentation; on-the-spot decision making, and warning signal presentation. An MOS Technology 6502 8-bit microprocessor was used because of its availability, low total cost, simplicity, programmability, and strong I/O capability. The 1-Hz real-time clock is derived from the 60-Hz power line. The system has 2 kbytes of PROM and 1 kbyte of RAM. A control for the obstetrician is being developed and an engineering console is provided for system processing and program debugging. In case of a system malfunction, a LED display provides a diagnostic error code. D/A converters provide outputs of raw signals or diagnosis data on a multichannel oscillograph or an x-y plotter.

A cross assembler for the 6502 written in PDP-11 MACRO generates the machine code, which is directly programmed into a UV EPROM chip (Intel 1702 or 2708) through an Intel universal PROM programmer (UPP) under the program control of the PDP-11.

Gibbons and Johnson (1976) have developed an Intel 8080 microprocessor-based fetal monitor. The system includes 4 kbytes of RAM and 512 bytes of EPROM. Modularity has been considered in the design of the system. For instance, a bedside module can be added to the system at a parts cost of about $600. The total hardware cost of the system is less than $4000 for all components plus a Tele-type. Different programs may be stored in preprogrammed ROM modules, selectable with pushbuttons. The device works in real time, taking 30 ms for calculations between each two heart beats. The tasks of the device are to calculate and display on a CRT screen the cumulative dip area of the FHR for each 10-min epoch, together with an R-to-R-interval histogram. Figure 5.14 shows the FHR and its dip area together with the IUP curve.

Neonatal apnea monitoring

A number of companies sell monitors for apnea detection and alarm for the neonate. All these products have significant problems with false-positive and false-negative alarms because of artifacts. No practical artifact-free technique exists for monitoring respiration. Approaches that have been used include motion detection using ultrasound or an air-filled mattress, impedance pneumography, and heart-rate analysis.

Flax and Yount (1978) developed a microprocessor-based apnea monitor that

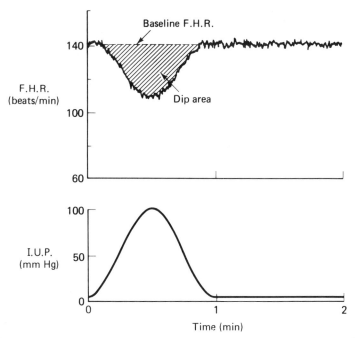

FIGURE 5.14 Fetal heart rate (FHR) and intrauterine pressure (IUP). Dip area is indicated. (From Gibbons, D. T., and Johnson, F. 1976. Microprocessors in fetal monitoring. Dig. Int. Conf. Med. Biol. Eng., pp. 556–557.)

attempts to overcome the artifact problem by using pattern-recognition techniques. Although their device is a research tool, their approach deserves further exploration for its commercial potential. They use a modest single-board microcomputer (MOS Technology KIM-1) interfaced to a mercury-in-rubber strain gage transducer which encircles the thorax of the infant. The microcomputer monitors the resistance changes caused by length changes of the mercury transducer during respiration and compares these patterns to patterns defined by an algorithm as normal. The microcomputer classifies the signals into (1) expiratory movement, (2) inspiratory movement, (3) lack of activity, and (4) noise. Thus the microcomputer algorithm ignores hiccups and other artifacts that do not follow a normal respiratory pattern. Only when lack of activity persists beyond a predetermined interval does the microcomputer signal apnea. When apnea is detected, the operator simply manipulates the infant to restore respiration, thus preventing death.

Katona et al. (1977) have developed a system for continuous monitoring of high-risk infants. The system consists of an Intel 8080 microprocessor operating as a memory drive. In conjunction with commercially available vital-sign monitors (Beckman 100B or KDC vital sign monitor), it is capable of making strip-chart records of potentially life-threatening episodes in continuously monitored infants. The system records each of these episodes for 90 s, of which 60 s is prior to the occurrence of the episode.

The memory device consists of a memory subsystem and a trigger subsystem. The inputs to the memory subsystem are the physiological signals obtained through the vital-sign monitor. The outputs are the same physiological signals after a desired time delay. The inputs to the trigger subsystems are the alarm signals from the vital-sign monitor. The trigger subsystem then provides signals to (1) turn on the recorder for a preselected period, (2) provide a marker to indicate the origin of the alarm, and (3) blank a length of strip chart to separate different episodes.

The Intel 8080 microprocessor sequentially samples four input channels through a multiplexed 8-bit A/D converter and stores the information in a 32-byte RAM, which serves as a circular buffer. After the desired delay, the microprocessor outputs the information through four D/A converters. The 334-byte-long program is stored in two 256-byte PROMs. The sampling frequency for each of the four input signals is individually selectable using pushbuttons. The delay is automatically adjusted to provide a full circular memory of 30,720 samples, regardless of the sampling rate.

For example, assume that the first channel (ECG) is sampled at the rate of 256 samples/s, the second and third channels (two respiration waveforms) are sampled at 128 samples/s, and the fourth channel is inactive. Then the total time delay is obtained by dividing 30,720 samples by the sum of all the sampling rates used for the channels (512 samples/s). Therefore, the total delay time is 60 s (30,720/512).

The advantages of using a microprocessor over other conventional devices are the following. The longest delay obtainable utilizing commercially available shift registers is about 15 to 20 s, with a sampling rate of at least 200 samples/s. This delay is insufficient for apnea monitoring. Tape loops suitable for producing long delays are not a good choice for the clinical environment because of the necessity of maintenance. While a special-purpose system could have been built using discrete devices and shift registers, the use of a microprocessor and RAMs provides an opportunity to use the memory subsystem as a general-purpose controller. The other special features that can be added to the system are classification and counting of different types of alarms, keeping track of the time of occurrence of alarms, and storing the sampled waveforms for further computer-aided analysis. The cost of the components is approximately $2000, of which half is for the RAM.

Animal monitoring

Several microcomputer-based instruments have been developed for use in physiology laboratories. Schoenfeld et al. (1977) describe several microcomputer-based instruments developed for biologists by their engineering support group. The instrument shown in Fig. 5.15 uses an M6800 microprocessor, 512-byte RAM, and 128-byte ROM to simultaneously detect movement or licking in 12 animal cages. Processed activity is printed out on paper tape and includes time of day, trial number, and number of licks or movements.

Hathaway et al. (1976b) used an Intel 4004 microprocessor, UV EPROMs,

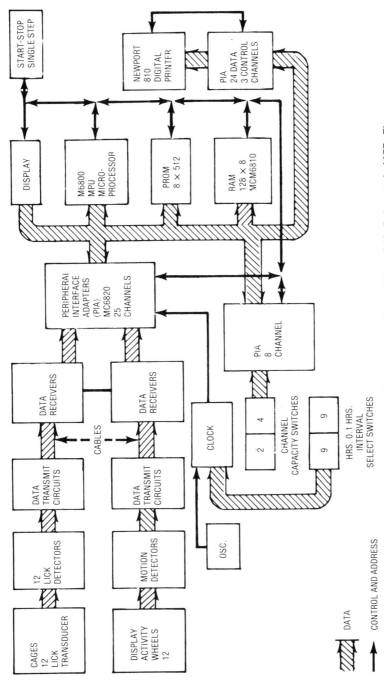

FIGURE 5.15 24-channel activity data recorder. [From Schoenfeld, R. L., et al. 1977. The microprocessor in the biological laboratory. Computer 10(5): 56–67.]

and RAMs to build a general-purpose data acquisition and processing system. Its applications include trend plotting during animal surgery and measurement, calculation, and plotting of data from experiments.

Hosek (1976) developed a microprocessor-based physiological data recorder for long-term monitoring of monkeys. The data recorder follows changes in systolic, diastolic, and mean blood pressure; maximum and minimum left ventricular pressure; interbeat interval (heart rate); and the integral of a signal obtained from an electromagnetic flow probe at the aorta. The Intel 8008 microprocessor handles sampling of the analog signals as they come from processing circuitry for conversion to digital form. A system monitor allows the user to execute any of the following software packages: an editor-assembler and loaders and routines for sampling, calibration, tape handling, and for interaction with a large-scale computer, the Univac 1106. Data may be stored on cassette or transmitted to the Decwriter or Univac. The microprocessor simplifies the hardware design and relieves the large computer of much of the control work.

Alexander and Hosek (1978) utilized an 8080 with 32 kbytes of memory to build the laboratory physiological data system shown in Fig. 5.16. During animal experiments they acquired up to 16 signals, multiplexed them through an A/D converter, computed heart rate and cardiac output, averaged evoked potentials, and

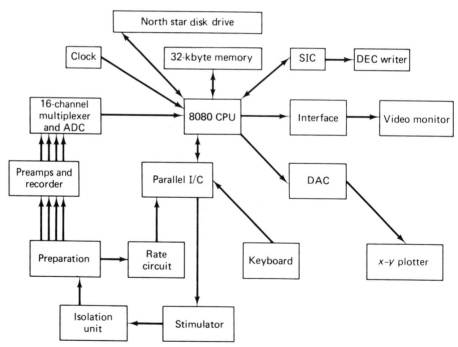

FIGURE 5.16 Animal physiological data recorder. (From Alexander, G., and Hosek, R. S. 1978. Microprocessorized laboratory physiological data system. Proc. Annu. Conf. Eng. Med. Biol. 20 : 157. Used with permission.)

printed, plotted, or recorded output. They used machine-language subroutines for rapid data acquisition but the easier-to-use BASIC interpreter for most programming.

Valvano et al. (1978) used an Intel 8080 in a research data acquisition system for measuring local tissue blood flow. A heated thermistor probe is cooled by increased blood flow. The microcomputer permits flexible operator control, permits sophisticated plotting routines, and utilizes mass storage on magnetic tape. It allows (1) measurement of baseline tissue temperature, (2) application and measurement of power supplied to the thermistor, (3) simultaneous operation of four thermistor probes, and (4) operation in either the transient or continuous mode. Either allows the determination of effective thermal conductivity and hence local tissue blood flow.

Another microprocessor-based device (Dennis and Cywinski, 1976) uses a signal-averaging technique to record a low-level preventricular electrical signal related to the activity in the cardiac conduction system. The device uses an Intel 8080 microprocessor together with analog circuits which provide high amplification, automatic gain control, and analog filtering. A 12-bit A/D converter, together with automatic gain control, provide a dynamic range of 12 μV to 2 mV. A memory buffer containing 24-bit words stores the accumulated data sum. Up to 256 signal cycles can be averaged. This work demonstrates the potential for recording weak repetitive signals in the presence of noise using simple microprocessor-based instruments.

5.4 PULMONARY INSTRUMENTATION*

Research impedance pneumograph

Figure 5.17 shows the block diagram of an impedance pneumograph that utilizes an 8080A microprocessor (Schmalzel et al., 1977). The instrument uses a constant current drive and provides for selection of either a two-, three-, or four-electrode configuration (see Section 1.3). Use of a microcomputer permits selection of magnitude, frequency, and guarded electrode voltages. The instrument measures the magnitude and the phase angle of the detected signal with respect to the drive signal. The magnitude and frequency of the constant current drive can be varied from 0.02 to 1 mA, and from 1 to 99 kHz.

After amplification, the AM demodulator detects the magnitude of the amplitude-modulated impedance signal. Phase detection is achieved by gating a fast clock to a counter for a period equal to the time difference between the zero-crossing detector outputs of the drive and the detected signal. The count is then a linear function of the phase difference between the two signals.

An analog-to-digital (A/D) converter provides the interface between the demodulator and the microprocessor. The operator chooses the drive variables to

---

*Section 5.4 written by Dhruba P. Das.

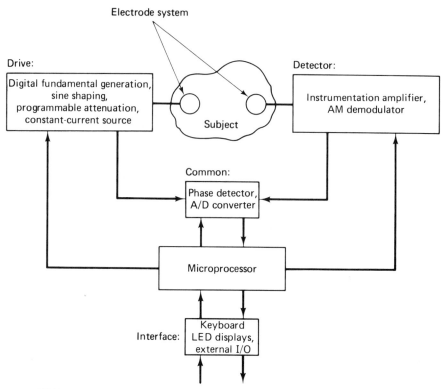

FIGURE 5.17 Impedance pneumograph block diagram. (From Schmalzel, J. L., et al. 1977. An impedance pneumograph utilizing microprocessor based instrumentation. Biomed. Sci. Instrum. 13 : 63–68. Used with permission of ISA.)

be displayed on the front-panel LEDs and the digital information to be communicated to an external I/O device. The microprocessor provides both control and communication functions.

The microprocessor is on a 3.5-in. by 4.5-in. card which also contains 512 bytes of UV EPROM, 128 bytes of RAM, separate 8-bit input and output ports, and all necessary timing circuits and control decoding.

The use of a microprocessor provides versatility and the ability to perform a programmed experimental procedure repeatedly with good reproducibility. This is particularly important in the case of impedance techniques when electrode geometry and placement are varied, and also when different subjects are used. The instrument took two worker-months for the software development, using hand coding in machine code. Hardware costs were about $2000.

Pulmonary function testing

General-purpose instruments. Honeywell (1978) uses General Instrument's CP-1600 microcomputer in their MEDDARS portable data-gathering/analyzing instrument. The system's clinical diagnostic applications include pulmonary-function lab activities and cardiac catheterization. Signal-conditioning modules detect biopotentials, pressures, and temperatures. On the nonfade display, the microcomputer shows alphanumeric characters, cursors, gridlines, and trace identification. It automatically calibrates each signal-conditioning module, stores protocols, controls I/O, and self-checks all key functions.

Gianunzio et al. (1978) use an Intel 8080 with 8 kbytes of PROM and 8 kbytes of RAM for assessing lung function. It acquires data from four analog inputs, processes it, and displays both x-y plots and printed copy. An audio cassette tape loads the BASIC language processor into RAM. The PROM contains the system monitor and routines for sampling, storing, and displaying the data. A cursor routine permits selection of portions of data for processing. The system processes standard lung function tests and also measures total pulmonary resistance and dynamic compliance.

Spirometry. Collins (1978) mates a conventional spirometer with a microprocessor to ease pulmonary function testing. It provides cueing lights to keyboard-enter patient data, time, and ambient temperature. From a forced vital-capacity maneuver and a maximal voluntary ventilation maneuver it calculates and prints 13 temperature-corrected test results.

Field testing. Slezak et al. (1978) use the MOS Technology 6502 microprocessor on the KIM-1 board to speed pulmonary function testing in the field. A potentiometer on a water-filled spirometer generates an electrical signal that drives the microcomputer. The microcomputer requests constants from the operator, stores the pulmonary volume data, and calculates and displays (1) vital capacity, (2) forced expiratory volume, (3) midmaximal flow, and (4) peak flow.

Flow-volume loops. Med-Science Electronics (1977) uses two 8080s to process lung-function data. The patient blows into a bellows spirometer as hard as possible and then sucks in the air just expired. Two 8080s then generate a flow-volume loop in real time as well as a brief statistical analysis. From these data doctors can determine the health of the patient's lungs and diagnose the severity of such diseases as asthma. One 8080 handles data-input routines and analyzes the data; the second performs housekeeping duties and formats the real-time graphics. The system uses 4 kbytes of static RAM, 8 kbytes of dynamic RAM, and 12 kbytes of EPROM.

Pulmonary compliance. Hsiao et al. (1978) use a 6502 microprocessor with 4 kbytes of memory to measure the elastic properties of the lung. In 250 ms they inject a 400 ml/s pulse of air into the airway. They monitor pressure and flow waveforms at the airway opening. The compliance is inversely proportional to the slope of the pressure ramp and proportional to the flow magnitude. The microcomputer calculates pulmonary compliance from a single pulse within a single respiratory cycle.

Whole-body plethysmograph

Dowling et al. (1978) use an 8080 microcomputer to acquire data from a whole-body plethysmograph (body box). The operator types the selected test on a keyboard. The instrument responds by loading the necessary program into memory and executing it. Software directs the operator through a calibration sequence for the variables: mouth flow, mouth pressure, and box flow. It compensates for amplitude and phase distortion and displays the results graphically and numerically.

Pulmonary edema detection

Wax et al. (1978) use the MOS Technology 6502 microprocessor on the KIM-1 board to study the production, detection, and prevention of pulmonary edema of dogs. From airway pressure and flow transducers, the microcomputer detects inspiration. It sums the flow signal at a 180-Hz rate, thus calculating tidal volume. They multiply each flow reading by the pressure reading and sum these products to yield total work. Other calculations yield dynamic compliance and elastic work. Changes in these results detect early increases in interstitial fluid.

Ventilator monitoring systems

Figure 5.18 shows a simplified diagram of a ventilation monitoring system (Hathaway et al., 1976a). Analog signal inputs are tidal volume, flow, and pressure. In addition, there is a fourth logic signal which tells the microprocessor whether the ventilator is in the inspiratory or expiratory phase.

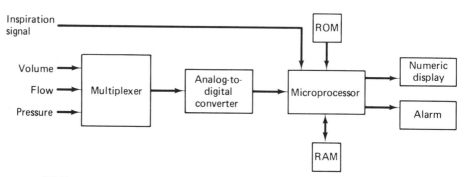

FIGURE 5.18 Block diagram of a microprocessor-based ventilator-monitoring system.

The system uses a 4-bit CPU (Intel 4004), 80 words of RAM, and 512 words of program memory (ROM) for storing various subroutines for signal processing and display. Various subroutines are used to (1) control the sampling sequence and start A/D conversion of the sampled data, (2) process the pressure signal to obtain peak pressure during inspiration, (3) determine minute volume (volume expired in 1 min) and minute leak (difference between the inspired and the expired volumes over 1 min), and (4) display the data on front-panel LEDs. The parameters that are displayed are inspired tidal volume, minute volume, minute leak, and peak inspiratory pressure. Alarm signals are triggered whenever an input signal crosses a set limit.

The microprocessor permits system flexibility with reduced hardware complexity. Also, the system has potential for further development, since functions can be added or changed by reprogramming.

Automated rodent respiratory monitor

Decker et al. (1976) developed a microprocessor-based data recording and retrieval system to determine the effects of cigarette smoking on Fisher rats. Figure 5.19 shows the system block diagram. The system monitors total inhaled volume (V), tidal volume (V_T), and respiratory frequency of Fisher rats before, during, and after exposure to cigarette smoke.

The V_T and V are both obtained by integrating the tidal flow rate ($\dot{V}$) detected by the pneumotachometer. A strip-chart recorder continuously displays both $\dot{V}$ and V. The system is also sensitive to small changes in V_T and respiratory frequency in order to evaluate the effects on rats of exposure to smoke from different types of

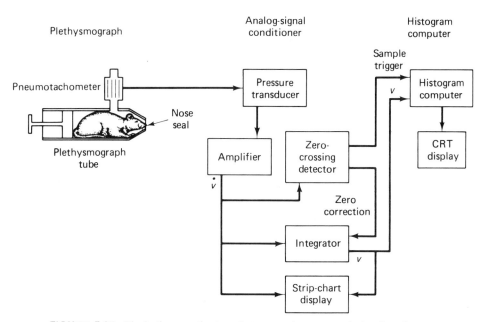

FIGURE 5.19 Block diagram of rat respiratory monitor system depicted as three subsystems: plethysmograph tube, analog signal conditioner and display, and histogram computer display. (From Decker, J. R., et al. 1976. Automated rodent respiratory monitor and histogram computer. Biomed. Sci. Instrum. 12: 7–13. Used with permission of ISA.)

experimental cigarettes. The microprocessor computes and the CRT displays both the tidal volume and respiratory period as histograms.

The output of a zero-crossing detector resets the volume integrator at the end of each exhalation, which is also used as a zero reference to allow measurement of V_T. The zero-crossing detector also supplies a sample trigger to the histogram computer and triggers a breath counter to count the number of breaths during a recording period.

The functions of the histogram computer are controlled by an Intel 8008-1 (ProLog model 8111) CPU. The sample trigger initiates the A/D conversion of the volume integrator output. The resulting digital value which represents V_T is stored in a memory array in a histogram representation of tidal volume. The time duration between two successive sample triggers is stored as a histogram of respiratory period. Both histograms are displayed simultaneously on the Tektronix 603 CRT monitor. For V_T, the cell size of the histogram can be varied from 0.01 to 0.08 ml and has its maximum resolution of 256 cells with the smallest cell size. The cell size of the period histogram can also be varied from 0.01 to 0.08 s. The most significant cells for each case are 2.56 ml and 2.56 s, respectively. The histogram computer also computes the average tidal volume (number of breaths times average tidal volume). The estimated overall error in recording volume is within $\pm 5\%$ of the correct volumes, and in recording respiratory period less than 1%.

5.5 ANESTHESIA MACHINE*

We present an example of the flexibility afforded by incorporating a microcomputer into an anesthesia machine for the delivery of inhalation anesthetics.

Boston anesthesia system

Developed at Massachusetts General Hospital, the Boston anesthesia system makes extensive use of the digital "on–off" design philosophy to enable the microcomputer to control gas flows and anesthetic concentrations. While the breathing circuit remains essentially unaltered, electronic digital control of these functions increases the system reliability by requiring fewer moving parts. They chose a microprocessor for this control because of the inherent flexibility and the ease with which they could modify the prototype. Figure 5.20 shows the overall system.

Gas flow control.   Digital valves in the prototype system replace the needle valves and rotameters of conventional anesthesia equipment. Each valve is composed of eight orifices that open or close under microcomputer control. A sonic nozzle in each orifice allows the calibration of gas flow through the orifice as a function of upstream pressure, orifice cross-sectional area, and temperature. The cross-sectional areas of the individual orifices have flows that are related in a binary manner; that

*Section 5.5 written by Gary V. Sprenger.

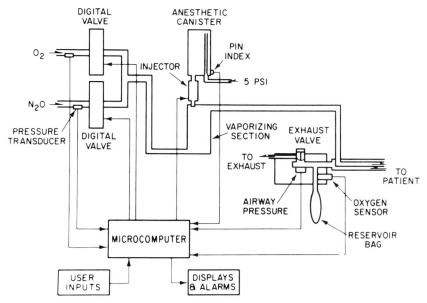

FIGURE 5.20 Overall system diagram of the Boston anesthesia system. [From Cooper, J. B., et al. 1978. A new anesthesia delivery system. Anesthesiology 49(5) : 310–318. Used with permission.]

is, each successively larger orifice allows twice the flow of the previous one at the same upstream pressure. After the user enters the desired flow via the display and control panel, the microcomputer measures the upstream pressure (via pressure transducer) and opens the appropriate orifice(s). The two gases then mix and make up the total fresh gas flow.

Control of liquid anesthetic vaporization.   A digital injector system that resembles the fuel injection system found in some automobiles replaces the vaporizer of the conventional anesthesia machine. To enter the fluid dynamics, the user reads a code found on the anesthetic agent reservoir and enters it into the microcomputer. The user then enters the desired anesthetic concentration. Since the fluid pressure and dynamics are known, the microcomputer calculates the injector on–off periods (pulse width) required to achieve the desired concentration at the current total fresh gas flow. A thermistor placed in the injection flow ensures the actual injection of anesthetic agent. A copper vaporization coil completely vaporizes the anesthetic after the injector nozzle atomizes it. A major advantage of this system is that temperature compensation is no longer required because the vaporization process does not lower the temperature of the remaining liquid anesthetic.

Microcomputer controller.   An Intel 8080 microprocessor controls the system. At the time the project was undertaken, it was the only microprocessor with available hardware and software support (Trautman et al., 1976). The control functions are:

1. Read sensors.
2. Compute effector settings from operator commands and sensor readings.
3. Set effectors.

The communication functions are:

1. Interpret user commands from the control panel.
2. Display current control settings and measured values.
3. Display alarms of unsafe or inappropriate conditions.

Display. A bar-graph display (Burroughs BG 16101-2) displays current control settings and sensor readings for airway pressure and expired oxygen. Increment/ decrement switches scanned by the microcomputer change the control settings. Two ranges of resolution correspond to high and low flow rates. For example, at high flow rates the total gas flow display range is 0 to 10 liters/min. At low flows the display reads 0 to 1 liter/min. It also displays various user alarm and warning messages. Currently, it displays 16 such messages one at a time, in order of decreasing priority. An audio alarm signals the user of an inappropriate setting or dangerous equipment dysfunction once every 5 s. Depending on the severity of the problem, the microcomputer also readjusts dangerous settings if not rectified by the user after a predetermined amount of time. Figure 5.21 shows the control and display panel.

System development and cost. Hardware for the anesthesia delivery system was developed on an Intel 8080 development system. Software was developed on the MIT MULTICS computer system in PL/M language (a higher-level language developed for microcomputers by Intel Corp.). Total development costs to date are estimated at $150,000. Prototype duplication cost is estimated at approximately $15,000. Commercial manufacturing should lower costs to a level competitive with conventional anesthesia equipment (Cooper et al., 1978).

5.6 OPERATING ROOM MONITORING*

Anesthesia monitoring and control

Blom et al. (1979) have developed a compact anesthesia monitor and controller. Every 20 ms it samples up to 32 channels of data from regular physiological monitors and converts to 12-bit accuracy. It monitors signals from the ventilatory system (concentrations of O_2, CO_2, and halothane; flow; pressure; and ventilator settings) and the circulatory system (ECG, arterial and venous pressures, core and skin temperature, and earlobe plethysmogram). It preprocesses these data as follows. It determines maxima and minima of respiratory flow, pressure, and gas con-

---

*Section 5.6 written by Gary V. Sprenger.

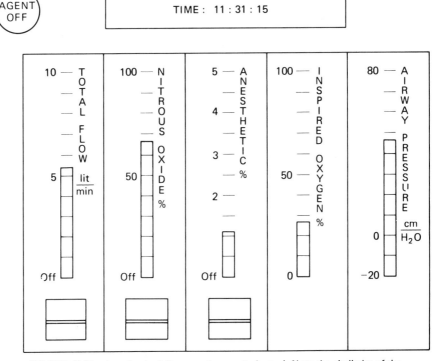

FIGURE 5.21 Anesthesia delivery system control panel. Note the similarity of the plasma displays to conventional rotameters. (From Trautman, E. D., et al. 1976. A new anesthesia delivery system using microprocessors. Proc. Electro 76 Prof. Prog., 13–4.)

centrations. From central venous pressure it calculates the mean pressure. It also calculates parameters based on two or more input signals. For example, from respiratory flow and pressure, it calculates airway resistance and respiratory work.

If there is a sudden change in the input signals, it automatically detects an error and classifies it. Errors may be caused by equipment problems such as transducer malfunction or by changes in the state of the patient.

The microprocessor is a 16-bit LSI-11, chosen because there were several other PDP-11 computers available locally with excellent edit and assembler facilities. An 8-kword core memory permitted construction of a more compact unit than would have been possible with a floppy-disk unit. An ASCII keyboard permits typing commands for calibration; then the system prompts the user through all the procedural steps.

A video display terminal provides feedback for tasks that require user intervention and also displays specific error messages.

A custom-built display unit displays 16 three-digit numbers, which are updated every second. A display channel flashes if software detects an error. A 1200-baud custom-built modem transmits by FSK a complete record-keeping log of a 4-h operation to a cassette tape recorder.

Advantages of the system are: (1) all information for the anesthesiologist is grouped on one numeric display unit, (2) more information is available to the anesthesiologist, (3) calibration is easier, (4) it signals sudden changes by flashing the display, and (5) it performs automatic recordkeeping.

Because of the flexibility of the microcomputer, the system is easily expanded. For example, the group is currently developing a model that will predict the most probable future state of the patient and signal significant deviations from this prediction.

Physiological trend monitoring

Rampil and Flemming (1978) use a Z80 microcomputer to collect, format, and display physiological parameters monitored during surgery. Previously, the anesthesiologist monitored and recorded the data every 5 min or whenever he or she detected the need. The new system automatically plots the data on a television screen so that the anesthesiologist can observe trends and reconstruct incidents.

From commercial monitors, the system acquires data such as (1) arterial blood pressure, (2) heart rate, (3) venous pressure, (4) intercranial pressure, (5) nasopharyngeal temperature, and (6) end tidal CO_2. Figure 5.22 shows that it uses a Z80 microcomputer with 26 kbytes of RAM and audio-cassette bulk storage. The formatted data update 8 kbytes of additional RAM that drive the point-plotting video graphics display on a television monitor. The Z80 plots alphanumeric data through a separate controller. The hardware cost was $2500.

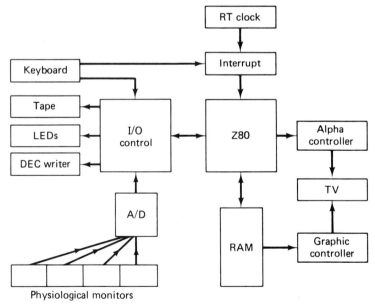

FIGURE 5.22 Hardware block diagram of surgical trend-monitoring system. (From Rampil, I. J., and Flemming, D. C. 1978. An inexpensive microcomputer trend monitoring system. Proc. New. Engl. Bioeng. Conf. 6:67–70.)

Clinical use has demonstrated the following advantages: (1) it recognizes events such as brief hypotensive episodes that were completely missed by conventional techniques; (2) it stores data during crises when the anesthesiologist is totally occupied by emergency management; and (3) it establishes responses to test doses of hypotensive drugs and thus assists in determining therapeutic doses.

5.7 ELECTROENCEPHALOGRAPHY*

Until recently, electroencephalographers have analyzed EEG tracings visually and have only just begun to employ automatic methods. Historically, there have been four methods of EEG analysis. One method separates the EEG into five frequency bands: delta, theta, alpha, beta, and gamma. In addition to the normal frequencies, there is spikey, impulse-noise-like, abnormal EEG activity associated with epilepsy. EEGs are also examined for abnormalities related to interhemispheric asymmetries and low-frequency (delta) wave sources. Analysis of frequency-to-amplitude ratios is another method used to discriminate normal EEGs from abnormal ones.

Automated EEG analysis methods in most respects are enhancements of the traditional methods mentioned above and fall into five groups: (1) power spectral analysis, (2) zero-crossing analysis, (3) pattern recognition, (4) amplitude histogram analysis, and (5) heuristic methods for detecting spikes.

Power spectral analysis

Power spectral analysis requires that 8 to 16 channels of EEG data be digitized and analyzed using a fast Fourier transform program. The resulting components are smoothed and plotted. Bickford et al. (1972) provide more information on this type of analysis.

Butler (1977, 1978) uses a TI 990/4 16-bit microcomputer to process EEG signals of surgical patients. To maximize the EEG signal without A/D converter saturation, the microcomputer determines maximum signal excursions of previous data. Then it sets the gain of a digitally controlled gain stage. Thus 8-bit A/D conversion is adequate for EEG signals. A 60-Hz sample rate synchronized to the power frequency reduces 60-Hz interference. Four-second epochs of data are fast-Fourier-transformed in 160 ms and rapidly displayed on a monitor. An x-y plotter also presents 2 h of side-by-side compressed spectral arrays with hidden line suppression. Both rapid individual spectra and the slower trend record are used in monitoring during anesthesia.

Zero-crossing analyses

Electroencephalographers often employ zero-crossing analysis, also called "period" or "wavelength" analysis. The analysis involves determining the number of zero crossings in a specified time interval, usually 1 s. Although this information is use-

---

*Section 5.7 written by Peter D. Gadsby.

ful, the amplitude information concerning the EEG process is discarded. Doyle (1976) reported a method of EEG analysis using a microcomputer. He amplified the potential difference between the two electrodes 10,000 times and fed it into a 1-bit quantizer. The output of the quantizer is in the logical 1 state whenever the instantaneous EEG signal is positive, and is in the logical 0 state otherwise. The quantizer is sampled every 5 ms. When the quantizer changes state, the system records a zero crossing.

The analysis system is composed of an 8-bit microprocessor (MOS Technology 6502), 1 kbyte of static RAM, 2 kbytes of ROM as well as a keyboard/display facility, an audio cassette for mass storage, a programmable interval timer, and an input port.

Figure 5.23 shows the basic system flowchart. The software supports six keyboard commands. It continuously displays the average zero-crossing rates over the last 10, 80, and 640 s. The 80-s average measurement is the mean of the last eight 10-s-interval rates. The 640-s average measurement is the mean of the last eight 80-s interval rates. Programs may be loaded into the RAM from cassette tapes using the system's ROM monitor program. The cassettes can also be used to store EEG data.

The whole system is relatively low in cost (under $500) and is expected to be used by neurologists and anesthesiologists in the assessment of brain function.

Keane (1978) has used an 8080A to detect EEG zero crossings. When playing back an 8-h-sleep EEG recording, the system operates in $\frac{1}{32}$ real time and controls three channels. Each zero crossing causes an interrupt, which is serviced in 128 μs. The system detects alpha, beta, delta, sleep spindles, and movement artifact. Advantages of the system are that program control of detection parameters makes hardware changes unnecessary.

Keane et al. (1978b) analyze the EEG in real time with an Intel 8748 single-chip microcomputer. Figure 5.24 shows that the EEG zero crossings interrupt the microcomputer. It monitors three frequency bands: slow-wave activity, 4 to 8 Hz; sensory motor rhythm activity (SMR), 12 to 16 Hz; and EMG activity, 20 to 30 Hz. Three LED readouts display the percent of time each type of activity is present. It is used to monitor EEG activity of epileptics during biofeedback training sessions.

Keane et al. (1978a) have built a portable unit using the Intersil 6100 12-bit CMOS microprocessor. An analog voltage proportional to the time SMR activity met or exceeded criteria over the preceding 2 s is provided by a D/A converter to drive the visual and audio feedback circuits.

Spike detection

Johnson and Smith (1978) describe a method to detect petit mal seizures using microprocessors. A petit mal seizure is an abnormality that has characteristic waveforms that each consist of a spike and slow wave coupled together. Individually, a spike or a slow wave can be present as a normal component of the EEG. The detection criteria utilize a microcomputer to perform pattern recognition based upon a

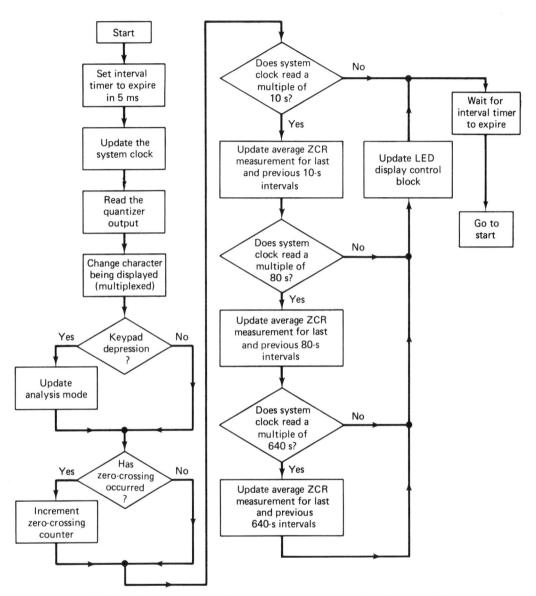

FIGURE 5.23 Flowchart for EEG brain function monitoring. (From Doyle, J. 1976. EEG brain function monitoring using a microcomputer. Proc. MIMI Symp. Mini Microcomput., pp. 213–216.)

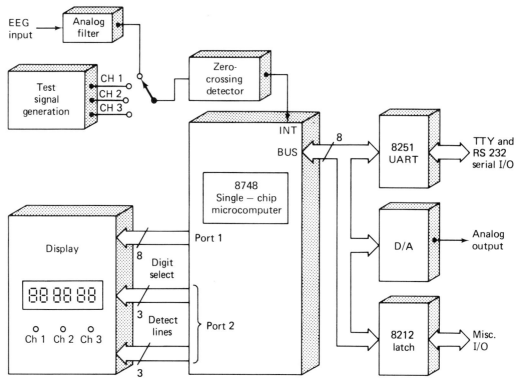

FIGURE 5.24 EEG analysis. The Intel 8748 single-chip microcomputer contains memory, I/O, CPU, and timing circuitry in a single 40-pin package. (From Keane, B., et al. 1978b. Real-time analysis of bioelectric data using a single-chip microcomputer system. Proc. Ann. Conf. Eng. Med. Biol. 20:321. Used with permission.)

series of algorithms modeled after the observed three-per-second couplet that is described as a fast spike waveform followed by a slow wave. Analog bandpass filtering initially separates the EEG into two narrow-frequency-range segments. Threshold detection adds an additional criterion for identification.

The microprocessor looks for a match with the preassigned pattern criteria. The pattern selected consists of a minimum of four spike and wave couplets. A further constraint is that the occurrence of the pattern must be synchronous in at least two separate channels. This instrument is being used to help identify the effectiveness of anticonvulsant drugs.

Programmable visual stimuli

Jorgens and Gilman (1978) used an Altair microcomputer to generate programmable visual stimuli for evoked potential research. The microcomputer sets up display patterns in 2 kbytes of memory. A Cromemco Dazzler two-board color-generating system uses direct memory access to cycle steal the pattern into a color video signal. The television monitor displays the pattern in one of four modes, with up to eight possible colors, two intensities, 128 × 128 picture elements, and various durations.

Nonlinear filtering

When linear filters are inadequate, nonlinear filters may provide improved performance. Johnson et al. (1979) noted that the EEG frequently has unwanted muscle spikes that contaminate the signal. Conventional 3-pole active low-pass filters that pass the desired EEG do not remove these muscle spikes. Their nonlinear filter examines a 19-sample window and decides if a muscle spike is present. If a muscle spike is present, the algorithm finds its polarity and amplitude and subtracts out a stored replica. This eliminates the muscle artifact while preserving the basic EEG. While the nonlinear filter requires more computation than a conventional filter, a dedicated microcomputer for each channel should be able to handle the task.

5.8 BLOOD PRESSURE*

Blood-pressure measurements find application in three clinical areas: during the physical exam, during surgical procedures, and in research. We describe an example of a microprocessor-based blood-pressure measurement system designed for application in each of these areas.

Auscultatory method

During routine physical examinations the physician uses blood-pressure measurement as a means to assess the patient's gross cardiovascular function, including the initial diagnosis of abnormalities, such as hypertension. Approximately 10% of the U.S. adult population has hypertension, and the majority are undiagnosed. The current technique for screening possible hypertension cases uses a sphygmomanometer, as described in Section 1.6. The physician or nurse performs the test in the clinical setting.

Figure 1.42 shows a standard sphygmomanometer. This type of screening procedure has three drawbacks. Personnel are required to perform the testing and to train other people to perform the testing. The sphygmomanometer auscultatory method is quite subjective, and different persons making blood-pressure measurements on the same patient often obtain dissimilar results. Patients who wish to have their blood pressure tested must travel to the location of the physician or nurse within some restricted time period.

Ramsey (1977) has developed a microprocessor-based blood-pressure testing machine that is completely self-administered and coin-operated. In this device an

---

*Section 5.8 written by Stephen L. Paugh.

Intel 4040 microprocessor chip takes the place of the decision-making process of the physician, and a sensitive microphone replaces the stethoscope.

To use the machine, the subject sits facing the console and inserts the left arm through the deflated blood-pressure cuff loop. After coins are inserted into the device an automated sequence of events occurs which snugs the cuff around the subject's biceps. Then it turns on a pump that inflates the cuff to 160 mm Hg. The cuff microphone then monitors the Korotkoff sounds (KS). If any are detected, the pump continues to inflate the cuff in 20-mm Hg increments until the KS are no longer detected.

Cuff deflation occurs in 6-mm Hg decrements until the first KS is detected. At this time, the microprocessor stores the cuff pressure in memory as systolic pressure. Cuff deflation continues and when the KS disappear, it stores the cuff pressure present in memory as diastolic pressure. Then a second set of automated events occur which purge the cuff, display the results, and ready the machine for the next user.

The control program for the machine's operation requires 1.2 kbytes of PROM. An 8-bit A/D converter digitizes the microphone analog output. Artifacts caused by subject motion are detected by requiring a period of silence after each KS. If the machine does not observe the expected silence, it assumes that the subject has moved and pauses momentarily before resuming the determination. In this manner it rejects most motion artifact. If the subject moves excessively, the machine "tilts" and turns on a "please start over" sign.

The machine's designer compared the results of blood-pressure determinations by the computer with those of a trained human observer to show that the computer results are quite consistent with those of the human operator. The major difference is that the computer has a 6-mm Hg resolution.

Oscillometric method

During surgery the anesthesiologist constantly monitors the patient's mean arterial pressure (MAP) to detect circulatory failure. If the MAP becomes too low, it could be an indication of too much anesthesia or hemorrhage. Ramsey (1976) developed a MAP computer for use during surgery. Cullen (1974) showed that a knowledge of pulse pressure does not provide significant usable information about anesthesia, and for this reason MAP was chosen as the parameter to be monitored.

Figure 5.25 shows the basic principle of the MAP computer (Yelderman and Ream, 1978). Figure 5.26 shows that the maximum cuff oscillations occur at a cuff pressure equal to the MAP. The system originally developed used an Intel 4040 microprocessor to monitor the cuff pressures and compute the MAP. Applied Medical Research developed the system under the trade name Dinamap, using the technique of oscillometry shown in Fig. 5.26.

Figure 5.27 shows the architecture of the microcomputer, which serves as the system controller. The microprocessor samples the cuff baseline pressure and the oscillation magnitude, controls the cuff pressure, makes the required logic decisions, and outputs the results.

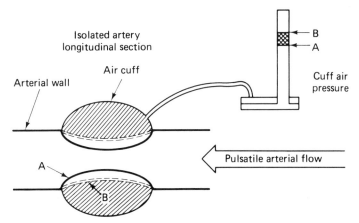

FIGURE 5.25 Cross section of air cuff encircling an isolated artery. Pulsatile arterial flow induces displacement of the arterial wall, thus influencing the cuff air pressure. Artery wall movement is reflected in the manometer readings. Arterial position A corresponds to pressure shown at A, and position B corresponds to pressure B. (From Yelderman, M., and Ream, A. K. 1978. A microprocessor-based automated non-invasive blood pressure device for the anesthetized patient. Proc. San Diego Biomed. Symp. 17: 57–64.)

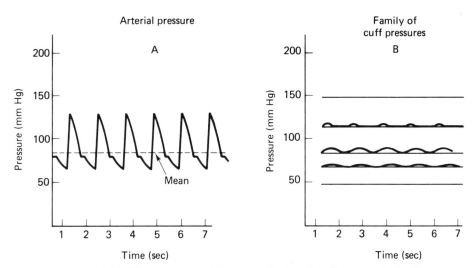

FIGURE 5.26 Time versus arterial pressure in A and cuff pressure in B. Five different cuff pressures are shown. Note that the baseline cuff pressure (thinner lines) which allows the largest oscillation above the baseline cuff pressure is closest to the arterial mean pressure shown in A. (From Yelderman, M., and Ream, A. K. 1978. A microprocessor-based automated non-invasive blood pressure device for the anesthetized patient. Proc. San Diego Biomed. Symp. 17: 57–64.)

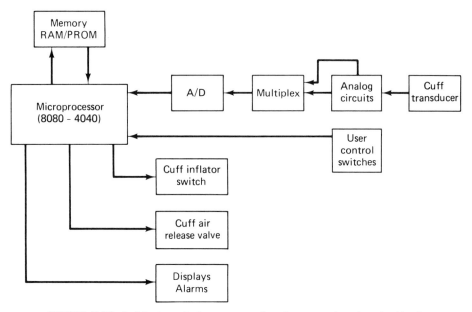

FIGURE 5.27 Architecture of microprocessor-based automated noninvasive blood pressure device. (From Yelderman, M., and Ream, A. K. 1978. A microprocessor-based automated non-invasive blood pressure device for the anesthetized patient. Proc. San Diego Biomed. Symp. 17 : 57–64.)

The program for the MAP computer is stored in less than 2 kbytes of PROM, with an additional 80 bytes of RAM used for temporary data storage. The cuff pressure transducer uses an 8-bit A/D converter. The output display consists of three seven-segment LED displays.

The total system development time was about 3 years, with the initial target selling price of $1950 per unit. Subsequent units developed by Applied Medical Research add additional features, such as heart rate and separate displays of systolic and diastolic blood pressure, in addition to the MAP display. These more-advanced units incorporate as the system controller the Intel 8080 microprocessor, which was chosen for its size, cost, and versatility. The Prolog PLS-881 microprocessor evaluation kit assisted the hardware development. A minicomputer cross assembler eased the software development.

Arterial tonometer

The Nicolet ML-105 arterial tonometer (Bahr and Dhupar, 1977) is a microprocessor-based application of the basic tonometry principles discussed in Section 1.6. A Z80 microprocessor was chosen for this system as it was the most powerful chip on the market at the time of the system development. A clock rate of 2.4576 MHz was used for microprocessor time base.

Standard Intel 8080 software was used along with the upward-enhanced instructions that are unique to the Z80. The Z80 system-compatible parallel input/

output chip family was used to keep the total system chip count down and to enhance the interrupt-handling capabilities. The 8-bit A/D converters used have their gain and offset under microprocessor control to keep the display on the screen of a CRT. The CRT is part of a Tektronix 5100 oscilloscope mainframe, which also serves as the system package.

Figure 5.28 gives an example of a typical output display. Note the use of both analog and alphanumeric information on the same display. The serial output port is standard ASCII format compatible for both the RS-232C and the 20-mA current loop printer interface.

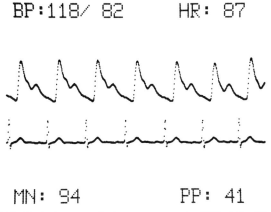

FIGURE 5.28 Typical output display as seen on the CRT of the ML-105 arterial tonometer. Sweep speed is 25 mm/s. (From Bahr, D., and Dhupar, K. 1977. A microprocessor-based arterial tonometer. Proc. 1st Ann. Symp. on Comp. Appl. Med. Care, pp. 90–98.)

Figure 5.29 shows the hardware organization for the system. The 5-kbyte PROM stores the instructions for the CPU as well as a look-up table for the on-screen messages. The 8-kbyte RAM stores analog ECG and tonometer data prior to display and the data manipulation. The analog display consists of a 256×375 matrix of discrete points. The 4-kbyte utility RAM provides for alphanumeric data buffering to the display. Fast, hardwired logic interfaces the RAM to the display CRT. A digital data port on the tonometer feeds a hard-copy output. Front-panel switches and a keyboard allow calibration information to be entered into the CPU. The front-panel controls also allow the operator to perform data manipulation.

5.9 CLINICAL CHEMISTRY*

Automation and computerization have reduced the need for technical personnel in the clinical chemistry laboratory (Aikawa, 1974). There have been improvements in accuracy and precision of the analyses, and in legibility, storage, and retrieval

*Section 5.9 written by Peter D. Gadsby.

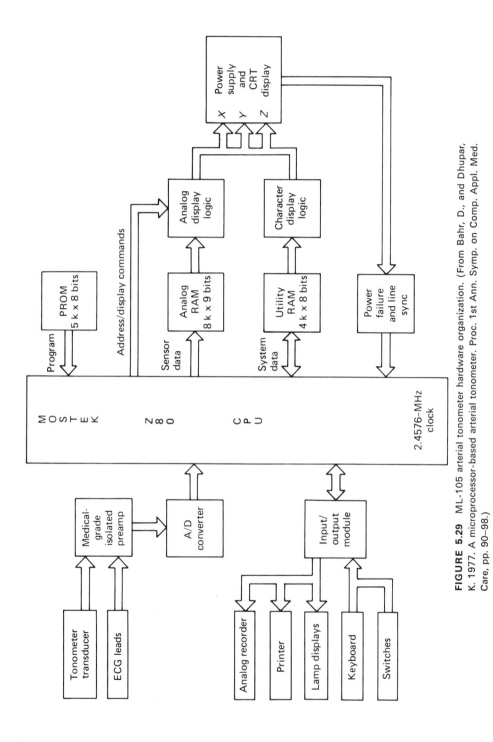

FIGURE 5.29 ML-105 arterial tonometer hardware organization. (From Bahr, D., and Dhupar, K. 1977. A microprocessor-based arterial tonometer. Proc. 1st Ann. Symp. on Comp. Appl. Med. Care, pp. 90–98.)

of information. The microcomputer is part of instrumentation that performs numerous tasks, such as measurement of net charge transport and weighing of samples. This section briefly describes some of the more recent innovations.

Measurement of net charge transport

Measurement of net charge transport is a new method for the direct determination of oxygen tension. Zick (1977) has shown that the magnitude of the net charge transport is proportional to the oxygen tension level of whole blood when the sensor is polarized for a duration as short as 1 ms. There are three separate units: the head stage, the controlling microprocessor system, and the external interfacing hardware.

A Texas Instrument 990/4 microprocessor provides timing, control, and waveform analysis. The software provides variable frequencies and pulse durations. The system integrates the resulting currents from the polarization potential of the differential electrometer and determines the net charge transport. Results can be displayed and transmitted to a cassette or another computer for storage. This system can also be used for other pulsed and dc polarographic measurements.

Specific ion or pH meter

Figure 5.30 shows the Ionanalyzer/901, developed by Orion Research (1977). This system has an analog amplifier with high input impedance, followed by an A/D converter. The output of the A/D goes to the microcomputer, which is preprogrammed with equations for calculating pH and concentration. The operator enters needed parameters for the different electrodes and tests with switches and pushbuttons on the front panel. Every 30 s the instrument displays the most recently

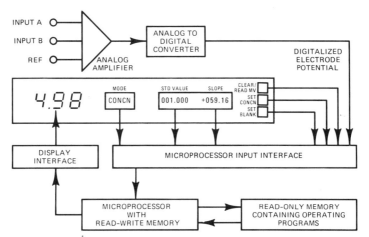

FIGURE 5.30 Block diagram of the microprocessor-based ionanalyzer. (Compliments of Orion Research, Inc. 1977.)

computed electrode potential. The precision of the instrument is on the order of 0.001 pH unit, depending upon initial calibration.

Automatic features of the instrument include pushbutton standardization and blank correction. The blank correction method automatically subtracts the background noise level from the result.

Blood gases

Margalith et al. (1977) have reported on a microcomputer-based system for *in vitro* measurements of pH, PCO_2, and PO_2. It samples the analog output of each electrode amplifier to determine when the reactions in the electrode chamber have reached steady state. Then the electrode signals, together with body temperature (T) and hemoglobin concentration (Hb), are used to calculate PO_2, PCO_2, pH, bicarbonate concentration $[HCO_3^-]$, base excess (BE), and percent oxygen saturation (% sat. O_2). A ticket printer generates three copies of the results, for filing and distribution.

The microcomputer includes an Intel 8080 microprocessor, less than 3 kbytes of EPROM, and 256 bytes of RAM. Thumbwheel switches provide for inputting the values of T and Hb. Calculations are performed by a floating-point mathematics package incorporating an 8-bit exponent and a 16-bit mantissa represented in sign-magnitude form. Included in this package are two subroutines that approximate 10^x and $\log_{10} x$. Although highly automated, the instrument requires a technician to clean and calibrate the system.

Radiometer Copenhagen has developed a microcomputer-based system similar to the one described above, called the ABL2 acid–base laboratory system. Capillary or syringe samples of arterial blood are injected into the sample inlet. The liquid sensor indicator lights when the blood reaches it. The patient's temperature is entered into the system via thumbwheels on the front panel. When the inlet flap is closed, the main pump draws the sample through the heat exchanger and into a chamber, where pH, PCO_2, PO_2, and Hb are measured. This system provides for temperature correction, automatic rinsing, and completely automatic calibration every 1.75 h.

The ABL2 is capable of analyzing 18 samples/h. The system comes complete with special test programs that check the liquid sensors, temperatures, valves, and computer hardware. This instrument sells for about $15,000.

Clark (1978) describes an *in vivo* automatic calibrating blood-gas monitor for measuring PO_2 and PCO_2. A probe microsensor unit containing a bicarbonate liquid comes to equilibrium with the blood gases through a gas-permeable membrane. The bicarbonate liquid serves as a common electrolyte for both the PO_2 and PCO_2 microsensors. The microsensor elements lie outside the region where equilibrium takes place. Probe monitoring is accomplished by movement of the equilibrated electrolyte to the sensors and then into the microtonometer. After measurement, the electrolyte flows back to the microsensors and then back to the tip to establish a new equilibrium.

The output of the microsensors controls the electronic gas proportioner, which supplies the microtonometer with gas. This method matches the gas proportioner gas fraction with that of the gas tensions of the patient. So far the results have indicated that this method of *in vivo* monitoring of PO_2 and PCO_2 has greater accuracy than standard blood-gas analyzers.

Developers of this instrument used a Mostek Z80 software development board, which included a Z80 CPU, a 2.5-MHz clock, 16 kbytes of dynamic RAM, 256 bytes of static RAM, 2 kbytes of ROM, 4 kbytes of EPROM, a Z80 counter-timer circuit, and four 8-bit parallel I/O ports with handshake lines. The software is written in Z80 assembly language. The program begins by calling up several subroutines. One starts up the hardware timer, which generates six interrupts every 2 s. A second displays the current gas-flow ratios. A third permits the operator to specify an initial gas mix. A fourth makes sure that both O_2 and CO_2 concentrations are at least 2% of the mixture. A fifth is used as the first part of a two-point calibration system. When the sensors are near the patient's values, a sixth does a one-point calibration. It sets the pump direction, monitors the sensors until they are stable, stores voltages and gas mixtures, and prints them out. A seventh prints header information on the operator terminal. An eighth calculates and stores the gain of the CO_2 sensor. A ninth takes sensor readings at intervals specified by the operator. Calculations are performed using the floating-point package.

Automatic analyzers

Lewis and Davis (1975) developed a controller for the Technicon SMA multichannel chemistry analyzer. The system uses an Intel 8080 microprocessor. The controller is plug-compatible with the existing controller and requires no modifications. The microprocessor software incorporates extensive self-checking techniques for its entirely solid-state design. The controller has doubled the sample throughput and halved the reagent volume needed. Provisions have been made for automatic recalibration of the instrument while running. The advantage of this controller is its saving of both time and money.

The new ChemResearch Model 1560 sample processor was developed by Instrumentation Specialties. The system was designed to do almost every wet chemical process that can be done manually, but with better repeatability and in less time. Keyboard programming is fast and simple with an annunciator display, which gives options for the next entry. Applications of this instrument are far more comprehensive than for other available chemical analyzers. This instrument is suitable for such diverse purposes as tissue culture growth, automatic control of complex process reactors, such as peptide synthesizers, biochemical processing, and various simple chemical analyses. Using manual methods it is often impractical to completely characterize all the effects on a chemical reaction of changing experimental parameters, such as reaction or incubation times and concentrations of reactants or buffers.

This system combines a simple and versatile mechanical sample-handling system with a microprocessor-based controller. A variety of external devices, such as pumps, valves, a spectrophotometer, a data printer, and other devices, may be used to complete the system.

The devices can be controlled in one of three ways. There are eight separate general-purpose accessory channels which can be used to provide timed on–off control. They can also be programmed to respond to a feedback signal or can be controlled with a 16-bit BCD code. There are also 40 on–off channels to control or select valves, recorder-chart drives, and other accessories that do not require return signal feedback. Up to 210 samples can be programmed on an individual basis, using up to 960 available program steps per run. This system provides flexibility that has not been seen before in a chemical analyzer. The basic system package costs $9000.

Microcomputer interfaces

The method described by Terdiman et al. (1977) will enable higher automation of a large number of older automated instruments. The older instruments typically do not have provisions for limit checking, calibration, and quality control. This method provides an intelligent front end for a basic laboratory instrument when a new automated laboratory system is far more complex and costly than is required. This system uses an Intel 8080 microprocessor and stores programs and limits within an EPROM. In one implementation, the microcomputer and an alarm were interfaced to a Coulter Model S blood-cell counter. The alarm alerts the technician whenever abnormal test results are detected. The system was programmed to control a variety of output devices, check calibration, perform quality control, and transmit data to a central computer. The advantages of using a dedicated microprocessor with each laboratory instrument are low cost, flexibility, simplicity of design, and independence from a central computer.

A similar method is proposed by Lynn et al. (1977). They implement an intelligent interface between several devices and the main computer. This method helps to reduce the interface cost per device. The system performs some preprocessing to reduce the load on the main computer, buffers incoming data indefinitely, provides error checking, and executes high-speed data transfers to the central computer on a low-priority basis. Thus it increases the number of devices that the central computer can handle.

At present an American Monitor KDA Automated Clinical Chemistry Analyzer is interfaced with the central computer. The interface includes a MOS Technology 6501 microprocessor. Modifications are under way for adding another clinical chemistry analyzer to the interface. The system is believed to be capable of handling from five to six devices.

Electronic balances

Sartorius Balances, a Division of Brinkmann Instruments, has designed a new top-loader balance with a built-in Texas Instruments microprocessor. The balance is designed around an electromagnetic force compensation system, with electronic damping which eliminates high-frequency vibrations encountered in factories and laboratories. The *g* symbol read after the digital numbers indicates when the system has achieved stability. This method provides a very stable readout. The electronic scales can be configured with several different types of data keyboards, including a universal keyboard and an animal keyboard, which provides variable integration times for mobile animals. The balance can be interfaced with printers, calculators, data logging equipment, and remote station digital displays. Several models are available, ranging in price from about $2000 to $4000, depending upon the functions desired.

Liquid scintillation counter

Radioactive samples are placed in vials and emit gamma rays of various energies. A liquid scintillator absorbs the gamma ray and emits a light flash, which is detected by a photomultiplier tube. The liquid scintillation counter classifies gamma rays by energy and stores their counts.

LKB-Wallac (1978) markets a microcomputer-based liquid scintillation counter. The teleprinter permits conversational control of the operations. Full program editing capability permits the operator to change count parameters such as count windows, preset count, time, background subtraction, low-count reject, and standardization time. The operator can change the printout format, which includes various counts and the standard error of each count.

5.10 SENSORY MONITORING AND AIDS*

Microcomputers have been utilized in instrumentation for diagnosis and treatment of neurological and sensory disorders. The ability of the microcomputer to aid in acquisition, formatting, and display of data is a common theme throughout the applications presented.

Ophthalmology

Perimetry. Drawn from the field of physiological psychology, the techniques of perimetry and campimetry quantitate and define the limits of a patient's visual field. With one eye covered the patient fixes his or her sight on a central point and a visual target or stimulus is presented at varying distances from the point. The patient then subjectively reports the perception of the visual target and the examiner manually records it on graph paper. Varying the position of the visual target at the same intensity produces an isocontour or isopter (kinetic perimetry). Increasing the stimulus intensity until perception occurs at a fixed location and then repeating the process at other locations on a straight line (meridian) in the visual field yields a profile of retinal sensitivity (static perimetry). Campimetry is a variation of peri-

---

*Section 5.10 written by Gary V. Sprenger.

metry using a tangent plane as a stimulus background rather than the interior of a hemisphere.

Hartz (1977) developed an on-line microcomputer-based system that acquires and stores the visual field information normally recorded by hand. Based on the Motorola M6800, the device interfaces to a conventional perimeter and allows the examiner to interact with the microcomputer during the course of the examination. A floppy disk stores patient demographic data as well as visual field data. A storage oscilloscope displays the stored visual field data to the examiner. User commands entered via the keyboard and panel display allow the data to be stored or deleted. Deleted data points are blanked from the oscilloscope display.

System expansion is envisioned to include an x-y plotter for hard copy of test results. A serial interface has been implemented to allow data transmission to a minicomputer with a larger data-base capability and a greater computational power. Statistical and temporal studies on the visual field data are currently being considered in this distributed computer system. Prototype development encompassed 4 to 5 worker-months for hardware and more than 12 worker-months for currently implemented software (Hartz, 1978).

Campimetry. Frugone et al. (1977) have also employed the distributed computing concept in an automated campimeter developed in Italy. Based on the Intel 8080, the system allows the examiner to enter pertinent patient and test data via keyboard and alphanumeric CRT. The microcomputer then controls the examination in real time after choosing one of 24 meridians to present the visual target. A pushbutton interrupt-driven routine indicates perception of the visual target. This routine stores the visual target location, intensity, and size and proceeds to present the visual target at the next location. At the end of the examination either the cathode-ray-tube display or x-y plotter presents the collected data for evaluation. If required, the mass-storage system of the minicomputer stores the data or the examination is repeated.

Nystagmus. Involuntary rhythmic movements of the eye(s) called nystagmus are present in many neurological disorders and, in some cases, identify the disease state (Thorn et al., 1977). The examination for nystagmus is done by first observing the eyes in the central position and then during upward, downward, and lateral movements. In certain neurological diseases, nystagmus-type movements can be elicited by movements of the head (vestibular nystagmus) or a visual field (optokinetic nystagmus), and/or by thermal or electrical stimulation of the auditory system (labyrinthine nystagmus). In conventional nystagmus analysis these eye movements are amplified with electrooculography (EOG) or photoelectric nystagmography (PENG). Parameters of interest are then estimated from the raw data recordings by hand.

Michaels and Tole (1977) have developed a semiautomated device for analysis of nystagmus and control of vestibular stimuli. Based on the Intel 8080, the device automatically corrects the data for EOG error and includes a calibration sequence for the direction of eye movements. After calibration, the device interrogates the user as to the stimulus required. The device then starts the stimulus and begins collection of eye displacement data for processing and output. Figure 5.31 shows a flowchart of these major tasks.

Software for the nystagmus analyzer was developed in a high-level language called STOIC (stack-oriented interpretive compiler) designed especially for micro-computer software development (Sachs, 1976). Total development time took approximately 36 worker-months for software and hardware.

If rapid eye movements overshoot the fixation point, this indicates cerebellar disease. Physician observation of overshoot is inaccurate. Analysis of recordings of the electronystagmogram is slow. Freeman et al. (1978) use an Imsai 8080 micro-computer with 32 kbytes of RAM to speed up the test and improve its accuracy. An 8-bit ADC provides 0.4% resolution. The operator uses an initialization routine if he or she wishes to run with threshold levels, noise tolerances, sampling rates, or timer and counter settings other than the default values.

The system calculates the percent overshoot and converts the parameters to ASCII code for cathode-ray-tube display.

Vestibular testing.   Tole et al. (1978) developed an 8080 microcomputer-based examination chair for use as part of a vestibular function test battery. The operator inputs commands via either a terminal or pushbutton front panel. The motor-driven chair responds with complete test protocols in rotation, pitch, and head-rest movement. The rotation servo system duplicates the function of a stepping motor by use of a motor, tach, encoder, and control board. To assure smooth operation, uniform spacing of pulses is necessary over a wide range of frequencies. Hence a rate multiplier generates the command frequency. An update clock interrupts the microcomputer at 25 Hz, requesting new data for the rate multiplier. The micro-computer calculates the data for simple velocity profiles at each interrupt. For complicated velocity profiles it constructs a table of data before the run and reads it sequentially during the run. Subroutines limit velocity and acceleration.

Visual contrast-sensitivity functions.   Measurement of the contrast-sensitivity func-tion helps to diagnose defects of the visual system. The contrast-sensitivity function is the minimum luminance contrast of a spatial sinusoidal grating necessary to perceive the grating as a function of the spatial frequency of the grating.

An M6800 microcomputer with 256-byte RAM and 1024-byte ROM permits test automation so that paramedical personnel can run the test (Keemink et al., 1979). The microcomputer controls an electronic attenuator to increase modulation of the sine-wave grating on a TV monitor. When the subject perceives the grating, he or she presses a response switch, which interrupts the microcomputer and decreases the modulation. When the subject does not perceive the grating he or she responds again and the modulation increases. The microcomputer stores these 16 contrast reversal limits on each side of perception threshold, averages them, and plots the average modulation. Then it selects a new spatial frequency and repeats

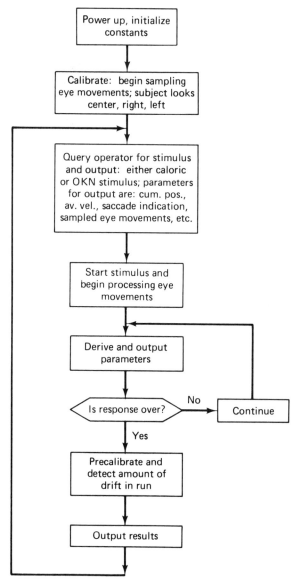

FIGURE 5.31 Flowchart of major tasks performed by nystagmus analyzer. (From Michaels, D. L., and Tole, J. R. 1977. A microprocessor-based instrument for nystagmus analysis. Proc. IEEE 65: 730–735.)

for nine spatial frequencies. Through DACs, it plots the complete contrast sensitivity function on an *x-y* recorder. It also plots the ratio of these functions for the two eyes.

Glaucoma diagnosis. Glaucoma results in elevated intraocular pressure, erosion of the optic nerve head, and characteristic patterns of visual loss. Shapiro et al. (1978a) use a MOS Technology 6502 (KIM-1) microcomputer to reduce errors and speed data analysis for early diagnosis of glaucoma. They project a striped pattern onto the optic nerve head through one side of the dilated pupil. Photographs taken through the opposite side of the pupil reveal the optic nerve head topography as deviations of the stripes from their original straight line. The microcomputer controls movement of the microscope stage, which contains the resulting negative, in a raster pattern perpendicular to the stripes. The operator stops the stage at each stripe. The microcomputer counts the number of steps between each stopping point. It tape-records these for later transmission to and data analysis by an IBM 370 computer.

Eyeglasses. Instruments designed to prescribe eyeglasses also incorporate microcomputers. Developed and marketed by Acuity Systems of Reston, Virginia, an instrument called an auto-lensmeter measures a lens simply and precisely and displays the exact prescription. The instrument employs a modulated laser and linear optical detector to obtain lens data. After A/D conversion the instrument statistically filters, expands, and converts the data from *x-y* coordinates to the polar coordinates used in lens prescriptions. The TI9900 microprocessor provides the required 16-bit multiply and divide calculations. The use of a microprocessor increases flexibility at lower cost than hardwired logic. Disadvantageous is the fact that the TI9900 is a relatively new microprocessor. Hence it is not thoroughly debugged and has little available software support (McDevitt, 1978).

Artificial vision. A system for artificial vision in the blind is under development at the University of Utah Institute for Biomedical Engineering (Electronics, 1973; Science, 1974; Electronics, 1974). A miniature semiconductor image array is mounted in the eyesocket. A microprocessor scans the array elements in a serial manner and processes and formats the data for transmission to circuitry implanted in the skull. This stimulates an associated electrode array chronically implanted in the visual cortex. Power is supplied to all implanted circuitry via inductive coupling. Although far from completion, these design concepts are envisioned to be useful in the development of prosthetic devices for the deaf (Dobelle et al., 1973).

Training devices and other applications

Microcomputers are employed for hand–eye coordination experiments with primates (Calma and Johnson, 1976). In this application the microcomputer aids personnel with data collection and in estimating performance and progress.

5.11 COMMUNICATION AND TRAINING AIDS FOR THE HANDICAPPED*

This section describes several microprocessor-based devices designed for handicapped individuals. Since the size of the market for such devices is comparatively small and the design costs high, these aids are usually developed by small research groups rather than corporations.

Manual skills training aid

Rehabilitation for mentally retarded individuals often includes training to perform simple tasks to allow them to work constructively in society. This training involves frequent one-to-one contact with a supervisor, who must evaluate trainees in terms of quality of work. Because of the number of required contact hours, a supervisor can effectively train only a limited number of clients. Since any technological solution to this problem must be cost-effective, the microcomputer has been used in these training aids rather than more expensive minicomputer systems.

In 1976, Portland State University began working on a training aid that is now used at the Salem Rehabilitation Facility in Salem, Oregon (Flax, 1977a, 1977b). This application involves training handicapped individuals to prepare precut, large-gage, insulated wire for use in transformers. The microprocessor monitors proper insertion of the wire into a cutting tool and times the manual process. If the trainee completes the task in a predefined length of time, he or she receives positive feedback (a reward); otherwise, the microprocessor notifies the supervisor that the cable was inserted wrong, the process took too long, or the trainee provided a false indication of insertion (too short a time). Figure 5.32 shows the flowchart of the software. In addition, trend analysis of learning or fatigue levels is available by plotting the production count as a function of time.

The system evolved around a KIM-1 microcomputer with 1 kbyte of RAM for program and data storage. A programmable timer produces a basic timing interval of 0.25 s, which the program converts to seconds to keep track of insertion time. Microswitches on the cutting jig are closed if the wire is inserted properly. The switches are interfaced to the microprocessor through input ports.

System development continues with an ultimate goal of defining a specialized microprocessor language for rehabilitation applications, which will facilitate the development of future monitoring and training aids by rehabilitation centers.

AUTOCOM portable communication aid

The AUTOCOM shown in Fig. 5.33 was initially developed at the University of Wisconsin–Madison to provide a young cerebral-palsied boy with a means of communication. This individual was nonvocal and did not have the manual control to write or type. Design constraints were that the communication aid must be porta-

---

*Section 5.11 written by James D. Woodburn.

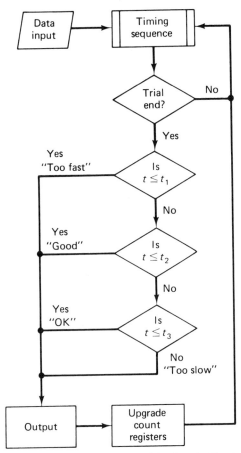

FIGURE 5.32 The logic system flowchart used for the rehabilitation system. (From Flax, S. W. 1977b. A microcomputer application for training the mentally retarded. IEEE Region 6 Conf. Rec., pp. 79–82.)

ble, durable, and controllable by spastic movements. In addition, it should have hard-copy capability for printout of selected letters, words, or phrases, as well as output interfaces to connect to a television monitor, a Teletype, a telephone, or a computer. Meeting these criteria would allow the device to be more useful to other handicapped individuals in addition to the person for whom it was designed. Because of the limited market, two problems involved in development of specialized communication aids are the high initial cost and the lack of adequate maintenance facilities. To overcome these problems, the highly flexible universal control system shown in Fig. 5.34 was developed to serve as a major basic hardware element in a wide variety of adaptable aids. Since the universal control system is a major component in a number of different communication aids, the cost per aid is lowered by the benefits of mass production. Versatility is preserved by including a repro-

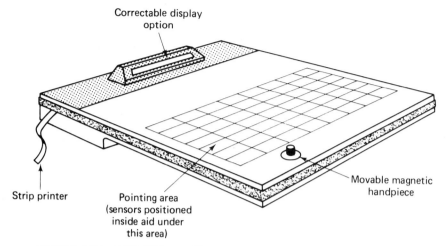

FIGURE 5.33 AUTOCOM portable communication aid. (From Vanderheiden, G. C., et al. 1976.)

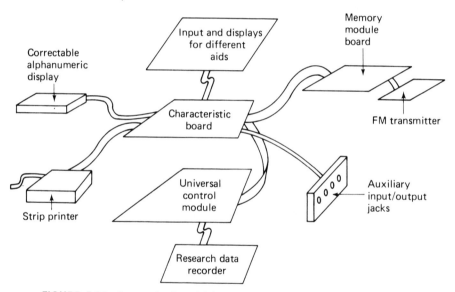

FIGURE 5.34 Communication aid based on a universal control module. The AUTOCOM is one of a family of aids each with its own characteristic board. (From Vanderheiden, G. C., et al. 1976.)

grammable microprocessor in the control system and providing for interfacing a number of different input devices. Maintainability is improved by including self-test software and subcomponents and modules.

The AUTOCOM shown in Fig. 5.33 has an 8 × 16 matrix of magnetic reed switches arranged in groups of five located beneath the tray surface. Holding a handpiece containing a magnet over a desired square for a length of time (which is adjustable) causes the underlying reed relay to close. The character or word printed in the selected square is then presented on a 32-character self-scanning alphanumeric display. Each square encodes up to seven different data strings that can be a single character, a word, a phrase, or a control function. The AUTOCOM has a total of about 50 subroutines, which perform such functions as initialization, input selection, and display.

Universal Control Module (UCM). The UCM, which comprises about 90% of the electronics in the device, includes the COSMAC CDP1802 microprocessor with associated CMOS digital logic for the external functions. Also on this board are 512 bytes of CMOS RAM, which has a battery backup power supply and also the main program memory, which consists of 2 kbytes of UV EPROM (Intel 2708). The data string selected by the user resides in 256 bytes of RAM, which then serves as an editing area for the 32 displayed characters. The editing is done on the data in RAM and then redisplayed to show the corrections. The AUTOCOM also has a hardwired stop command, which enables a flip-flop to stop the processor clock and hence power down the entire system to extend battery life until it is reactivated by a reed switch closure. One of the reed relays acts as an on–off switch to disable all other reed switches so that the board can be used for other purposes, such as a wheelchair lunch tray, without paying attention to the position of the handpiece.

Memory module board. The memory module board accepts plug-in memory modules, each containing an EPROM (Intel 2708). These modules store the data strings accessed by the main program and are removable and reprogrammable so that each individual can store any desired vocabulary. The usual vocabulary set requires 2 kbytes of EPROM.

Power supply. The AUTOCOM is powered by rechargeable nickel cadmium batteries and has internal circuitry for recharging the batteries from a 120-V-ac wall outlet.

Strip printer. The thermal strip printer has a print head consisting of a 5×4 matrix of metal pads which heat up to produce visible spots on thermally sensitive paper. The processor controls the printing by activating the appropriate metal pads in the print head. It then moves the paper strip to the next print location by activating a solenoid.

LED display. The self-contained alphanumeric LED display displays up to 32 characters at a time and requires 600-mA maximum current. The user corrects typographical errors on the display before printing the message on the strip printer. The printer operates only when the display is full or a special function square is selected to print the displayed character string.

Initialization. The initialization routine is a short subroutine which presets the 16 dedicated microprocessor registers. It includes setting up the address for the memory module containing the data strings for each of the reed switches.

Input selection. The system usually rests in the low-power state with the clock stopped and power down on the PROM. An interrupt awakens the processor when a reed relay closes, and the process of selecting the correct switch begins. The switches do not always encode meaningful data. In different text-square configurations a fraction of the switches are nonactive (not encoding data) but not disconnected (the processor will still sense the magnet over an unused square and provide visual feedback to the user). The selection process must also keep track of the length of time the magnet is over the reed relay. By comparing this time to a preselected limit the processor prevents very rapid, spastic motions over other reed relays from selecting those squares. The more uncontrollable the arm movement of the handicapped individual, the longer the required time delay for reliable square selection. Once a valid switch closure is established, the text corresponding to the switch is located in the EPROM. The processor then fetches 1 byte from the EPROM and tests to see if it is a character or a control function. The program then continues into the display section as follows.

Display. Each of the bytes selected from EPROM is either sent to the output device as a character (ASCII display, strip printer, Teletype, or television screen) or executed as a subroutine if it is a control character. The external output of the AUTOCOM is 110-baud, 8-bit ASCII code. The character in EPROM is not in ASCII format but rather is encoded in such a way that the average character length is only 4 bits. The processor must then decode into ASCII before transmission.

Speech communication aid

Vartanian and Groesberg (1978) use an Intel 8080 to enable aphonic (without speech), motor-deficient patients to communicate. The system displays alphanumeric messages on two opposite-facing screens so that user and respondent can maintain eye contact. The screens display up to 20 characters and a thermal printer provides hard copy. In the scan mode, the patient waits for the correct character to be lighted and then actuates a SPST switch by a motion such as head tilt or elbow touch. Patients with reasonably good motor control select characters by activating proximity switches on a 16-square message board. Changeover between modes is effected by replacing EPROMs, which contain messages. Messages available are single characters or complete sets of stored characters (e.g., I AM HUNGRY). Additional characters provide for control operations, such as delete, print, clear, or beep the attention-getting buzzer.

Communication for the severely disabled

A quadriplegic cannot move his or her limbs but can close one of two normally open switches by puffing or sipping on a tube. Doubler and Childress (1978) use these switch closures as inputs to a Motorola M6800 microcomputer with 3 kbytes of EPROM and 4 kbytes of RAM. The display presents 10 characters with a cursor over the first character. Puffing advances the cursor one character at a time along the list, resetting to the beginning when the end of the line is reached. A sip input when the cursor is positioned over a character causes that character or the action associated with it to be selected. Five of the characters are used for message building. The remaining five characters are used for command/editing. For example, if the desired letter or symbol is not in the displayed group, a sip with the cursor in the first position will produce a new group of letters. The system takes advantage of the syntax rules of letter occurrence to decrease the number of actions required for the letter selection.

Vocal Communicator

The Votrax Division of the Federal Screw Works manufactures two portable, battery-powered, hand-held speech synthesizers called Handi Voice. One model uses 128 touch-sensitive squares with 373 words, 16 short phrases, 20 letters, and 45 phonemes, from which any word can be formed. By touching the appropriate square, each of which contains up to four different words, spoken words or phrases are produced by a speech synthesizer. The second model has 893 words in addition to the other items listed above, and the operator selects the words by pressing a series of keys on a 16-pad keyboard. The stored words and phrases are listed on a separate sheet of paper with their respective code numbers.

The Handi Voice uses a Motorola M6800 microprocessor. It was developed using an in-circuit emulator. The development time was about 2 to 3 worker-months for the hardware and about 4 worker-months for the software involved.

Diagnosis and treatment of aphasics

Brain damage and stroke victims may lose the ability to recognize or correctly interpret visual or auditory cues and may not speak (aphasia). Searle and Kissock (1978) use a PRO-LOG PLS-443 (Intel 4040) microcomputer to control a random-access slide projector and tape recorder. The operator selects a test or therapeutic program by a control keyboard. After tape-recorded instructions, the test stimuli are presented with varying sequences and durations. The system measures the latency and accuracy of the patient response. It can repeat the stimuli, pause, or branch to a simple program if the frequency of errors is excessive. It dispenses tokens to provide positive reinforcement for therapeutic programs. A printer lists correct and incorrect responses, response times, and cumulative totals. Hardware costs were $3000 for the computer, $3000 for the peripherals, and software hand coding in machine code took 4 worker-months.

5.12 DIAGNOSTIC ULTRASOUND*

Much work has been done on imaging internal body structures using ultrasound. Unlike x rays, ultrasound at low levels is nondestructive to body tissues. Unfortunately, the resolution of images obtained with this technique has been generally

---

*Section 5.12 written by Michael J. Yanikowski.

poor, and considerable skill has been required to operate the equipment. Improvements in video-scan converters and ultrasonic transducers, together with the addition of the microprocessor to the instrumentation, are improving diagnostic ultrasound, both in ease of use and in quality of image.

Digital systems

The analog versions of diagnostic ultrasound instruments work very well, but with the introduction of digital circuitry and microprocessors the original capabilities have been improved and some new abilities have been implemented. Several limitations of an analog instrument that can be improved with a digital approach are:

1. Positional accuracy and registration of the ultrasound scanning arm.
2. Acoustic dynamic range.
3. Image resolution and writing-speed limitations due to scan converters.
4. The lack of quantitative data concerning scan parameters and acquired images.
5. Pre- and postimage processing.

Positional accuracy and registration. A phased-array transducer can give real-time displays without transducer motion, but a transducer on a scanning arm can provide better resolution and a wider field of view. Using a transducer arm requires that the position sensing be very accurate. Errors in position produce reduced spatial resolution or a distorted image. The original transducer arms used potentiometers as the positional sensors in the arm joints. Potentiometers have a number of problems, including excessive wear, inaccuracies, and frequently errors in the wire coupling. Instead of potentiometers, microprocessor-based systems use optical shaft encoders as the angle-sensing device. (See Section 2.3 for a description of shaft encoders.) All the calculations of position are done by the microprocessor using sine and cosine look-up tables. Digital circuits provide long-term positional stability that results in an angular accuracy of 0.015 degree.

Dynamic range. As the beam of ultrasound travels into the body, it is attenuated exponentially within a given tissue. One purpose of the equipment is to compensate for this, but no commercial electronic device can perform an accurate correction. The beam is also focused so that the microcomputer can digitally correct for attenuation of the beam and also adjust for differences in beam intensity because of focusing. It is possible to store beam profiles for given transducers so that a number of different transducers can be used.

Image resolution and writing speed. Probably the greatest use of the microprocessor in ultrasonic imaging is to improve the resolution of the image. Scan converters have resolution characteristics and writing speeds that are inversely proportional. For better resolution, the image must be written more slowly. With a digital approach, the video signal is digitized and stored so that it can be processed later, thereby eliminating writing speed limitations.

Quantitative data. The microprocessor is able to store and display front-panel settings and alphanumeric data on the output screen so that they can be recorded on film with the scan.

Pre- and postimage processing. In an analog instrument the scan is recorded only on the video screen. With the microprocessor approach, the signal is digitized and stored. The data can be processed before or after storage. In this way, image enhancement and noise reduction are possible.

Stanford system. As an example of the foregoing, Stanford University uses Cromemco's Z-2 microcomputer as the main component of an ophthalmic ultrasound system (Garland and Ahlgren, 1978). Physicians punch relevant patient information into front-panel switches for display of the images. The scan data are stored in shift registers for slow playback later. The ultrasound image appears on the front-panel TV screen along with an annotation, which includes information such as patient number, date, and photograph number. As part of the user-oriented design objective, the system also has a teaching component built in to facilitate system use by physicians, who can call up this instructional program when needed.

5.13 PACEMAKERS*

Pacemakers are used in the treatment of heart block. Partial or complete heart block may exist because of such factors as cardiac surgery, cardiac infarction, and coronary atherosclerosis. Heart block can be subdivided into first-degree AV block, where only the conduction time is prolonged; second-degree AV block, where some of the pulses are conducted from the atrium; third-degree AV block, where the atria and the ventricles beat asynchronously; and bundle branch block, where the stimulus is not conducted normally to the ventricle served by a conduction system branch.

A more complete understanding of pacemaker technology is provided in Thalen et al. (1970), Furman and Escher (1970), and Siddons (1974). At present, we have found only four published applications of microprocessors in the field of pacemakers.

Battery testing

Creitz and Schneider (1976) devised a microprocessor-controlled testing system for the characterization of lithium pacemaker cells. This method utilizes the fact that lithium cells have an unusual electrochemistry. As the cell discharges, a

---

*Section 5.13 written by Peter D. Gadsby.

high-impedance solid electrolyte accumulates, which allows early detection of aberrant cells in a production lot by simple electrical measurements. The cells are maintained at 37°C under a 100-kΩ load for 2 months. Weekly measurements are made of cell voltage, ac and dc impedance. Abnormal slopes for any of these parameters are detected by statistical analysis. Using a microcomputer, a high-speed, high-accuracy automated system can perform these measurements for 1000 cells/h. This system outputs measurements on a $5\frac{1}{2}$-digit digital voltmeter and does a limited amount of raw-data checking. The results are put on magnetic tape for future computer analysis. This microcomputer approach allows flexible testing procedures through simple software changes.

Self-monitoring tester

Until recently, the only way a patient could determine that the pacemaker was still functioning was to use a transistor radio tuned to an unused frequency, place the radio by the implanted pacemaker, and listen to the impulses.

Bilgutay et al. (1976) have developed a self-monitoring pacemaker function tester with a pace-pulse tracer. This is a microcomputer-based unit capable of receiving and displaying pacemaker impulse rate and heart rate simultaneously. The pacemaker impulses are detected conductively by electrodes or by inductive coupling from the pacemaker by holding a coil over the implantation site. A photo-electric transducer obtains pulses from a fingertip and provides a sequential relationship of pacemaker impulses to pulse rate via signal lights. A logic circuit has been incorporated into the design so that the impulse and heart rates are given together with an indication as to whether the pacemaker is working. A green light indicates proper function, and a red light indicates a malfunction. Prior to this the patient had to determine from charts whether or not the pacemaker was working. Already used with over 300 patients, this method is very promising.

Performance evaluation

O'Desky et al. (1977) described a method utilizing a microprocessor for a pacemaker tracking system. The heart of the system is an Intel 8080A. There are 4 kbytes of ROM for bootstrapping to a floppy-disk controller and certain key routines. The 16 kbytes of RAM are used for program storage. One floppy disk contains the indices to the various patients and another contains all pertinent data for a particular patient. The signal analyzed is the patient's ECG. The whole system is interfaced with a Tektronix 4006 storage display terminal. The ADC samples at a rate of 50 ksamples/s and contains a signal slope-detection circuit. This method isolates the initiation of a pacemaker spike using a circularly stored RAM buffer of digital data. For more information on this technique, see Chapter 4. This technique allows the normalization of the spike within a time frame. The normalized spike is then recorded on the patient's floppy disk. This method enhances the physician's ability to review the pacemaker's performance over time, and evaluate its future performance more accurately.

Pacemaker control

Electronics (1979) reports that "although company officials refuse to discuss it, sources close to Medtronic Inc. say the Minneapolis manufacturer of medical electronics equipment is now testing a heart pacemaker containing a custom microprocessor. In addition to generating a pulse to stimulate the heart muscle to pump blood, the device in Medtronic's unit also transmits external signals about patient and pacemaker condition and can automatically change the unit's pulse width and rate to override a heart malfunction. A few patients already have the pacer installed, but the large-scale and lengthy clinical investigation that is necessary before commercial introduction of the system is not yet under way."

5.14 MEDICAL IMAGING*

Bone-mineral-measurement instrumentation

The measurement of bone mineral content and geometrical parameters is carried out by scanning a collimated beam from a monoenergetic gamma source of 25 to 75 keV energy across a given section of a bone and measuring the transmitted beam with a radiation detector (Alberi and Hardy, 1976). The total bone mineral content is obtained by computing the area under the corresponding absorption curve.

During the measurement, the source and detector move together across the patient's forearm, which is held fixed. The scanner carriage moves on linear ball bearings, with the start and end of each scan detected by limit switches. The radiation detector is a high-purity germanium [Ge(HP)] detector and the radiation source is ^{170}Tm.

Figure 5.35 shows the block diagram of the system. The output of the detector feeds the preamplifier which outputs to a single-channel analyzer for each photon energy specified. The output of a single-channel analyzer feeds a 16-bit scaler. The microcomputer incorporates 1 kbyte of RAM for data storage, 256 bytes for calculation, and about 4 kbytes of EPROM for the program.

The processor initiates the measurement under program control and the scalers are gated on from 0.25 to 2 s. The 8-bit status register containing start and halt request bits may be read by the processor at any time. Under program control, the processor may reset the hardware, which means resetting the status register and positioning the scanner carriage at the start limit switch.

Measurement of optic disk blood flow

Optic disk blood flow is measured by taking fluorescence photographs of the optic disk after the intravenous injection of a bolus of fluorescent dye in the patient's arm. The intensity of fluorescence may be obtained using a microdensitometer, which measures the optical density of the film at various locations. The measurement

---

*Section 5.14 written by Handayani Tjandrasa.

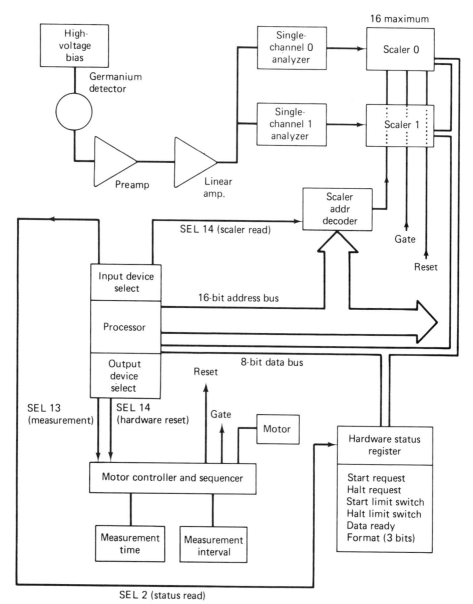

FIGURE 5.35 Block diagram of a bone scanning apparatus with its digital implementation. (From Alberi, J. L., and Hardy, W. H. 1976. An instrument for home mineral measurement using a microprocessor as the control and arithmetic element. IEEE Trans. Nucl. Sci. NS-23 : 645–650.)

process is automated using a KIM-1 microcomputer based on the MOS Technology 6502 microprocessor. The automatic process involves the following operations: driving a stepping-motor-controlled x-y stage, measuring and storing the optical densities, advancing the film, and returning control to the operator. The optical density data are stored on a tape and transmitted to a large computer. The time of peak fluorescence (dye-dilution curves) may be obtained by using curve fitting done on the large computer. The measurement result is used to study the effects of glaucoma.

Microdensitometer

A microdensitometer is a device that detects and analyzes the transmission and reflection properties of a small specified area of photographic film. It measures the optical density of black-and-white photographs of the optic disk. A photograph is mounted on the microscope stage, which rotates to allow the area of the image measured to be scanned. A light beam from a high-intensity light source beneath the stage is projected through the film; the light passing through a pinhole is received by a photomultiplier. The analog electrical output of the photomultiplier is processed by a medical laboratory computer. The processor has 8 kbytes of core memory to store data and operate programs. Interfacing to the computer are a Teletype, an oscilloscope, and an x-y plotter. The photograph is scanned in polar coordinates, starting at the center of the sample, and the computer is triggered to count revolutions. The frequency-distribution curve of optical densities of the optic disk may be used as a means for the diagnosis of glaucoma.

Microdensitometer for x-ray image analysis

The system used by the Radiology Department of New York University Medical Center is a modified Joyce–Lobel 3CS microdensitometer. This system scans a strip of film up to 25 cm long with a 1-μm slit and gives up to 1000 density measurements per scan. The microdensitometer is controlled by a Wavemate Jupiter II computer system with a Motorola MC6800 and 8 kbytes of RAM. The information gathered is transmitted to a large time-sharing computer, which is used to do the extensive calculations. The information of the position and density are digitized using optical shaft encoders. The software to control the microdensitometer is written in BASIC. A dual audio cassette is used to store the data from each complete scan, and the microprocessor transmits the accumulated scans from this tape to a large time-shared computer. The results are transmitted back and presented as a cathode-ray-tube display or a printout.

5.15 STIMULATORS*

If we wish to cause involuntary muscle activity in a subject, we apply an electrical stimulus. Externally applied electrical stimuli are also used to identify nerves and the extent of nerve damage, to treat muscle disorders, and to measure nerve conduc-

---

*Section 5.15 written by Stephen L. Paugh.

tion velocities. A typical physiological stimulus system incorporates two pulse generators, whose outputs are summed, controlled by a single trigger. By controlling the polarity and amplitude of the individual pulse generators, we can obtain a stimulus waveform of any desired shape. The pulse rate and waveshape are controlled by an external trigger coupled to a waveform generator.

Programmable stimulator

In the microprocessor-controlled stimulator we replace the waveform generator by a microprocessor and the trigger by a computer program. Figure 5.36 shows such a microprocessor-controlled stimulator (Guardo and Bertrand, 1976). In this system an 8080 microprocessor simulates 255 pulse generators, each with individually adjustable amplitude, period, duration, and initial delay. This flexibility allows the user to produce almost any desired waveform. The pulse amplitude is adjustable from 0 to 1 V in 4-mV steps, with a scaling factor of either 1 or 10. The pulse duration is adjustable from 1 ms to 32.8 s.

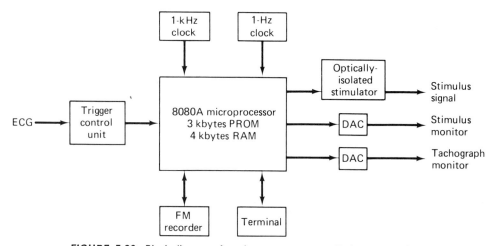

FIGURE 5.36 Block diagram of a microprocessor-controlled programmable physiological stimulator. (From Guardo, R., and Bertrand, M. 1976. A programmable physiological stimulator. Proc. Annu. Conf. Eng. Med. Biol. 18:191. Used with permission.)

This system is part of a programmed cardiac stimulator, of which there are a number of non-microprocessor-controlled commercial units currently available. The microprocessor-controlled stimulator reduces the time required for the clinical investigation performed during a catheterization procedure. The microprocessor allows the procedure protocol to be defined in advance and preprogrammed for automatic execution during the catheterization. The stimulus sequence is now programmed via an input terminal keyboard, which eliminates extensive equipment interconnected by cables and wires.

The only disadvantage of this system is the real-time constraint due to the 1-ms clock-timing rate. This parameter is suitable for cardiac stimulation studies but not for neurological studies.

The microprocessor is not totally occupied with the task of producing stimulus waveforms. Considerable processor time is available to perform other tasks. The software generates time codes using the 1-s interrupt. A UART transmits the time code serially as three 8-bit values (hours, minutes, seconds). The time codes are stored on the logging tape as event markers. To recall an event, the operator need only type in the time of the event and the microprocessor searches the tape until the desired event time is located.

Also included in the software is a stopwatch function based on the 1-ms clock interrupt. These additional functions show the extreme versatility and power of a microprocessor when it is incorporated into laboratory instrumentation.

The hardware development of this stimulator was implemented on an Intel SBC 80/20 microprocessor evaluation kit. The software was developed on an MDS-800 in-circuit emulator. The hardware development took approximately 12 worker-months and the software development 18 worker-months.

Stimulus programmer

An alternative to the previous approach is to use a number of commercial stimulators and build a programmable stimulus controller. Such a system was designed and built at the University of Wisconsin–Madison (Wilson, 1978).

The system is capable of controlling up to eight stimulators simultaneously. The operator manually presets the output signals of the individual stimulators as desired. Their outputs sum to produce the desired stimulus waveform. The operator enters a program to control the stimulators in the desired sequence via a hexadecimal keyboard. A 1-kHz interrupt clock establishes system timing.

This design incorporated a Motorola MC6800 microprocessor and the 6800 series support chips. The EPA MICRO 68 evaluation kit assisted the hardware development. Total parts cost was approximately $200, not including the CRT display. The hardware took about 6 weeks to complete. An EPROM programmer at a cost of $800 programmed the system controller instruction set. The cost of purchasing an EPROM programmer rather than renting one was based on the usefulness of having in-house EPROM programming capabilities for future projects.

The software development required about 16 weeks using an MC6800 cross-assembler and simulator running on a Harris Datacraft computer. Total development time was $1\frac{1}{2}$ years of part-time work, with the total development cost for hardware and software estimated at $10,000. A major problem encountered was the lack of adequate documentation throughout the development of the project. This became painfully apparent when the person who started the project left abruptly midway through the project. Much time was lost reconstructing what had already been done.

A second problem was trying to design software to do functions that could have been implemented in hardware at lower cost. The software development represented the major cost of this system. It is frequently reasonable to increase the complexity of the hardware to simplify the required software. It is often easier to troubleshoot hardware than to debug a long, complicated program that no one but the original programmer can understand. Many people tend to overlook the software development stage of the design process. After the hardware is functioning, it may be months before the software operates as desired.

5.16 PROSTHETICS*

One of the first modern prosthetic devices was the "NU-VA-Fidelity hand" developed at the Northwestern University in 1969. Later the "Boston arm" was developed at M.I.T. (Allan, 1976). It was inevitable that computers would be used to emulate at least part of the sophisticated control provided by the human brain. Microprocessors seem tailor-made for filling this need. They provide fairly sophisticated control for prosthetic devices and can still be made part of the device itself. A number of research workers have tried to take advantage of this potential. However, most of their efforts are still in the development stage, and no commercial ventures have yet been undertaken. Difficulty in deriving a reliable control signal from the body (and thus ensuring reliable operation of the device) is one of the prime bottlenecks (Klig, 1978).

A number of microprocessor-based prosthetic devices are currently under development. Freedy et al. (1975) at the Biotechnology Laboratory at UCLA are developing an upper-arm prosthesis using the RCA COSMAC microprocessor. Graupe et al. (1976) at Colorado State University are using the Intel 8080 to control an artificial upper-extremity prosthesis for above-elbow amputees. While the foregoing approaches use the EMG for control, a stored-program microcomputer using the F8 microprocessor has been developed at the University of Wisconsin (Grundmann and Seireg, 1976; Kautz, 1977). Howers and Rowell are developing a prosthetic knee joint using a microprocessor (Computer News, 1978). Next, we review some of these systems in detail.

University of Wisconsin lower-limb prosthesis

Figure 5.37 shows the schematic diagram of the control system for the prosthetic limb. A minicomputer (Computer Automation Alpha) was used for initial development work. This was subsequently replaced by the F8 microprocessor. The computer, through the A/D acquisition module, samples both the instantaneous desired knee angle (θ_{DES}) as indicated by the electrogoniometer (K) and the instantaneous actual knee angle (θ_{PROS}) sensed by the feedback potentiometer (J) mounted on the prosthetic knee axis. Using the control software given in Fig. 5.38, the

*Section 5.16 written by Nitish V. Thakor.

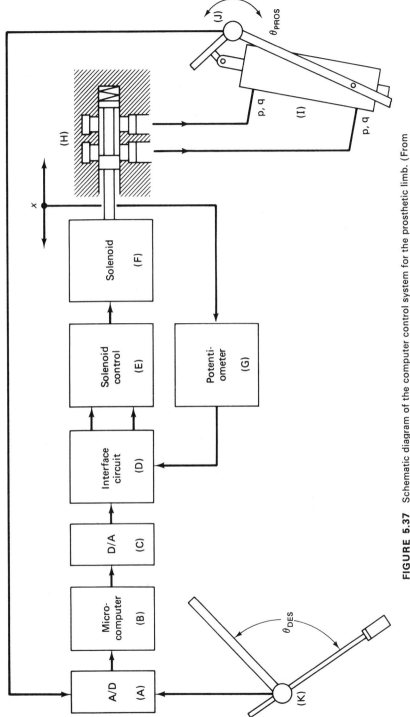

FIGURE 5.37 Schematic diagram of the computer control system for the prosthetic limb. (From Kautz, T. O. 1977).

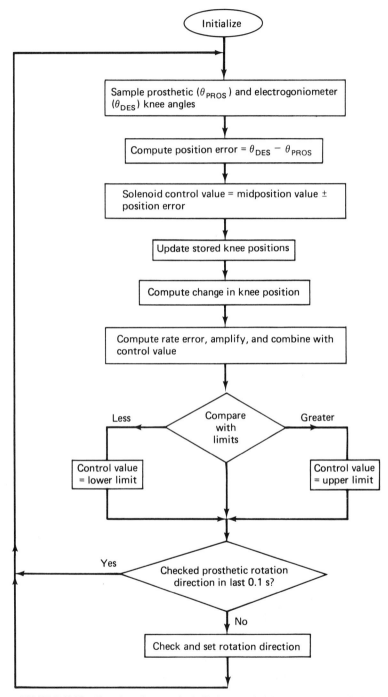

FIGURE 5.38 Flowchart for prosthetic limb control. (From Kautz, T. O. 1977.)

computer immediately calculates prosthetic position and rotational velocity errors. It determines a change in the valve (H) position necessary to attain the desired rotational position. This feeds through the DAC (C) via an interface circuit (D) to a solenoid controller (E). The solenoid controller instructs the proportional solenoid (F) to move the valve spool to the new position. The limb responds by either rotating faster or slower, thus achieving a new rotational position closer to the desired position. The whole process repeats roughly 930 times/s, thus closely responding to desired limb control pattern.

Colorado State University system

The Colorado State University system is based on an Intel 8080 microprocessor, which is interfaced through its input/output ports and with a 4-kbyte semiconductor memory (Fig. 5.39). To increase the speed of the multiply and divide operations (which are very time consuming with a microprocessor), the microprocessor is interfaced with a hardware multiply unit. It is based on Fairchild 9344 × 2-bit multiplier modules. The multiplication time is 350 ns, compared to 1 ms for the microprocessor itself.

The system is based on EMG signals. A 12-bit data acquisition system samples the EMG at 5000 samples/s and delivers the digital data to the microprocessor system. The control algorithm is based on time-series identification techniques for parameter discrimination (Graupe et al., 1976).

UCLA arm prosthesis

The UCLA upper-limb prosthesis was initially developed using a Teledyne TDY-52 microcomputer but has been subsequently replaced by an RCA COSMAC micro-computer. The computer interprets myoelectric signal patterns from nine electrodes. A pattern-recognition algorithm maps control signals from electrodes into coordinated motions for any possible combination of arm motors. The computer and the pattern-recognition subsystem fit into a complete control system organized in a fashion similar to the human brain.

The microcomputer uses a COSMAC microprocessor and 1 kbyte of RAM for program storage. An analog multiplexer (CD4067) selects the electrode input for the ADC. The microprocessor controls three motors—elbow, wrist, and hand—in various combinations.

Design example

We desire to build a microprocessor-based forearm prosthetic device. We wish to implement three degrees of freedom at the wrist joint, as described below:

1. Clasping–unclasping control.
2. Up–down motion of the hand.
3. Sideways motion of the hand.

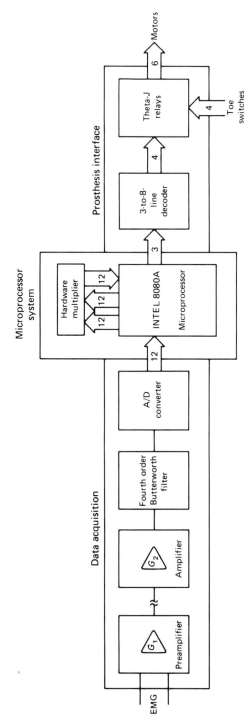

FIGURE 5.39 Colorado State University prosthetic limb. (From Graupe, D., et al. 1976. A micro-processor prosthesis control system based on time series identification of EMG signals. Proc. IEEE Int. Conf. Cybern. Soc. 6 : 680–684.)

From a series of experiments we find that eight electrodes, placed at various locations on the arm to record the EMG, will be needed to achieve the required control. Assume that through the interfacing analog circuitry a series of pulses are derived from each electrode. That is, a constant stream of pulses is generated for the time interval that EMG recorded from that electrode exceeds a preset threshold value. Using the COSMAC microcomputer, implement this system.

A very efficient way to implement this prosthesis would be to use the four flag lines to sense the eight control signals. To accommodate eight control signals on four flag lines, we must use a multiplexer. The Q line commands alternate switching of the four electrodes. We obtain the three degrees of control by three stepper motors connected to the three output lines, N0, N1, and N2. A monostable stretches the output pulse (8 μs) to that duration required by the stepper motor.

Figure 5.40 shows the schematic for implementing this. Figure 5.41 shows the flowchart for this prosthetic system. We should ascertain that sufficient time is available to do the job. For example, each input channel receives pulses (when the EMG is present) at the rate of 10/s. Maximum pulse rate to stepper motors is 50/s. The CPU clock rate is 2 MHz.

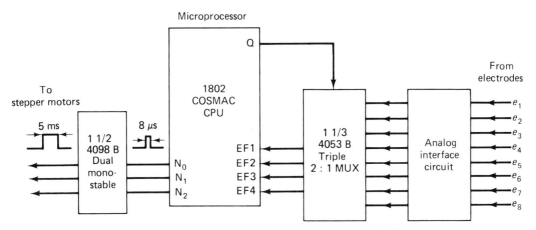

FIGURE 5.40 Microprocessor-based control of prosthetic arm.

Making the worst-case calculations: with all eight channels active, the number of flags to be tested $= 8 \times 10/s = 80/s$. (Note that to select the multiplexer, an instruction pair SEQ and REQ is necessary.) A typical flag testing sequence would be B1 Addr [i.e., short branch to Addr if flag EF1 $= 1$ (two machine cycles)]. This would be followed (or preceded) by condition BN1 Addr [i.e., short branch if flag EF1 $= 0$ (again, two machine cycles)]. Hence the minimum time required to test all the flags would be

$$\underset{\text{number of flags}}{8} \times \underset{\text{B1, BN1 instructions}}{(2 + 2) \times 8 \,\mu s} + \underset{\text{SEQ, REQ instructions}}{(1 + 1) \times 8 \,\mu s}$$

$$= 256 + 16 = 272 \,\mu s$$

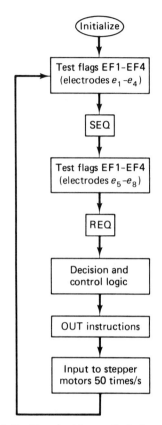

FIGURE 5.41 Flowchart for prosthetic forearm example.

After testing all the flags (272 μs), decision logic determines which stepper motor to turn on, at what rate. Let us say that 100 instructions are executed. Then the time required is

$$100 \times 8 \times 2 \ \mu s = 1600 \ \mu s$$

Hence the total time consumed between each output command is

$$1600 + 272 = 1872 \ \mu s = 1.872 \ ms$$

But since output commands have to be repeated at the rate of

$$3 \times 50 = 150/s$$

the available time is 7 ms. Hence there is sufficient time available to do the necessary control function. In fact, the decision logic may be allowed to execute approximately 400 instructions.

5.17 GENERAL MICROPROCESSOR-BASED MEDICAL DEVICES*

This section on presently available microcomputer medical instrumentation contains several devices that do not fit into any of the other categories. Some of these instruments are a spinal-curve-tension monitor, a psychometric tester, an intra-aortic balloon timer, a programmed exerciser, and a jogging computer.

Microprocessor cable-tension monitoring for spine-curve correction

Scoliosis is a spinal deformity that causes the spine to curve laterally (toward the side of the patient). For 90% of the patients, an external brace is sufficient to correct the condition, but in the remaining cases more drastic surgical procedures are necessary. One of the new techniques involves attaching a cable to the vertebrae in the affected area which have had the material between them removed. The surgeon then tightens the cable. This jams the affected vertebrae on top of each other and leads to a straight but rigid backbone in the area. The microprocessor-based device developed at M.I.T. monitors the tension applied to the cable after surgery.

The implanted strain-gage transducer changes resistance proportional to the amount of tension it undergoes from the titanium cable. A second strain gage is located on the load-cell neutral axis. This compensates for temperature variation and provides a reference from which the actual tension can be calculated. This implant contains no energy sources. It transmits the resistance value by changing the load impedance of an external electromagnetic source, as shown in Fig. 5.42. This external source couples inductively to the implanted rectifier, which provides a dc voltage to the relaxation oscillator. The strain-gage resistance is a part of the oscillator circuit that determines the rate of oscillation. Since the amount of power drawn from the external electromagnetic source changes as the frequency of the implanted oscillator changes, we can deduce the resistance of the strain gage controlling the oscillator. The two different strain-gage circuits can be selected by applying a magnetic field that activates a reed switch to change the circuit configuration.

The detector and processor provide the microprocessor with a digital representation of the period of the power oscillation of the external source. This is caused by the changing load impedance of the implant, which is proportional to the strain-gage resistance.

The Motorola MC6800 microprocessor has 512 bytes of ROM and 128 bytes of static RAM. The tension is read out on a four-digit LED display. An analog output of tension can be recorded on a tape recorder. The two four-digit thumbwheel switches are used to enter two load-cell parameters, which are needed to compute the tension and are determined before implantation.

There are three operating modes available in this instrument. The reference

---

*Section 5.17 written by James D. Woodburn.

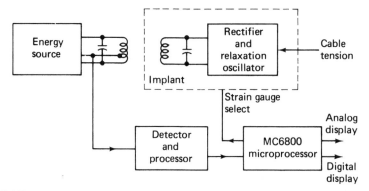

FIGURE 5.42 Implantable μP-based biotelemetry system measures the tension in a titanium cable attached to a patient's backbone to correct lateral curvature of the spine. Inputs from active and reference strain gages sequentially modulate the period of the implant's relaxation oscillator; the ratio of the two periods is proportional to the cable tension. [From Digital Design. 1976. © Benwill Publishing Corp. μP-based system monitors cable tension in spine-curvature-victim treatment. 6(5): 28–32. Used with permission.]

mode checks the reference strain gage and the active mode checks the active strain gage. These two modes can be selected manually or the processor can be switched into the automatic mode, which does both reference and active load-cell updating. The hardware provides the period timing pulses, which the processor uses as stop and start markers. It counts the number of clock pulses over a predetermined number of periods to form an average time interval, from which the microcomputer computes and displays the tension.

Testing soft tissue

Vito et al. (1978) use a single-board microcomputer to control arterial diameter during longitudinal stretch. A light-sensing charge-coupled phototransducer monitors arterial diameter and feeds data to the microcomputer. The microcomputer commands a digital servo that longitudinally stretches the artery at a constant rate. The microcomputer also controls a stepping-motor-powered pump that increases arterial pressure to maintain constant diameter. The program requires 2.5 kbytes of EPROM and 256 bytes of RAM. A larger computer takes data for plots of pressure and force versus time.

Penile tumescence

Researchers wish to measure the duration and amount of penile tumescence during sleep research. Underwood (1978) acquires these data using an Intel SBC 80/10 single-board microcomputer which contains an 8080, 1 kbyte of RAM, and 4 kbytes of ROM. An Intel SBC 104 Memory and I/O Expansion Board contains 4 kbytes of RAM and 4 kbytes of EPROM. A data acquisition module contains a

32-channel multiplexer and 12-bit A/D converter. A touch-tone key pad provides data entry and a thermal printer provides output.

Mercury strain gages encircle the penis and increase resistance during penile erection. The microcomputer takes 8000 samples during 1 s, averages them, and stores the average. The program scans a least-squares approximation of a straight line of the past 60 averages. If the present average deviates from the line by more than a threshold and a slope criteria is exceeded, it declares a tumescence event. A standard serial computer terminal provides monitoring capability and a cassette tape recorder provides data storage.

A cross assembler on an Intel MDS-800 computer assisted in software development, which took 1 worker-month. Hardware development took $\frac{1}{2}$ worker-month.

Esophageal manometry

To investigate diseases of the esophagus, the patient swallows a bundle of three catheters, with tips spaced 5 cm apart. Water perfuses the catheters and strain gages measure the pressures while the catheters are withdrawn through the esophagus. Fotland et al. (1978) analyze these data using an Intel 8080 microcomputer with 32 kbytes of RAM, 4 kbytes of ROM, a real-time clock, 12-bit A/D converters, two floppy-disk drives, a color CRT, and a high-speed printer.

The software is divided into four parts: calibration, pattern recognition, calculation, and output. The program determines the location of each tip; recognizes onset, peak, and end of contractile responses; and distinguishes responses from respiratory artifacts. During the test the color CRT displays a bar graph that indicates the location of each tip within the esophagus and indicates the distance from the incisors. The printer provides immediate hard copy that summarizes the parameters for the five regions of the esophagus. The system saves 2 h of manual data reduction per test.

Intraaortic balloon timing

Two microprocessor-based devices control the inflation/deflation cycle of an intra-aortic balloon. Inflation of the balloon aids a patient's circulation by increasing the systolic blood pressure after the closing of the aortic valve. The balloon is inflated at a generally accepted, fixed time interval after aortic valve closure. But users desire the ability to adjust the deflation timing. The two devices allow flexible timings so that an efficient deflation time interval may be established.

The first device was developed by a team from the Cardiovascular Engineering Laboratories in the Department of Surgery at Baylor College of Medicine (Cooper et al. 1977). It allows two modes of deflation control: (1) deflation occurs at a preset time interval before the next systole, or (2) deflation occurs after a preset percentage of diastole. A Motorola MC6800 calculates the deflation point by using a 1-kHz clock rate and counts the number of pulses between the detection of QRS complexes. It calculates either the percent diastole or the preset time and compares this value to the current count to deflate the balloon, as shown in Fig. 5.43. The system begins in a reset subroutine. The operator presses a pushbutton, which clears the peripheral interface adapters and the processor. Then the system goes into a wait state. After an interrupt generated by the occurrence of an R wave, a clock pulse, or a data input, the program executes the proper subroutine and returns to the wait state. If the interrupt was an R wave, it stores the time interval from the last QRS to the present R wave and uses it to calculate the new resultant (R) that will be used to control deflation. If a clock pulse occurred, it increments the interval counter (PC) and compares it to the resultant. If the counter exceeds the resultant, the balloon deflates; otherwise, the program returns to wait. If the front-panel button generates the interrupt, then the program enters into memory the information on the front-panel thumbwheel switches that corresponds to the pre-systolic time, percent diastole, and systolic duration time. Two LEDs indicate deflation and an error condition.

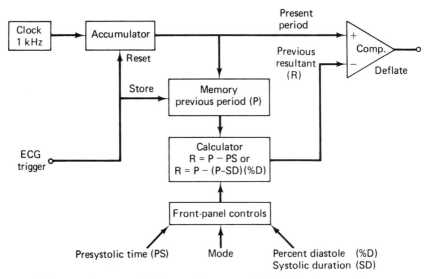

FIGURE 5.43 Schematic diagram of intraaortic balloon inflation controller. (From Cooper, J. B., et al. 1977. Microprocessor control of intra-aortic balloon timing. Proc. Annu. Conf. Eng. Med. Biol. 19:351. Used with permission.)

The second microprocessor device was developed by the Avco Everett Research Laboratory for their AVCO Intra-Aortic Balloon Pump. It uses an Intel 8008 and 4 kbytes of ROM. The software implements a more sophisticated ECG detection algorithm, which allows greater detection, reliability, and artifact rejection. The detection algorithm averages recent QRS complexes. Then it establishes a threshold that the current R wave must exceed. When the signal exceeds this threshold, it must reverse polarity (as the QRS complex does) and fall to another threshold voltage later than 15 to 20 ms and sooner than 125 ms. This device has been effective in handling spike artifacts, depressed S-T segments, PVCs, abrupt T waves, and baseline drifts. The resultant proper timing has prevented obstructing the blood flow or exceeding the pump characteristics.

Infusion pump

The infusion pump infuses liquids, nutrients, and medications into patients through catheters at rates up to 1 liter/h. IVAC (1979) incorporates a microcomputer into their infusion pump to prompt setup procedures, indicate flow and volume, and reveal alarm situations. During setup it displays sequenced messages that will not advance until step completion: LOAD SET, CLOSE DOOR, OPEN CLAMP, SENSOR, SET RATE, and START. The operator sets the rate by thumbwheels and the LED displays the total volume infused.

During operation other displays reveal alarm situations: BOTTLE (container is empty), CLAMP (flow is restricted), OCCLUDED (excessive back pressure), LOW BATT (use power cord), DOOR (close door), RATE = 000 (no pumping), SET OUT (IV set removed from pump), and FIX ME (call technician). The memory provides a sequential history of the past 16 alarm situations—a helpful in-service tool.

Programmed exerciser

The programmed exerciser monitors exercise rate and provides feedback to indicate the desired level of conditioning (*Electronic Design*, 1976). The programmed exerciser consists of an exercycle (a stationary seat with pedals like a bicycle) that controls its load on the pedals by electronically switching in a braking torque. The Rockwell PPS-4/2 4-bit microcomputer contains a CPU, an I/O chip, a 4-kbyte ROM, and a 128-byte RAM. A rechargeable battery initially powers the electronics. The pedals operate an alternator that drives the electronics, recharges the battery, and drives the resistive pedal load. The rider enters personal data such as sex, age, or weight into a keyboard and a display echoes the input. A warm-up load level starts the exercise period, and after a few minutes, the microprocessor switches the load to a higher conditioning level. It also monitors the heart rate picked up by a solid-state sensor clipped onto the ear or three chest electrodes. It lights one of three LEDs to indicate warmup, proper, or overconditioning levels. The rider can instruct the computer at any time to display on a four-digit LED display the parameters of calories expended, elapsed exercise time, exercise units, actual heart rate, target heart rate, workload, or a review of the initial entries. During the final 3 min of the exercise period, the microprocessor compares the user's performance with the average value of the group of same sex, weight, and age. The final result gives a score that corresponds to the individual's overall physical condition.

X-ray control

The General Electric Company has incorporated an 8080A microcomputer in its MPX x-ray system. A ROM provides permanent storage for the main program. The RAM provides storage for extensive look-up tables and has a nickel–cadmium battery backup. The service person can easily update these look-up tables as required.

The operator selects the desired technique by pushing several pushbuttons. He or she must pick (1) patient size (small, medium, large) and (2) anatomical part (skull, ribs, hand, feet, etc.); and may pick (3) lateral or oblique and (4) specialized techniques (pediatric torso, etc.).

Each pushbutton interrupts the microcomputer and transfers updated tube parameters from the look-up tables to the technique registers. The technique registers set parameters on the x-ray tube, such as peak voltage, current, and current–time product. LED displays provide tube parameter information to the operator.

Microprocessor system for psychometric testing

A microprocessor-based system that creates, administers, monitors, and grades a psychomotor test has been developed at Vanderbilt University. The scores give an indication of the amount of nitrogenous wastes in the blood, since patients with high levels of these bases have a poorer response to the test than do normal subjects. The microcomputer generates four types of tests: reaction time (two different ways), scanning ability, and short-term memory.

This system uses an 8080-based Intelligent Systems Corp. Model 8001 terminal to store the program and display the various patterns on the screen. The manual response consists of hitting a button switch. The system has only one peripheral device (the switch) other than the terminal. This shows that minimal hardware can be used to perform a very useful function.

The microprocessor generates the following test. It randomly selects and displays one character out of four possible characters. If the character is the chosen one, the subject presses the switch. The microcomputer measures reaction time by two different methods. It measures scanning ability by having the individual pick out the one character that is displayed three times in an array of 16 characters. The final test of short-term memory consists of deciding whether or not a computer-selected character had been displayed earlier in a string of characters. The software generates a random number for each of the tests, displays the individual test, and produces a statistical mean of the responses for grading. The program is presently down-line-loaded into RAM from another computer.

Independent living for the elderly

Loss of short-term memory frequently accompanies advancing age. This is a significant threat to the continued ability to live independently for individuals who require dietary restrictions or self-administered medications. Houge (1979) used a

6502 microcomputer with 4 kbytes of RAM to develop a low-cost prompting and information retrieval aid.

The individual presses a start button and on his TV screen receives a list and times for the day's schedule; for example:

1. Take insulin injection.
2. Breakfast menu.
3. Four capsules of medicine.
4. Take and record blood pressure.
5. Receive home visit from nurse.
6. Dentist appointment.
7. Meals on wheels delivery.

If he or she forgets to perform an item by the scheduled time or to cancel it, an alarm rings until it is canceled. A caretaker periodically enters new information into the system.

A second-generation system will use notebook storage for the instructions. The battery-operated CMOS microcomputer system will display notebook page numbers on a LCD. Rather than viewing messages on a TV screen, the user will then look up the information in the notebook.

Physician's office

Cameron (1978) shows that a $5000 microcomputer has potential for helping the single physician or small group practice. He used a Processor Technology SOL-20, which includes a CRT, a North Star Mini-Floppy Disk System, and an Okidata printer. Using BASIC, he designed, implemented, tested, and debugged a problem-oriented medical record (POMR) system in about 24 worker-hours. The programs are interactive and self-prompting and follow the following outline.

1. Enter new patient:
   a. Identification.
   b. Initialize record.
2. Update patient record:
   a. Add new problem.
   b. Resolve old problem.
   c. Remove any entry (edit).
   d. Add new allergy.
   e. Add new prescription.
3. Examine patient record:
   a. CRT.
   b. Printer.
4. List patients on disk.

The typical patient record requires about 200 to 800 bytes of floppy disk storage.

REFERENCES

AIKAWA, J. K. 1974. The cost-effectiveness of the C. U. computerized clinical laboratory system. Biomed. Sci. Instrum. 10: 89–92.

ALBERI, J. L., AND HARDY, W. H. 1976. An instrument for bone mineral measurement using a microprocessor as the control and arithmetic element. IEEE Trans. Nucl. Sci. NS-23: 645–650.

ALEXANDER, G., AND HOSEK, R. S. 1978. Microprocessorized laboratory physiological data system. Proc. Annu. Conf. Eng. Med. Biol. 20: 157.

ALLAN, R. 1976. Electronics aids disabled. IEEE Spectrum 13(11): 36–40.

BAHR, D., AND DHUPAR, K. 1977. A microprocessor-based arterial tonometer. Proc. 1st Annu. Symp. Comp. Appl. Med. Care.: 90–98.

BERTRAND, M., GUARDO, R., MATHIEU, G., BLONDEAU, P., AND LeBLANC, R. 1975. A microprocessor-based system for ECG encoding and transmission. Proc. Annu. Conf. Eng. Med. Biol. 17: 435.

BICKFORD, R. G., BILLINGER, T. W., FLEMING, N. I., AND STEWART, L. 1972. The compressed spectral array (CSA)—a pictorial EEG. Proc. San Diego Biomed. Symp. 11: 365–370.

BILGUTAY, A. M., BILGUTAY, I., AND GARAMELLA, J. J. 1976. Self-monitoring pacemaker function with pace-pulse-trace. Proc. AAMI Annu. Meet., pp. 46–47.

BLOM, J. A., VAN DER AA, J., JORRITSMA, F. F., BENEKEN, J. E. W., NANDORFF, A., SPIERDIJK, J., AND VAN BIJNEN, A. 1979. A research-oriented microcomputer based patient monitoring system. Dept. Elec. Eng., University of Technology, Eindhoven, Netherlands.

BURKOWSKI, F. J., AND TRENHOLM, B. G. 1978. Design of a microprocessor-based physiological data averager. Proc. AAMI Annu. Meet. p. 270.

BUTLER, L. A. 1977. EEG signal processing during surgery. Biomed. Sci. Instrum. 13: 89–92.

BUTLER, L. A. 1978. A real-time microprocessor system for EEG spectral analysis. Proc. Annu. Conf. Eng. Med. Biol. 20: 5.

CALMA, I., AND JOHNSON, F. 1976. Using a microprocessor to provide automatic control of hand–eye co-ordination experiments in primates. Proc. J. Physiol. (Lond.) 258(1): 6P–7P.

CAMERON, J. M. 1978. Microcomputer medical information system. Proc. Annu. Conf. Eng. Med. Biol. 20: 320.

CHEMETRON. 1977. RICS II respiratory intensive care system. St. Louis, MO.

COLLINS. 1978. Eagle one. Braintree, MA.

COMP-U-MED. 1977. Computer-assisted ECG service. Los Angeles, CA.

Computer News. 1978. Micro-controlled knee customizes artificial leg. 4(7).

COOPER, T. G., SADLER, C. R., AND NORMANN, N. A. 1977. Microprocessor control of intra-aortic balloon timing. Proc. Annu. Conf. Eng. Med. Biol. 19:351.

COOPER, J. B., NEWBOWER, R. S., MOORE, J. W., AND TRAUTMAN, E. D. 1978. A new anesthesia delivery system. Anesthesiology 49(5):310–318.

COX, J. R., JR. 1965. Special purpose digital computers in biology. In R. W. Stacy and B. D. Waxman (eds.), Computers in biomedical research, Vol. 2. New York: Academic Press.

CREITZ, W. W., AND SCHNEIDER, A. A. 1976. Characterizing lithium–iodine pacemaker cells with a microprocessor-controlled testing system. Proc. AAMI Annu. Meet., p. 54.

CULLEN, D. J. 1974. Interpretation of blood pressure measurements in anesthesia. Anesthesiology 40(1):6–11.

CUPAL, J. J. 1977. A transmitter identifier for use with wildlife biotelemetry. Biomed. Sci. Instrum. 13:13–17.

DECKER, J. R., HOF, P. J., AND PHILLIPS, R. D. 1976. Automated rodent respiratory monitor and histogram computer. Biomed. Sci. Instrum. 12:7–13.

DEHART, W. R., AND BARCLAY, M. L. 1978. Birth from the uterus: parameters by commercial microcomputer. Proc. Annu. Conf. Eng. Med. Biol. 20:181.

DENNIS, J. H., AND CYWINSKI, J. K. 1976. The use of microprocessor for non-invasive recordings of electrical activity from the conduction system of the heart. Proc. Annu. Conf. Eng. Med. Biol. 18:187.

DEUTSCH, L. S., ENGELSE, W. A. H., VAN DER VOORDE, F., AND HUGENHOLTZ, P. G. 1977. The unibed patient monitoring system: a new approach for a new technology. Med. Instrum. 11:274–277.

Digital Design. 1976. μP-based system monitors cable tension in spine-curvature-victim treatment. 6(5):28–32.

DOBELLE, W., MLADEJOVSKY, M., STENSAAS, S., AND SMITH, J. 1973. A prosthesis for the deaf based on cortical stimulation. Ann. Otol. Rhinol. Laryngol. 82:445–463.

DONATI, F., GUARDO, R., BERTRAND, M., LAPOINTE, A., AND ROBERGE, F. A. 1978. A micro-computer system for monitoring hemodynamic variables. Proc. AAMI Annu. Meet.

DOUBLER, J. A., AND CHILDRESS, D. S. 1978. Applications of microcomputer technology to rehabilitation problems of severely disabled persons. Proc. Natl. Electron. Conf. 32:271–274.

DOWLING, N. B., McFADDEN, E. R., SYKES, T. W., BURNS, S. K., AND MARK, R. G. 1978. Microcomputer-controlled operation of a whole-body plethysmograph. Proc. Annu. Conf. Eng. Med. Biol. 20:229.

DOYLE, J. 1976. EEG brain function monitoring using a microcomputer. Proc. MIMI Symp. Mini Microcomput., pp. 213–216.

Electronic Design. 1976. Pedal exerciser with built-in μP quickly reveals your fitness level. 24(17):38.

Electronics. 1973. An electronic link to the visual cortex may let blind "see." 46(26):29–39.

Electronics. 1974. Data processing, LSI will help to bring sight to blind. 47(2):81–86.

Electronics. 1979. Medtronic tests pacemaker run by a microprocessor. 52(4): 33.

ELECTRONICS FOR MEDICINE. 1979. SMART ECG amplifier. Pleasantville, NY.

Electronics Test. 1979. Digital scopes. 2(1): 68–75.

ELLIS, R. C., JR. 1976. Signal averaging and medical applications. Med. Electron. Data 7(2): 41–43.

FENG, C. H., LIN, W. C., AND NEUMAN, M. R. 1976. A microprocessor-based data acquisition and preprocessing system for obstetrical patient monitoring. Proc. Annu. Conf. Eng. Med. Biol. 18: 189.

FLAX, S. W. 1977a. An experimental utilization of microcomputers in training the mentally retarded. Proc. Annu. Conf. Eng. Med. Biol. 19: 120.

FLAX, S. W. 1977b. A microcomputer application for training the mentally retarded. IEEE Region 6 Conf. Rec., pp. 79–82.

FLAX, S. W., AND YOUNT, J. E. 1978. A microprocessor based apnea monitor for the neonate. Proc. Annu. Conf. Eng. Med. Biol. 20: 71.

FLEMING, R. A., COLES, J. R., AND SMITH, N. T. 1976. Patient protection for a biomedical computer system. Proc. San Diego Biomed. Symp., pp. 67–74.

FOTLAND, D. A., JONES, R. D., CROSS, F. S., AND ALPERT, M. A. 1978. Real time microcomputer esophageal manometry analysis. Proc. Annu. Conf. Eng. Med. Biol. 20: 162.

FREEDY, A., SOLOMONOW, M., AND LYMAN, J. 1975. A microcomputer based arm prosthesis with two-channel sensory feedback. Proc. 1975 IEEE Conf. Decis. Control, pp. 92–98.

FREEMAN, J. J., HOLZHAUER, L. A., AND NOWAK, G. F. 1978. Microprocessor analysis of electronystagmographic signals. Proc. Annu. Conf. Eng. Med. Biol. 20: 99.

FRUGONE, G., GIANNOTTI, E., MORANO, P., TAGLIASCO, V., AND VERNAZZA, T. 1977. The use of mini- and micro-computers in eye clinical practice. Doc. Ophthalmol. 43(1): 31–44.

FURMAN, S., AND ESCHER, D. J. W. 1970. Principles and techniques of cardiac pacing. New York: Harper & Row.

GARLAND, H., AND AHLGREN, A. 1978. Personal computers go to work. Computer 11(6): 28–32.

GIANUNZIO, J. W., DENNIS, W. H., PEGELOW, D. F., AND WERNER, M. W. 1978. A microcomputer system for the pulmonary function laboratory. Proc. Annu. Conf. Eng. Med. Biol. 20: 233.

GIBBONS, D. T., AND JOHNSON, F. 1976. Microprocessors in fetal monitoring. Dig. Int. Conf. Med. Biol. Eng., pp. 556–557.

GRAUPE, D., BEEX, A. A. M., MAGNUSSEN, J. AND SOFFA, M. B. 1976. A microprocessor prosthesis control system based on time series identification of EMG signals. Proc. IEEE Int. Conf. Cybern. Soc. 6: 680–684.

GRUNDMANN, J., AND SEIREG, A. 1976. Computer control of multitask exoskeleton for paraplegics. In A. MORECKI, AND K. KEDZOIR (EDS.), Theory and practice of robots and manipulators. New York: Elsevier, 1978.

GUARDO, R., AND BERTRAND, M. 1976. A programmable physiological stimulator. Proc. Annu. Conf. Eng. Med. Biol. 18: 191.

HARTZ, R. K. 1977. A microprocessor-based system for the acquisition of visual field data from a Goldman perimeter. M.S. thesis. Washington University, St. Louis.

HARTZ, R. K. 1978. Personal communication.

HATHAWAY, J. C., ASCHE, D. R., COOK, A. M., AND ZUMSTEIN, R. R. 1976a. Microprocessor implementation of ventilation-patient monitoring. Med. Instrum. 10(1): 69.

HATHAWAY, J. C., COOK A. M., AND SMITH, W. D. 1976b. A versatile microprocessor based instrumentation system for use in biomedical engineering instruction. Biomed. Sci. Instrum. 12: 1–5.

HONEYWELL. 1978. MEDDARS physiological data system. Denver, CO.

HOSEK, R. S., AUGENSTEIN, J. S., SCHNEIDERMANN, N., AND PETERSON, E. A. 1976. A microprocessor-based physiological data recorder. Proc. Annu. Conf. Eng. Med. Biol. 18: 190.

HOUGE, J. C. 1979. A microprocessor-based prompting and information system for support of the elderly in independent living situations. Instrumentation Systems Center, University of Wisconsin, Madison, WI.

HSIAO, H. S., HARRY, R., AND WILLIAMS, S. 1978. A microcomputer-based instrument to measure pulse compliance. Proc. Annu. Conf. Eng. Med. Biol. 20: 322.

IVAC CORP. 1979. The IVAC 630 volumetric infusion pump. San Diego, CA 92121.

JENKINS, J., COLLINS, S., AND ARZBAECHER, R. 1978. Two-channel microprocessor arrhythmia analyzer. Proc. Annu. Conf. Eng. Med. Biol. 20: 61.

JOHNSON, A. S., AND SMITH, J. R. 1978. Automatic detection of petit-mal seizures. Proc. AAMI Annu. Meet, p. 139.

JOHNSON, T. L., WRIGHT, S. C. AND SEGALL, A. 1979. Filtering of muscle artifact from the electroencephalogram. IEEE Trans. Biomed. Eng. BME-26: 556–563.

JOLDA, J. G., AND WANZEK, S. J. 1978. Prototype inflight physiological data acquisition system. Proc. Annu. Conf. Eng. Med. Biol. 20: 165.

JORGENS, J., III, AND GILMAN, R. 1978. Microcomputer generated stimuli for evoked potentials research. Proc. Annu. Conf. Eng. Med. Biol. 20: 318.

KATONA, P. G., DURAND, D., STERN, K., FLEMING, D. G., AND MARTIN, R. J. 1977. Microprocessor-controlled memory for cardiopulmonary monitoring of high risk infants. IEEE Trans. Biomed. Eng. BME-24: 536–538.

KAUTZ, T. O. 1977. Feasibility study of a computer-controlled hydraulic above-knee prosthetic limb. M.S. thesis, University of Wisconsin, Madison, WI.

KEANE, B. 1978. EEG phasic event detection by microcomputer. IEEE Trans. Biomed. Eng. BME-25: 297–299.

KEANE, B., SINGH, G., AND NELSON, A. V. 1978a. Microprocessor-based portable EEG conditioning unit. Proc. AAMI Annu. Meet., p. 146.

KEANE, B., HENKE, J., AND BISCHOF, G. 1978b. Real-time analysis of bioelectric data using a single-chip microcomputer system. Proc. Ann. Conf. Eng. Med. Biol. 20: 321.

KEEMINK, C. J., VAN DER WILDT, G. J., AND VAN DEURSEN, J. B. P. 1979. Microprocessor-controlled contrast sensitivity measurements. Med. Biol. Eng. Comput. 17: 371–378.

KEIMER, M. L., JOHNSON, D., AND WELLS, M. 1978. A microprocessor-based system for the implementation of psychometric testing. Proc. AAMI Annu. Meet, p. 128.

KLIG, V. 1978. Biomedical applications of microprocessors. Proc. IEEE 66: 151–161.

KROUSE, C. T., FLAX, S. W., YOUST, J. E., AND SHENAI, J. P. 1977. A research apnea monitor based on microcomputer technology. IEEE Region 6 Conf. Rec., pp. 1–4.

LEWIS, J. W., AND DAVIS, J. E. 1975. Improving the throughput and efficiency of a multichannel clinical chemistry analyzer with a microprocessor controller. Proc. AAMI Annu. Meet, p. 56.

LIN, W. C., FENG, C. H., AND NEUMAN, M. R. 1977. A microprocessor-based data acquisition and processing system for studying the kinematics of labor. Proc. IEEE. 65(5): 722–729.

LKB-WALLAC. 1978. RackBeta series of liquid scintillation counters. Stockholm.

LOONEY, J. 1978. Blood pressure by oscillometry. Med. Electron. Data 9(2): 57–63.

LYNN, D. E., PEARSON, J. R., AND PINFIELD, E. R. 1977. Design of a microprocessor-based intelligent interface. Biomed. Sci. Instrum. 13: 59–60.

MARGALITH, A., PRIMIANO, F. P., AND MERGLER, H. W. 1977. Automation of an existing blood gas analyzer using a microprocessor. Proc. AAMI Annu. Meet., p. 85.

MARQUETTE ELECTRONICS. 1978. MAC-1 microcomputer augmented cardiograph. Milwaukee, WI.

McDEVITT, H. 1978. Personal communication. Reston, VA: Acuity Systems.

Med-Science Electronics. 1977. Microprocessing lung analyzer minimizes analog signal handling. EDN. 1977 (Oct. 5): 33–34.

MICHAELS, D. L., AND TOLE, J. R. 1977. A microprocessor-based instrument for nystagmus analysis. Proc. IEEE. 65: 730–735.

MIDWEST ANALOG AND DIGITAL. 1978. M.A.D. color video data system. New Berlin, WI.

MOORE, B. J. 1970. Signal averaging. Med. Electron. Data 1(2): 65–70.

MORITZ, W. E., AND MURDOCK, D. B. 1975. Microprocessor based patient monitoring system. Proc. Annu. Conf. Eng. Med. Biol. 17: 438.

NEUMAN, M. R. 1978. In J. G. WEBSTER (ED.)., Medical instrumentation: application and design. Boston: Houghton Mifflin.

NICOLET INSTRUMENT. 1978. Instruction manual for series 2090 Explorer digital oscilloscope. Madison, WI.

NORLAND INSTRUMENTS. 1976. NI 2001 programmable calculating oscilloscope user reference manual. Fort Atkinson, WI.

O'DESKY, R. I., NELMS, G. E., AND WEISBROD, S. P. 1977. Hardware considerations for a microprocessor-based pacemaker tracking system. Proc. Annu. Conf. Eng. Med. Biol. 19: 130.

ORION RESEARCH. 1977. Guide to electrodes and instrumentation. Form 1 and EB/776. Cambridge, MA.

RAMPIL, I. J., AND FLEMMING, D. C. 1978. An inexpensive microcomputer trend monitoring system. Proc. New. Engl. Bioeng. Conf. 6: 67–70.

RAMSEY, M. 1976. Device for indirect noninvasive automatic mean arterial pressure. Proc. Annu. Conf. Eng. Med. Biol. 18: 99.

RAMSEY, M. 1977. Microprocessor-based blood pressure screening device. Proc. AAMI Annu. Meet., p. 57.

ROSS, D. T. 1957. Notes on analog–digital conversion techniques. Cambridge, MA: MIT Press.

SACHS, J. M. 1976. STOIC, an interactive language for microprocessors. Proc. Annu. Conf. Eng. Med. Biol. 18: 252.

SCHMALZEL, J. L., GALLAGHER, R. R., AND BARQUEST, J. M. 1977. An impedance pneumograph utilizing microprocessor based instrumentation. Biomed. Sci. Instrum. 13: 63–68.

SCHOENFELD, R. L., KOCSIS, W. A., MILKMAN, N., AND SILVERMAN, G. 1977. The microprocessor in the biological laboratory. Computer 10(5): 56–67.

Science. 1974. Artificial vision for the blind: electrical stimulation of visual cortex offers hope for a functional prosthesis. 183(412): 440–444.

SEARLE, J. R., AND KISSOCK, P. 1978. Microcomputer-assisted diagnosis and treatment of aphasics. Proc. Annu. Conf. Eng. Med. Biol. 20: 158.

SHAPIRO, J. M., KINI, M. M., AND PHILPOTT, D. E. 1978a. Early diagnosis of glaucoma: a microprocessor-based system. Proc. Annu. Conf. Eng. Med. Biol. 20: 161.

SHAPIRO, J. M., KINI, M. M., AND PHILPOTT, D. E. 1978b. A microprocessor-based system for non-invasive measurement of optic disc blood flow. Proc. San Diego Biomed. Symp. 17: 39–46.

SIDDONS, H., AND SOWTON, E. 1974. Cardiac pacemakers. Springfield, IL: Charles C Thomas.

SLEZAK, K. D., MOSTARDI, R. A., ATWOOD, G. A., WOEBKENBERG, N., AND AMBELANG, M. 1978. Microprocessor application in studies of pulmonary functions. Proc. Annu. Conf. Eng. Med. Biol. 20: 234.

TERDIMAN, J. F., SCHENKER, W., AND TUTTLE, R. 1977. Microcomputer interfaces with clinical laboratory instruments. Proc. AAMI Annu. Meet., p. 211.

THALEN, H. J. TH., BERG, J. W. VAN DER, HEIDE, J. N. H. VAN DER, AND NIEUEEN, J. 1970. The artificial cardiac pacemaker. Assen: Royal Van Corcum.

THORN, G. W., ADAMS, R. D., BRAUNWALD, E., ISSELBACHER, K. J., AND PETERSDORF, R. G. (EDS.). 1977. Harrison's principles of internal medicine, 8th ed. New York: McGraw-Hill.

TOLE, J. R., YORKER, J. G., AND RENSHAW, R. L. 1978. A microprocessor controlled multi degree of freedom chair for vestibular testing. Proc. Annu. Conf. Eng. Med. Biol. 20: 160.

TRAUTMAN, E. D., COOPER, J. B., AND NEWBOWER, R. S. 1976. A new anesthesia delivery system using microprocessors. Proc. ELECTRO 76 Prof. Prog., Paper 13-4.

UNDERWOOD, S. A. 1978. Use of micro-processors for medical monitoring in sleep research Proc. MIDCON, Paper 26/2.

VALVANO, J. V., WOODS, M., AND BOWMAN, H. F. 1978. A microprocessor-based thermal diffusion probe for blood flow. Proc. Annu. Conf. Eng. Med. Biol. 20: 163.

VANDERHEIDEN, G. C., KELSO, D. P., HOLT, C. S., AND RAITZER, G. S. 1976. Portable microprocessor-based communication aids for non-vocal severely physically handicapped individuals. Madison, WI.: Trace Center, University of Wisconsin-Madison.

VARTANIAN, M. M., AND GROESBERG, S. W. 1978. A microprocessor-based communicator for aphonic persons. Proc. Annu. Conf. Eng. Med. Biol. 20: 319.

VITO, R. P., WILLIAMS, T. V., AND NYGAARD, R. 1978. A microprocessor-based bi-axial tissue testing device. Proc. Annu. Conf. Eng. Med. Biol. 20: 259.

WAX, S. D., WEBB, W. R., AND OSBURN, K. C. 1978. Microprocessor-based pulmonary mechanics instrumentation. Proc. Annu. Conf. Eng. Med. Biol. 20:231.

WILSON, P. 1978. Wisconsin stimulus programmer (Personal communication). Medical Electronics Lab, University of Wisconsin-Madison, Madison, WI.

YELDERMAN, M., AND REAM, A. K. 1978. A microprocessor-based automated non-invasive blood pressure device for the anesthetized aptient. Proc. San Diego Biomed. Symp. 17:57–64.

ZICK, G. L. 1977. A microprocessor-based instrument for measurement of net charge transport. Proc. AAMI Annu. Meet, p. 84.

PROBLEMS

5.1 We wish to use the microcomputer to implement signal averaging of EEG data in evoked response experiments. The data are available in 8-bit samples. If we wish to average 100 such evoked responses and thus improve our SNR by 10, how much memory is needed for each data point?

5.2 A digital oscilloscope has a 10-bit ADC and 2 kwords of memory. The sampling period is selectable from 500 ns to 5 s in the standard 1, 2, and 5 steps (i.e., 500 ns, 1 μs, 2 μs, 5 μs, 10 μs, etc). Can this oscilloscope accurately record a 15-Hz signal with frequency components of 1 MHz? What sampling period would you select? What is the amplitude resolution?

5.3 Under ideal conditions, how many repetitions of a signal must be averaged to improve the SNR by 30 dB?

5.4 The ECG of a fetus is of diagnostic importance. It is impossible to externally pick up the fetal ECG without also picking up the ECG of the mother. However, the maternal and fetal ECGs are uncorrelated. Can signal averaging be used to record the fetal ECG? How?

5.5 With delta coding with threshold, assume that generated characters are three 6-bit differential amplitudes and the 6-bit elapsed time and the difference exceeds a threshold value 50 times/s. (a) What is the necessary baud rate to transmit ECG data with this method? (b) What is the data compression ratio?

5.6 What controls the priorities of maskable interrupt requests?

5.7 In Fig. 5.16, what is the function of the 16-channel multiplexer?

5.8 What are some of the advantages and disadvantages of using a common data bus for the GE and Spacelabs monitoring systems?

5.9 As engineers we are all familiar with the advantages of feedback. The Boston Anesthesia system uses a different form of control over gas flow with its digital valves. Can you identify what engineering principle is used?

5.10 What is one of the major problems with implanted circuitry?

5.11 If the arterial tonometer is developed to the point where it accurately reflects the pressure in the radial artery at the wrist, will it give accurate readings of a person's mean blood pressure as measured by more conventional means? Why?

5.12 Design a control system for a lower-limb, above-knee prosthesis for a subject with one leg intact. By means of switches placed below the feet, synchronizing timing pulses are provided by (1) a switch under a toe on each foot and (2) a switch under each heel. An electrogoniometer provides a signal proportional to the knee angle of the intact leg. Two motors in the prosthesis must be controlled: (1) knee rotation and (2) ankle rotation. Since the system must be mounted on the prosthesis and be battery-operated, use the COSMAC microcomputer.

5.13 (a) For the intraaortic balloon timer described in Section 5.17, draw an operational flowchart. (b) Assuming that the heart rate is 72 beats/min, duration of systole is 300 ms, and the balloon is to deflate at 30% of diastole, show the calculations that the computer must perform.

5.14 The thermal printhead in the AUTOCOM is a set of metal "dots" which heat up. They are connected in a 5×4 row-column (x-y) fashion that allows each pad or "dot" to be selected by driving the proper x and y lines. In the AUTOCOM, the nine lines are activated by driving power transistors from output ports. After a character is printed, a solenoid is activated which moves the thermal paper so that the head is above the next print position. Develop a flowchart for printing characters, assuming that the pads print as soon as they are selected.

6

A Detailed Design Example— Ambulatory ECG Monitoring

In this chapter we describe in detail a design example of a microcomputer-based biomedical system. We have picked a real-life project planned and implemented at the University of Wisconsin. Our approach in this chapter is to first develop a philosophy for the project based on real needs. We identify a physiological problem and our approach to solving it. We define the physicians' criteria for identifying arrhythmias and translate them into computer algorithms. Having worked out an approach to the problem, we set up detailed target specifications for our device— the arrhythmia monitor. We describe, at system and block-diagram level, the design of the entire monitor. Then we decide on the hardware needed to meet the specifications and discuss the detailed design of the system. We begin with analog circuit development and follow this by the design of the digital system, including the microcomputer. Subsequent to the hardware design we summarize work done on software development, an integral part being data-reduction algorithms. Finally, we describe system testing and evaluate the completed project.

6.1 PRESENT MONITORING METHODS— AN INTRODUCTION TO A PORTABLE ARRHYTHMIA MONITOR*

Physician's office ECG

A patient's prime contact with cardiac care before a heart attack is usually the family physician. Older individuals tend to visit doctors at more frequent intervals for physicals, minor complaints, and follow-up exams. It has become very common for a physician to take a patient's ECG in his or her office. Of course, the doctor will have a list of prime candidates for heart attack based on known cardiac risk factors, including high blood pressure, heavy smoking habits, and obesity. The family doctor may capture 10 s to 5 min of ECG data on any given day and not see the patient again for several months. Unless the patient happens to have some arrhythmia at the time of the ECG or complains about dizziness, minor chest pains, or other symptoms, the physician will not have any hint of developing heart trouble.

CCU monitoring

After a heart attack, the patient is normally placed in a coronary care unit for a few days. During this time he or she is usually monitored by a simple cardiotachometer, which alarms on high or low heart rates. Some of the more advanced hospitals may have a computer monitoring system in the CCU which analyzes the patient's ECG for a multitude of arrhythmias. Unfortunately, the CCU is very expensive and has a limited number of beds. Therefore, the patient is only extensively monitored for a few days until he or she is moved to a room where there is little or no monitoring.

Holter monitoring and the cardiologist

After the heart attack the patient will be under the care of a cardiologist. The cardiologist may gather ECGs several times a day while the patient is in the hospital in an attempt to determine exactly what is wrong with the heart. Of course, more than just ECGs are used to make a diagnosis. But after the patient leaves the hospital, there is no monitoring at all. A normal course would be to put the patient on a multitude of drugs and prescribe limited activity for several months.

A few patients may be monitored with a Holter monitor, a tape recorder that the patient carries around for a day. The monitor makes a tape recording of the ECG for a 12- to-24-h period. After the recording is taken, it must be analyzed. The analysis is generally performed by coronary care nurses, who view the recording played back at 60 times real time. An oscilloscope triggers on each R wave during playback so that single normal complexes almost superimpose, while abnormal complexes stand out because of their different shapes. When an abnormal complex is detected, the operator can back up the tape for another look, and if the arrhyth-

*Section 6.1 written by John P. Abenstein.

391

mia is considered interesting it can be played out on a pen recorder for permanent record and subsequent analysis by the cardiologist (Webster, 1978).

Alternative methods of analysis include both in-house and commercial scanning services that occasionally make use of computer systems. Although the Holter monitor can capture 24 h of ECG data, it has significant limitations. First is the assumption that the arrhythmia of interest will occur on the day of recording. Many patients have dangerous cardiac events that occur only once every few days or even weeks. Even if the arrhythmia is captured on tape, it must be found by the coronary care nurse. The nurse's job is tedious, time-consuming, and subject to a great deal of human error. Finally, after the recording is completed and analyzed by a nurse, it must find its way into the hands of the patient's physician for final diagnosis and subsequent action, a process requiring from 1 to 4 days. Recently, computer systems have been developed to analyze Holter tapes automatically, but the analysis is imperfect and there is still a significant time lag between recording and diagnosis.

An intelligent monitor

There is a need for a portable arrhythmia and conduction disturbance monitor to fill the gap in patient monitoring discussed above. It should detect arrhythmias and conduction disturbances, store samples of such arrhythmias, transmit them to a central computer for display and analysis, and generate alarms. It should be continuously worn for up to 1 month without the need to change batteries. It should only respond to programmed abnormal ECGs and be flexible in terms of alarm criteria so that it can be both patient- and physician-specific.

This chapter discusses our development of a device that meets these criteria. We have designed it to monitor cardiac patients that normally would have little diagnostic information gathered for their specific cardiac problems. Finally, the device has a general-purpose computer as its heart; therefore, it is reprogrammable, thus providing for implementation of other applications.

6.2 DEFINING THE PHYSIOLOGICAL PROBLEM*

Before hardware and software design can begin, we must define the problem to be solved. Our device must monitor the ECGs of ambulatory patients living and working outside the hospital. This demands that the device be relatively light and conveniently worn for many days at a time in order to record those abnormalities that might occur only once every several weeks. A microcomputer seems the best choice to analyze the ECG. Since there is a limited amount of computing time available to reliably detect arrhythmias, our monitor must be restricted to recognizing only life-threatening and premonitory arrhythmias.

---

*Section 6.2 written by John P. Abenstein.

This intelligent monitor must alarm on catastrophic arrhythmias that pose a direct threat to the patient's life. These include:

1. Extreme tachycardia.
2. Extreme bradycardia.
3. Sinus arrest.
4. Ventricular fibrillation.
5. Asystole.

The device must also detect premonitory arrhythmias that indicate a serious threat to the patient. These include:

1. Premature ventricular contractions (PVCs).
2. Interpolated PVCs.
3. Bigeminy.
4. Trigeminy.
5. R-on-T phenomenon.
6. Skipped beat.
7. Atrial premature beats (APBs).

Each arrhythmia must be defined in mathematical terms so that the microcomputer has the capacity to detect it in real time.

Variations among cardiologists

Development of the arrhythmia-detection algorithms consisted of examining strip charts of identified arrhythmias and discussing the subject with cardiologists. The cardiologists we consulted had one thing in common; they did not agree. What is extreme and dangerous bradycardia to cardiologist A is a slow and normal heart rate to cardiologist B. Cardiologist A wants to know of every occurrence of a skipped beat, but cardiologist B is only interested if the heart skips a beat more often than five per minute.

It became very obvious that each cardiologist has his or her own method of analyzing ECG recordings and utilizes past experience more than firm quantitative analysis of data. This is very understandable, for cardiology is a visual art, and the human eye and brain can analyze data by making use of many diverse bits of information. Unfortunately, the computer, especially a microcomputer, does not have this flexibility. We must define each arrhythmia mathematically and alarm on exact numerical criteria. The algorithms developed are compromises between the cardiologist's training and experience and the engineer's numerical constraints. These compromises are not insignificant because many physicians will not accept these criteria, either for detection or alarm. However, the device makes use of a general-purpose computer, and the software can and will be changed to meet the needs of individual physicians and patients.

Arrhythmia-detection algorithms

ECG data sampled at 200 samples/s are processed by a reduction algorithm and then stored (see Section 6.8). An R-wave detector is also an integral part of the device (Section 6.6). When an R wave is discovered by the detector, one of the computer's external flags goes high. The device examines this flag each time a sample is taken (every 5 ms). When the flag is high, the computer makes use of a real-time clock to calculate the R-to-R interval. The R-to-R interval is the primary piece of data the arrhythmia algorithms use for detection and alarm.

Bradycardia.   Extreme bradycardia is a critical reduction of heart rate; therefore, only ECG rhythm is needed to identify this arrhythmia. If one R-to-R interval is greater than 1.5 s (equal to 40 beats/min), the monitor alarms. If the average R-to-R interval (the average of the previous eight R-to-R intervals) is greater than 1.2 s (50 beats/min), the monitor alarms.

Tachycardia.   Tachycardia is a serious racing of the heart and is also detected by simple ECG rhythm analysis. An average R-to-R interval less than 0.5 s (120 beats/min) produces an alarm.

Asystole and ventricular fibrillation.   Asystole and ventricular fibrillation can be identified by the lack of a QRS complex for an extended period. If there is no detection of a QRS complex for more than 1.6 s, this triggers an alarm.

Criteria for identification.   The criteria to identify bradycardia, tachycardia, and asystole are subject to variation among physicians. The criteria for alarm are subject to even greater variation. Our numerical thresholds for each were determined by discussion with physicians and cannot be considered exact physiological definitions. Therefore, these thresholds can be changed to agree with an individual physician's analysis of ECGs in general or even as required for a specific patient.

Skipped beat.   Skipped beat can be detected by an R-to-R interval approximately equal to twice the previous average R-to-R interval and not following a premature beat. If the R-to-R interval is greater than twice the average but less than 1.5 s, sinus arrest is detected. Mobitz type I and II are also detected by the above criteria.

At present a single skipped beat causes an alarm. It is possible that clinical testing or the user's needs may demand that skipped beats cause an alarm at a specified rate. This additional criterion is easily included.

Premature ventricular contractions.   Premature ventricular contractions (PVCs) are detected by more complex criteria. A PVC can be identified if the QRS complex is premature and followed by a full compensatory pause, the QRS width is wider (i.e., the complex is broadened), the T wave is in the opposite direction from the T wave of a normal beat, and there is no P wave (Fig. 6.1). P and T waves cannot be

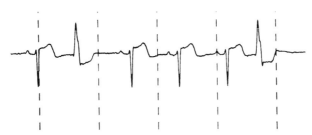

FIGURE 6.1 Electrocardiogram with PVCs (positive waves) and normal QRS complexes (negative waves).

reliably detected by our monitor since baseline artifact is large for ambulatory patients and there is not enough computing time. Also, at this stage of development we decided not to analyze the configuration of the QRS complex. Therefore, only rhythm analysis is used to detect PVCs.

Using only rhythm analysis for detection of PVCs has certain inherent problems. First is the detection of a premature beat. It is difficult to determine when a beat is premature and when it is only subject to sinus arrhythmia. We decided that if an R-to-R interval is less than 0.9 times the average R-to-R interval not incorporating the present beat, a premature beat is indicated. If a premature beat is detected, the R-to-R interval and previous average R-to-R interval are saved. It is difficult to exactly define a full compensatory pause. Examination of the strip-chart recordings of PVCs shows that the full compensatory pause plus the previous R-to-R interval does not exactly equal twice the average interval. Therefore, if the next R-to-R interval is added to the saved R-to-R interval (the premature beat) and this sum is about equal to twice the saved average, a full compensatory pause is indicated. We will determine what "about equal to twice" means during clinical testing. A premature beat followed by a full compensatory pause indicates a PVC. Clinical testing will determine the value of the premature threshold and full compensatory pause window that gives the greatest reliability for PVC detection. If PVCs occur more often than 10/min, the monitor alarms. The rate criteria for alarm can be adjusted.

R-on-T phenomenon. The R-on-T phenomenon is a very dangerous arrhythmia. It is a premature ventricular contraction that occurs during ventricular repolarization (the T wave). Since we have no way to detect T waves, we must depend only on rhythm analysis. The T wave occurs within the first one-third of the R-to-R interval. Therefore, if an R-to-R interval is less than one-third the previous average R-to-R interval and followed by a full compensatory pause, the R-on-T phenomenon is detected and the monitor alarms. A rate criterion can again be added to meet the needs of the user, although at this time the device is designed to alarm on one occurrence of R-on-T phenomenon.

Bigeminy. Bigeminy is a condition where PVCs come as alternate beats so that each normal beat is paired with a PVC. If two PVCs are detected in a row, bigeminy is found and the monitor alarms.

Trigeminy. Trigeminy is a condition where a normal beat is followed by two premature beats and a full compensatory pause. In this case a full compensatory pause is defined as follows: the two previous R-to-R intervals (RR_{t-2} and RR_{t-1}) are each less than 0.9 times the average R-to-R interval (before the first premature beat), and the present R-to-R interval added to the previous two R-to-R intervals approximately equals two times the average interval. If this is true, trigeminy is detected and an alarm sounds.

Interpolated PVCs. Interpolated PVCs are premature beats that are not followed by a compensatory pause. Therefore, the R-to-R interval of the premature beat added to the next R-to-R interval approximately equals the average R-to-R interval preceding the premature beat. If this condition is detected at a rate greater than 10/min, an alarm triggers.

Atrial premature beats. Atrial premature beats (APBs) are identified by a premature beat followed by a compensatory pause (not a full compensatory pause). The difference between a full compensatory pause and a compensatory pause is another factor that will be determined during clinical testing. The goal is to maximize the reliability of detection for all arrhythmias. If APBs occur at a rate greater than 20/min, an alarm sounds.

Formal algorithm definition

Following is a mathematical definition of each arrhythmia-detection algorithm. Two variables are used, RR and AR, where RR is the R-to-R interval and AR is the average of eight R-to-R intervals. Subscripts denote the time relations. RR_t is the latest R-to-R interval, RR_{t-1} is the previous interval, and so on. AR_t is the average over eight R-to-R intervals, including RR_t. Therefore, AR_{t-1} is the previous average.

Figure 6.2 defines the timing relations that we used to define catastrophic arrhythmias shown in Fig. 6.3 and premonitory arrhythmias shown in Fig. 6.4 (Abenstein, 1978):

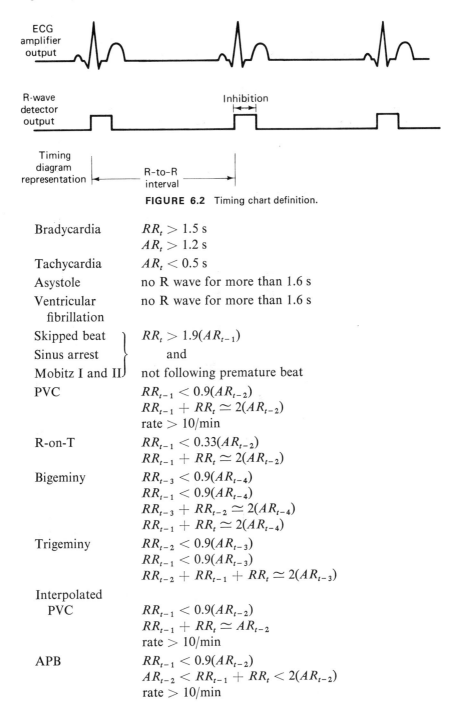

FIGURE 6.2 Timing chart definition.

Bradycardia	$RR_t > 1.5$ s
	$AR_t > 1.2$ s
Tachycardia	$AR_t < 0.5$ s
Asystole	no R wave for more than 1.6 s
Ventricular fibrillation	no R wave for more than 1.6 s

Skipped beat ⎫
Sinus arrest ⎬ $RR_t > 1.9(AR_{t-1})$
Mobitz I and II ⎭ and
    not following premature beat

PVC	$RR_{t-1} < 0.9(AR_{t-2})$
	$RR_{t-1} + RR_t \simeq 2(AR_{t-2})$
	rate > 10/min
R-on-T	$RR_{t-1} < 0.33(AR_{t-2})$
	$RR_{t-1} + RR_t \simeq 2(AR_{t-2})$
Bigeminy	$RR_{t-3} < 0.9(AR_{t-4})$
	$RR_{t-1} < 0.9(AR_{t-4})$
	$RR_{t-3} + RR_{t-2} \simeq 2(AR_{t-4})$
	$RR_{t-1} + RR_t \simeq 2(AR_{t-4})$
Trigeminy	$RR_{t-2} < 0.9(AR_{t-3})$
	$RR_{t-1} < 0.9(AR_{t-3})$
	$RR_{t-2} + RR_{t-1} + RR_t \simeq 2(AR_{t-3})$
Interpolated PVC	$RR_{t-1} < 0.9(AR_{t-2})$
	$RR_{t-1} + RR_t \simeq AR_{t-2}$
	rate > 10/min
APB	$RR_{t-1} < 0.9(AR_{t-2})$
	$AR_{t-2} < RR_{t-1} + RR_t < 2(AR_{t-2})$
	rate > 10/min

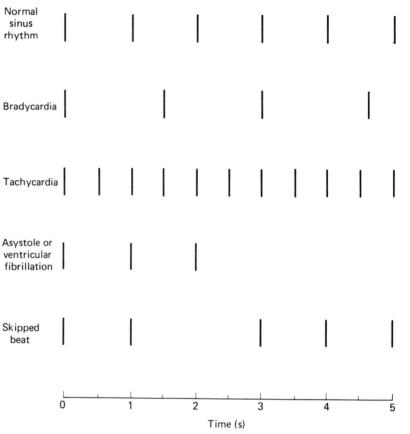

FIGURE 6.3 Catastrophic arrhythmias. (Each line represents the location of an R wave.)

The last step in the process before programming is to integrate these formal algorithms into a concise system of calculations and comparisons. This process produces a flowchart that can then be implemented on the microcomputer. Figure 6.5 shows the flowchart produced to implement the arrhythmia-detection algorithms.

The initial problems involved in meeting the diverse needs of the cardiologist have been solved by analysis, discussion, and patience. Interdisciplinary communication provides the solution to the problems of developing criteria for arrhythmia detection. Physicians are not taught to talk the engineer's language of mathematics and analysis, and engineers do not understand the complexities of biological problems. The goal in the algorithm development has always been clinical acceptance. Therefore, flexibility in design is very important.

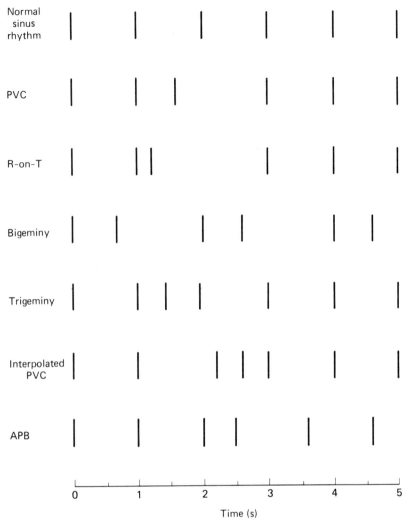

FIGURE 6.4 Premonitory arrhythmias. (Each line represents the location of an R wave.)

6.3 INSTRUMENT SPECIFICATIONS*

Our specific instrument needs for an intelligent monitor are:

> 1. A portable device that runs on batteries for up to 1 month without the need to change batteries.

---

*Section 6.3 written by Nitish V. Thakor.

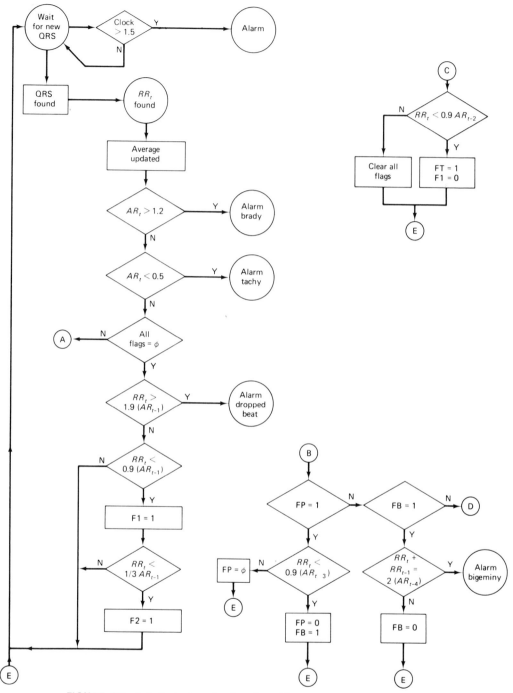

FIGURE 6.5 Arrhythmia detection flowchart. (From Abenstein, J. P. 1978. Algorithms for real-time ambulatory ECG monitoring. Biomed. Sci. Instrum. 14:73–79. Used with permission of ISA.)

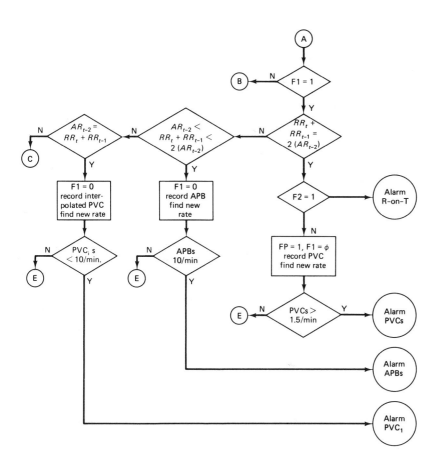

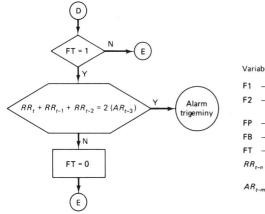

Variables for arrhythmia algorithm:

F1 — Flag notes that last R-R interval was premature

F2 — Flag notes that last R-R interval was premature and fell within the first one-third of an average R-R interval

FP — Flag notes that last two beats were identified as a PVC

FB — Flag notes that last R-R interval was premature <u>and</u> follows a PVC

FT — Flag notes that last two R-R intervals were premature

RR_{t-n} — R-R interval. Subscript n denotes time of R-R interval. $n = 0$ — R-R interval at t (or present), $n = 1$ — previous R-R interval, etc.

AR_{t-m} — Average, over 8 R-R intervals. Subscript m denotes time of average interval. $n = 0$ — average equals $(RR_t + RR_{t-1} + \ldots + RR_{t-7})/8$. $n = 1$ — average equals $(RR_{t-1} + RR_{t-2} + \ldots + RR_{t-8})/8$, etc.

FIGURE 6.5 (continued)

2. A general-purpose computer at the heart of the device, which is programmed to alarm on specified arrhythmias but which is also flexible in terms of alarm criteria, which can be modified if need be.

3. The ability to get in touch with a central station (a central computer) via telephone lines.

Our aim is to design a replacement for the existing Holter monitor but one that is superior by virtue of an integral, programmable microcomputer as its central element. We want to design a device that is approximately the size and weight of a Holter monitor and also with a cost in the range of a Holter monitor, that is, between $2000 and $5000. To satisfy these main objectives, we define a set of instrument specifications that are realistic in terms of available technology, meet our basic objectives, and serve as ultimate design targets.

General specifications

The general specifications describe the general structure of the instrument and its operating environment. Since we have decided to draw a parallel between this device and the Holter monitor, we specify the size and weight of a typical Holter monitor. Our first specific need is for a battery-powered device that can operate up to 1 month—the single biggest constraint on the design. Upon studying the size and the watt-hour capacities of a wide range of batteries that are presently available, we immediately realize the need for a device with ultra-low power consumption. For example, the best available lithium cells of reasonable size have a capacity of 10 A·h or 56 W·h (for two D cells in series). For 30 days of operation, this implies a permissible circuit power consumption of

$$\frac{56 \text{ W·h}}{30 \text{ days} \times 24 \text{ h}} = 78 \text{ mW}$$

We would put a realistic estimate for power consumption of our device at 150 mW in view of the large memory and complex circuitry we would like to support. This, of course, compromises the period over which the instrument can be used, so we revise our design target for continuous operation to be 7 days minimum and 30 days maximum. Finally, since this is necessarily a portable device, it should meet environmental specifications common to most portable electronic instruments, such as operation through a temperature range of 0 to 70°C. Figure 6.6 lists the instrument specifications.

Microcomputer specifications

In keeping with our primary objectives of low power consumption and small size, there should be a minimum number of IC chips to reduce power consumption and minimize the system size. In view of the sophisticated arrhythmia analysis it has to perform, a fairly large number of instructions will have to be executed by the

General specifications

Weight	1 kg (excluding batteries)
Size	13 x 11 x 8 cm (excluding batteries)
Average power consumption	150 mW
Operating life (until battery change)	
Min.	7 days
Max.	30 days
Power source	Lithium–mercury batteries
Operating-temperature range	0 to 70°C

Microprocessor specifications

CPU clock	2 MHz
Average instruction time	8 μs
Memory	
Program	2 kbytes
Data	2 kbytes
Display	
Visual	Liquid crystal
Audio	Beeper
Alarms	Arrhythmia, lead-failure, manual override

Analog system

Amplifier input impedance	
Differential	2 MΩ
Common-mode	2 MΩ
CMRR	60 dB
Bandwidth	0.5 to 40 Hz
QRS filter	
f_0	17 Hz
Q	3.3
QRS pulse width	200 ms
Lead-fail detection	Impedance between electrodes 10 kΩ at 100 kHz
Number of electrodes	3
Electrode type	Disposable foam pad–Ag/AgCl
A/D-conversion sample rate	200/s

Communication interface

Data rate	300 baud
Transmission time	30 s
Transmit frequency	
Mark (1)	1180 Hz
Space (0)	980 Hz
Receive frequency	
Mark (1)	2225 Hz
Space (0)	2025 Hz
Mode	FSK, half duplex
Transmitter	100-turn inductive coil or 8-Ω, 0.2-W loudspeaker
Receiver	2500-turn inductive coil or crystal microphone

FIGURE 6.6 Instrument specifications.

microcomputer—in real time. We specify an 8-bit microprocessor to restrict the width of the data paths, thereby limiting the number of required memory chips (e.g., 50% more chips would be required to provide the same number of words for a 12-bit microprocessor). The total number of memory chips is important in determining size, power, cost, and reliability. The choice of microprocessor is clear, since the only 8-bit microprocessor with sufficiently low power consumption is the RCA COSMAC (RCA, 1976b).

For reasons described subsequently, we decided on a sampling rate of 200 samples/s, with data storage for 16 s of the ECG. These two specifications indicate a RAM memory size of 3.2 kbytes. We decided to employ a data-reduction algorithm to reduce the amount of required memory space to save the ECG. We specified 2 kbytes of data storage to hold 16 s of data (Tompkins, 1978). Additionally, we specified 2 kbytes for program storage in a nonvolatile memory (e.g., UV EPROM or a battery backed-up RAM).

Two kinds of conditions should provide an audiovisual indication (alarm) to the patient—(1) arrhythmia and (2) lead failure. We specified an audible beeper and a liquid-crystal display—in view of its ultra-low power consumption—with at least four display segments to indicate four different alarm codes.

A/D conversion

The sampling rate of 200 samples/s ensures adequate fidelity of the ECG signal with a 40-Hz bandwidth (see Chapter 2). Since all computations on the signal must be done between samples, a higher sampling rate would put severe restrictions on real-time computing. The A/D converter must be a low-power device (preferably, CMOS) and operate on a single battery supply. We specify an 8-bit A/D converter, as this should provide adequate amplitude resolution for our application. For a 10-mV dynamic range of signal (ECG) as seen at the amplifier input, this would imply a resolution of

$$\frac{10 \text{ mV}}{256} \simeq 40 \text{ } \mu\text{V}$$

Also, an 8-bit A/D converter is directly compatible with an 8-bit microprocessor.

Analog circuit specifications

Since our application is for monitoring the ECG and detecting rates, we do not need a high-quality diagnostic ECG. Hence we specify an amplifier bandwidth of 0.5 to 40 Hz, which provides the advantages of reducing electrical interference and baseline drift. Because the battery-operated equipment does not have an earth ground, the requirements for input impedance as well as CMRR are lower than in normal medical instruments. We specified a QRS filter, as recommended by NASA (center frequency of 17 Hz and $Q = 3.3$), which produces a pulse with a width of 200 ms to prevent false triggering during the latency period.

Communication interface

The arrhythmia monitor must communicate with the central computer via a standard telephone. We specify a transmission rate of 300 baud, which is the maximum rate for acoustic coupling. The coupling to the telephone is to be inductive or acoustical. The mode of transmission is FSK (frequency-shift keying) and half duplex for reliable transmission, particularly since the communication is mainly unidirectional (from the arrhythmia monitor, which will transmit data to the central computer).

6.4 AMBULATORY ECG MONITORING SYSTEM*

The monitoring system consists of two computers. The first is a microcomputer contained within the portable monitor worn by the patient. This monitors the ECG and alarms upon detection of dangerous arrhythmias. The second is a central computer, which receives data from the portable monitor.

Portable monitor block diagram

Figure 6.7 shows that the monitor consists of an RCA COSMAC microcomputer and an interfaced set of specialized circuits. The COSMAC microcomputer uses CMOS circuitry and has the very low power consumption required for battery operation. These circuits provide for A/D conversion, audible and visual displays, hardware R-wave detection, lead-fail indicator, manual override, and bidirectional telephone communication.

A/D converter. The ECG amplifier provides a signal with a bandwidth of 0.5 to 40 Hz and a signal level compatible with the input of the 8-bit A/D converter. The A/D converter samples the analog ECG signal at a rate of 200 samples/s and interrupts the COSMAC every 5 ms, when a valid data byte becomes available. A software interrupt service routine updates the time of day and captures the new data byte by issuing an input command (INP). This causes the N1 line to go high and activates the A/D converter to put the data byte onto the data bus.

Audible and visual displays. An 8-bit output port is interfaced to the data bus and controls the audible beeper and liquid-crystal display (LCD). The output command (OUT) transfers a byte of data to the data bus and causes the N0 line to pulse high. This N0 signal strobes the byte into the output port, where it is latched. The bit pattern of the latched byte controls the operation of the audible beeper and the selection of one of four possible liquid-crystal display codes.

R-wave detector. A special circuit that follows the ECG amplifier provides reliable hardware R-wave detection (see Section 6.6). When the R-wave detector discovers

---

*Section 6.4 written by John P. Abenstein.

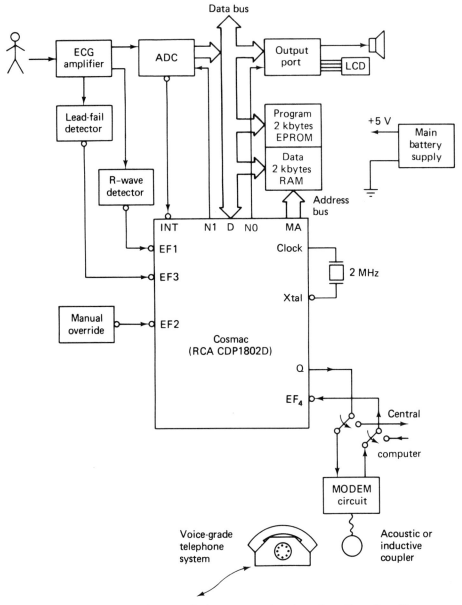

FIGURE 6.7 Block diagram of microcomputer-based monitor. (From Tompkins, W. J. 1978. A portable microcomputer-based system for biomedical applications. Biomed. Sci. Instrum. 14: 61–66. Used with permission of ISA.)

an R wave, it produces a 200-ms active-low pulse on the EF1 input flag of the COSMAC. The program running in the COSMAC checks the EF1 flag every time it is interrupted by the A/D converter. When the program discovers that an R wave has occurred, it calculates the time lapse since the last R wave (R-to-R interval). With this information, arrhythmia analysis can proceed. The program also does not detect another R wave until the flag goes high (the pulse is active-low). This effectively produces an absolute refractory period for R-wave detection, which reduces the possibility of triggering on an artifact or of multiple detection of the same QRS complex. The program also flashes the LCD each time an R wave is detected, to give the patient feedback that the monitor is working properly.

Lead-fail detector. If an electrode system failure occurs (i.e., the electrode or lead falls off), a separate circuit signals this problem to the COSMAC on the EF3 flag. Software then informs the patient of this fact by beeping the audible alarm and flashing the appropriate LCD signal.

Manual override. A manual override circuit is connected to the input flag EF2. This permits the patient to inhibit the automatic analysis and record 16 s of the ECG by pressing a button. This option permits manual recording when the patient experiences symptoms.

Telephone communication. When the monitor alarms, either from arrhythmia detection or manual override, the patient proceeds to a telephone and calls a central computer to transmit the recorded ECG data. Using inductive or acoustic coupling to the telephone handset, a modem circuit transmits and receives in a half-duplex mode over the voice-grade telephone system. The software-testable input flag EF4 and the software-settable output flag Q manage serial bit streams between the modem circuit and the COSMAC. Standard frequency-shift-keying (FSK) modem protocols provide a communication rate of 300 baud. These circuits require significant current in comparison with the rest of the monitor. Therefore, the COSMAC controls switches to turn off the communication circuit's power until it is needed.

Memory. We use 2 kbytes of CMOS UV EPROM for the program and 2 kbytes of CMOS static RAM for the ECG data and other dynamically varying parameters.

Central computer system block diagram

Figure 6.8 shows a block diagram of our central computer system. Included as peripherals are a Tektronix graphics terminal and hard-copy unit, a Centronics printer, a dual floppy-disk drive with high-density storage, and a laboratory interface with 16 A/D channels and two D/A channels. The operating system is Digital Equipment Corporation's RT-11. We use FORTRAN IV as the primary language for PDP-11 software development. For the COSMAC we have implemented a COSMAC cross assembler and a simulator written in FORTRAN, which are based on a software product developed by RCA. The cross assembler permits the resources of the PDP-11 to be used as a developmental system to write assembly-language

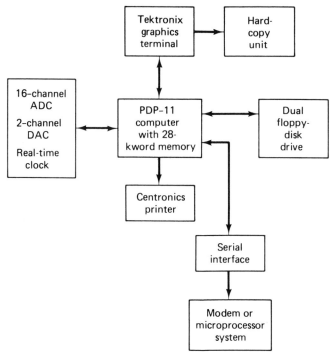

FIGURE 6.8 Central computer system block diagram.

routines in COSMAC source code and convert them to hexadecimal for direct use by our COSMAC-based system. Once written, the simulator can execute programs to determine if they run properly. After testing, a hardwired connection transfers the hexadecimal programs directly from the PDP-11 to the COSMAC system. Therefore, these powerful software tools, FORTRAN and the cross assembler/simulator, permit us to write and debug programs rapidly and efficiently for both the central computer and the COSMAC.

The PDP-11 was selected because it is part of a family of compatible computers, ranging in size from very small to very large. Therefore, those programs written for the prototype system will need minimal retooling when the system is transferred to a larger computer. This small computer is capable of processing only one telephone call from a monitor at a time, but we estimate that we will be able to support at least 100 portable monitors, since the probability of any 2 out of 100 portable monitors simultaneously requiring service is quite small.

6.5 CHOICE OF HARDWARE*

We selected the hardware to meet specifications, optimize the system performance, reduce cost, and minimize power consumption.

---

*Section 6.5 written by Nitish V. Thakor.

Selection of batteries

Most ICs and microprocessors operate on 5 V. Thus the battery should provide 5 V at 30-mA current drain. We calculate the required capacity of the battery as follows:

$$\text{capacity} = (5 \text{ V})(30 \text{ mA})(7 \text{ days})(24 \text{ h})$$
$$= 25.2 \text{ W} \cdot \text{h}$$

Figure 6.9 shows that lithium D cells provide the highest capacity, lowest weight, and have a sufficiently high voltage so that only two cells are required (Power Conversion, 1976). Nickel–cadmium cells have the lowest capacity of any cells on this list but have the advantage that they are rechargeable.

Battery type (D cell)	Voltage (V)	Capacity (W·h)	Weight (g)	Cost ($)
Zn–C	1.5	5.5	85	0.28
Alkaline	1.5	10.5	130	0.65
Mercury	1.35	19.0	165	5.00
Lithium	2.8	22.5	82.5	10.00
Ni–Cd (rechargeable)	1.25	5.0	125	6.00

FIGURE 6.9 Comparison of various battery types.

EXAMPLE

For our portable arrhythmia monitor, we have selected a sampling rate of 200 samples/s. Between each sample we must execute at least 500 instructions (rate calculations, data reduction, and data storage). Justify the choice of the COSMAC CDP 1802 microprocessor for this application.

Solution

Since the sampling rate is 200 samples/s, we have 5 ms between each sample. Hence the maximum available instruction time is 5 ms/500 = 10 μs.

Since the COSMAC has primarily single-byte instructions with an execution time of 8 μs at a 2-MHz clock rate (Section 4.6), it will be possible to execute the required number of instructions per sample interval.

Selection of a microprocessor

The microprocessor must meet the following needs:

1. Low power consumption; CMOS technology is implied.
2. Operation from a single 5-V supply.
3. Minimum supporting chip set.
4. Sufficient speed.

Only two currently available microprocessors, both CMOS, meet needs (1) and (2): RCA COSMAC CDP1802 and Intersil 6100. We selected the RCA COSMAC because of reason (3) as well as its 8-bit architecture. In contrast, the 12-bit architecture of the Intersil 6100 requires wider data paths and larger memories.

Selection of digital ICs

We selected CMOS technology because it has much lower power consumption than TTL, as shown by Fig. 6.10(a) (RCA, 1976a). CMOS has the added advantage of operation over wide voltage ranges. This permits us to select the following batteries (in proper combination): lithium batteries provide 5.6 V, mercury 5.4 V, and alkaline 6 V. We estimate the power consumption in the following example.

Characteristic (typical values)	7404	4069B
Supply voltage	4.75–5.25 V	3–18 V
Supply current	6 mA (o/p high) 18 mA (o/p low)	0.01 mA (static) 0.1 mA (dynamic)
Cost	$0.21	$0.45

(a)

Characteristic (typical values)	μA741	LM4250
Supply voltage	± 15 V	± 1.5 V
Supply current	1.4 mA	8 μA
Gain-bandwidth product	1 MHz	50 kHz
CMRR	90 dB	70 dB
Cost	$0.35	$1.75

(b)

FIGURE 6.10 Comparisons of specifications and cost of electronic components. (a) Digital hex inverter chips. The 7404 is TTL and the 4069B is CMOS. (b) Operational amplifiers. The 741 is a very popular type and the 4250 is a low-power, programmable device.

EXAMPLE

Estimate the power consumed by a memory system composed of 16 Harris HM6508 CMOS RAM chips (1024 × 1 bit) organized as four banks of 1 k × 8 bits (Harris Semiconductor, 1976). The standby power is 50 nW/bit and the operating power (when the chip is enabled) is 15 μW/bit.

Solution

Only 1 kbyte of the memory operates at a time; eight chips are "on" while the remaining banks are in standby mode. Hence the power consumed is

$$P = 8 \times 1024 \times 15 \ \mu W + 8 \times 1024 \times 50 \ nW$$
$$= 123.2 \ mW$$

If used with the COSMAC microprocessor, the memory is accessed only for one clock cycle (or $\frac{1}{8}$ instruction cycle) for the write operation and approximately $\frac{3}{4}$ instruction cycle for the read operation. Hence the average power consumption is lower than 123 mW.

Selection of an A/D converter

We narrowed the choice of a CMOS A/D converter down to the following:

1. Teledyne 8703 (Teledyne Semiconductor, 1976).
2. Analog Devices AD7570 (Analog Devices, 1976).
3. National ADC0816 (National Semiconductor, 1977).

All three are CMOS, have sufficient conversion speed to meet our 200 conversions/s requirement, and are microprocessor-compatible (Tristate outputs). The 8703 requires a dual power supply and hence we eliminated it. The 7570 was used in an initial design but is not very attractive for our application: it uses an external comparator that draws power and is difficult to use. In our current design we use the ADC0816.

Selection of analog ICs and transistors

Figure 6.10(b) shows that the 741 op amp is comparatively inexpensive. Many op amps are available in the market that yield far superior performance (particularly the bi-FET variety). However, our need to operate on low power supply voltages and low current drain requirements limits us to the use of programmable op amps such as the Siliconix L144 (Siliconix, 1973), National LM4250 (National Semiconductor, 1976), or Harris HA2735. We chose the L144 for its compactness (three op amps in one package) and the 4250 for its low bias current and better overall performance. Similarly, we selected transistors like the 2N5311, as they operate on ultra-low currents.

Miscellaneous hardware

For development purposes we assemble our circuit on Vector boards and mount all ICs in sockets. We make the connections by wire wrapping. We use $\frac{1}{4}$-W 5% resistors and ceramic, polyester, or tantalum capacitors throughout.

Choice of electrodes

Electrodes are critical components in acquiring the ECG. For reliable long-term monitoring, proper selection of electrodes is important. For artifact-free, long-term ECG recording, it is important (1) to select electrodes that have a long-lasting adhesive and low irritant gel, and (2) to select optimal electrode locations on the chest (Thakor, 1978; Tam and Webster 1977).

6.6 ANALOG CIRCUIT DEVELOPMENT*

The analog circuit is mounted on a single board. It consists of (1) a differential amplifier, (2) an R-wave detector, (3) a lead-fail detection circuit, (4) a sample-and-hold circuit, and (5) an A/D converter. Also on the same board is a modem circuit, which is described later.

ECG amplifier

Because the amplifier and R-wave detector are used on ambulatory subjects, we designed them for (1) operation from low battery voltages, typically 5.6 V from two lithium cells; (2) low power consumption for long-term operation; and (3) compact design and minimum component count. Figure 6.11 shows a functional block diagram which includes the integrated circuit (IC) packages used.

The ECG amplifier uses a single IC package consisting of three programmable op amps. We program each IC to draw less than 10 μA of current. The bandwidth of the amplifier is 0.5 to 40 Hz. Careful trimming results in a CMRR of

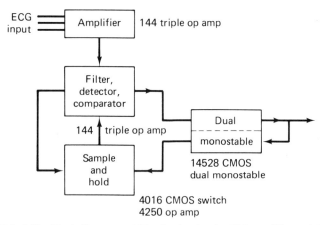

FIGURE 6.11 Block diagram and IC selection for the ECG amplifier and R-wave detector. (From Thakor, N. V. 1978. Reliable R-wave detection from ambulatory subjects. Biomed. Sci. Instrum. 14 : 67–72. Used with permission of ISA.)

*Section 6.6 written by Nitish V. Thakor.

10,000 (80 dB). The limited bandwidth and good CMRR result in low electrical interference and artifacts. A possible design variation may permit use of two electrodes instead of the usual three (Thakor and Webster, 1977).

R-wave detector

Various hardware R-wave detectors have appeared in the literature. Most use a filter that selects the frequencies present in the QRS complex to trigger a threshold detection circuit. There is a wide variation in the filter bandwidth, as reviewed by Brydon (1976). We have selected the NASA filter developed by Vogt and Hallen (1964).

Figure 6.12 shows that the circuit first passes the amplified ECG output through a pacer reject circuit. It consists of four forward-biased diodes that form a bridge, followed by a slew-rate-limiting capacitor. The bridge limits the capacitor current and hence the slew rate to 200 V/s. The filter has a center frequency of 17 Hz and a Q of 3.3. The filter uses a single op amp in a multiple-feedback bandpass filter configuration. Note that analog circuits use ± 2.8 V and digital circuits use 5.6 V. The half-wave rectifier provides an always-positive output for comparison with a threshold level set by an automatic threshold circuit (Fig. 6.13). The variable threshold level provides reliable R-wave triggering for a variety of QRS complex morphologies in the presence of artifacts and interference. The threshold varies according to the following criteria: (1) the minimum threshold exceeds the filter output caused by most baseline interference and most P waves; and (2) a sample-and-hold circuit stores the filter output from the previous R wave. This decays with a time constant of 10 s. Fifty percent of this decaying signal is added to the minimum threshold to serve as a variable threshold. This circuit functions as a fast-acting (beat-by-beat) automatic gain control, which is responsive to the size of the previous QRS complex; (3) the 200-ms monostable causes a 200-ms refractory period. This blocks possible incorrect triggering from the ringing output of the filter as well as triggering on T waves. The 50-ms monostable resets the stored filter output after each R wave, which permits rapid recovery from saturation and lead failures.

EXAMPLE

For the three-electrode ECG amplifier shown in Fig. 6.14, calculate the differential gain of the amplifier and its low and high corner frequencies.

Solution

The differential gain is given by

$$
\begin{aligned}
A_d &= \frac{R_2}{R_1} \times \frac{R_3 + R_4}{R_4} \times \left(1 + \frac{2R_6}{R_5}\right) \\
&= \frac{680 \text{ k}\Omega}{680 \text{ k}\Omega} \times \frac{82 \text{ k}\Omega + 4.3 \text{ k}\Omega}{4.3 \text{ k}\Omega} \times \left(1 + \frac{2 \times 120 \text{ k}\Omega}{10 \text{ k}\Omega}\right) \\
&= 501.7
\end{aligned}
$$

The low corner frequency,

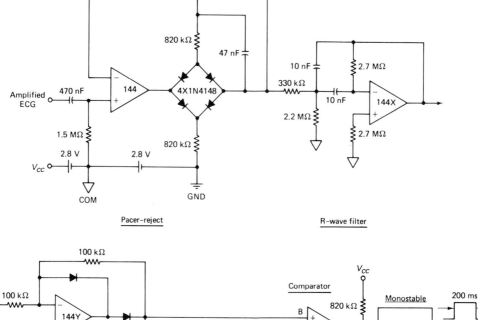

FIGURE 6.12 Circuit diagram of complete R-wave detector. (From Thakor, N. V. 1978. Reliable R-wave detection from ambulatory subjects. Biomed. Sci. Instrum. 14 : 67–72. Used with permission of ISA.)

$$f_L = \frac{1}{2\pi R_1 C_1}$$

$$= \frac{1}{2\pi \times 680 \text{ k}\Omega \times 470 \text{ nF}}$$

$$= 0.5 \text{ Hz}$$

The high corner frequency,

$$f_H = \frac{1}{2\pi R_3 C_3}$$

$$= \frac{1}{2\pi \times 82\ \text{k}\Omega \times 47\ \text{nF}}$$

$$= 41\ \text{Hz}$$

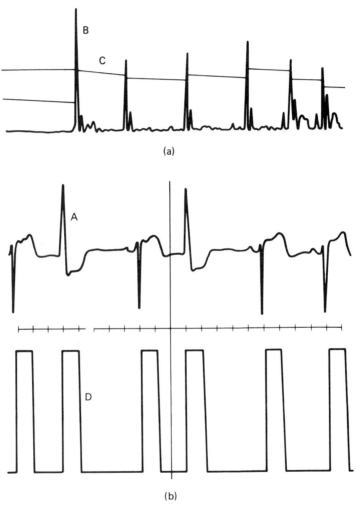

(a)

(b)

FIGURE 6.13 Signals in R-wave detector circuit of Fig. 6.12. (a) Signal B is the output of the R-wave filter and C is the output of the automatic threshold circuit. (b) Signal A is an amplified ECG with PVCs and D is the output of the R-wave detector which goes to the COSMAC. (From Thakor, N. V. 1978. Reliable R-wave detection from ambulatory subjects. Biomed. Sci. Instrum. 14: 67–72. Used with permission of ISA.)

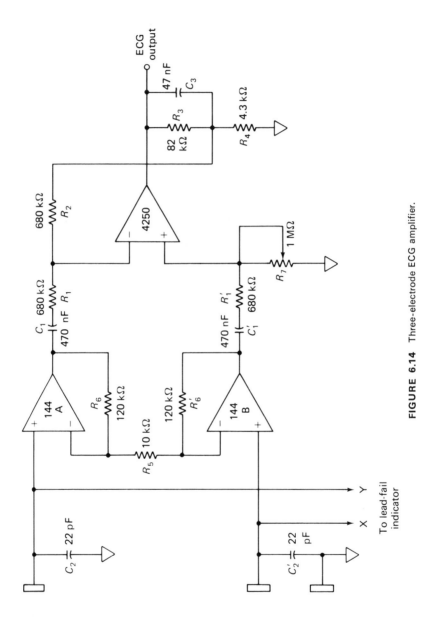

FIGURE 6.14 Three-electrode ECG amplifier.

Lead-fail detector

Since this arrhythmia monitor will be worn by ambulatory patients for periods longer than 7 days, we must inform the patient as to whether or not the electrodes are functioning properly. If an electrode falls off or if the electrode gel drys up, this causes excessively high electrode impedance.

Figure 6.15 shows the lead-failure-detection schematic. Op amp 144C is connected as a voltage follower, which provides high input impedance to the biasing circuit. Op amp 4250 is connected as a comparator. The inverting input of this comparator is connected to a fixed threshold of 1.25 V with respect to the amplifier common. The noninverting input switches between approximately the common voltage (0 V) if there is no lead failure and the supply voltage (+2.5 V) if there is a lead failure. The output of the comparator is 0 (−2.5 V) and 1 (+2.5 V) for the respective cases. This swing in the comparator input voltage (the noninverting input) is brought about because of the flow of op-amp bias current through the 100-MΩ resistors. In case there is no lead failure, the bias current flows through the body and hence the op-amp inputs are held at the amplifier common voltage. But if there is a failure of any lead, the bias current flows through the 100-MΩ resistor(s) to the positive supply. This raises the noninverting input of the comparator to the supply voltage and therefore flips the comparator. The output of the comparator signals flag EF2 to the computer.

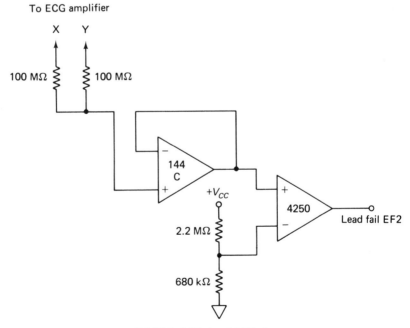

FIGURE 6.15 Lead-fail indicator.

Sample-and-hold circuit

The A/D converter samples data at the rate of 200 samples/s. Before each sample, the data must be held constant so that the analog signal input to the converter does not change during conversion. Figure 6.16 shows the sample-and-hold circuit. The CMOS switch passes the analog signal, but the switch is closed by the same signal that starts analog-to-digital conversion. The switch then opens and the data are held constant on a capacitor until the next sampling time.

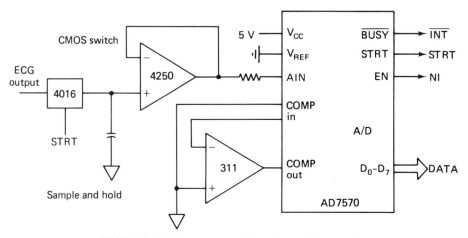

FIGURE 6.16 Sample-and-hold circuit and A/D converter.

A/D converter

A previous A/D converter design based upon the Analog Devices AD7570 is shown in Fig. 6.16. This CMOS device has a typical current drain of 200 μA and operates on a single $+5$-V power supply. Although it needs a negative reference voltage, this problem can be circumvented by connecting the reference to ground and giving a 2.5-V offset to the analog input signal. This scheme creates a "virtual" negative reference of -2.5 V and permits the analog signal (ECG) to swing from $+2.5$ V to $+5$ V and ground.

The maximum conversion time is 40 μs, which is more than sufficient for our application. One drawback of this A/D converter is that it needs an external comparator. Here we use an AD311 fast comparator. As comparators are susceptible to oscillation, a careful component layout is necessary. The A/D converter samples at a rate of 200 samples/s and outputs a pulse to the COSMAC interrupt pin (INT) every 5 ms, when a valid data byte becomes available. A software-interrupt service routine updates a register, which contains elapsed time and accepts each sampled data point by executing an input (INP) command. This command causes a control pulse on the N1 line of the COSMAC, which activates the A/D converter to gate the data byte to the data bus at the proper time during the instruction cycle.

Figure 6.17 shows our current A/D converter design using the National Semiconductor ADC0816 single-chip data acquisition system. We give details of this design in Section 6.7.

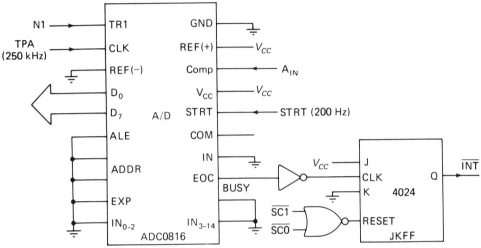

FIGURE 6.17 Interfacing the ADC0816 A/D converter to the COSMAC microprocessor.

EXAMPLE

Consider the two A/D converter types Teledyne 8700 and 8703. They are similar except that the 8703 includes tristate output buffers and the 8700 does not. How would you interface each of them to the COSMAC microprocessor? How are the tristate data outputs handled? Figure 6.18(a) shows the schematic for 8700/8703. Since the 8703 has tristate data output lines, it can be directly connected to the data bus and put in a high-impedance state until accessed by the microprocessor. On the other hand, the 8700 must be interfaced with the COSMAC data bus using separate tristate buffer chips or an I/O port. Figure 6.18(b) shows both A/D interfaces.

The data are read by the CPU in the case of the 8703, in the same manner as described in the text for AD7570. Data from 8700 are read by treating the I/O port as an input port and issuing an INP instruction. Figure 6.18(c) shows the sequence of timing operations as follows: (1) the system gives an "initiate conversion" command; (2) the A/D (8700 and 8703) starts conversion and sets its "busy" line; (3) the "data valid" line is set, thus interrupting the microprocessor after conversion is completed; and (4) the microprocessor issues the INP 1 instruction as part of the interrupt service routine. This sets the N1 line. In the case of the 8700, N1 latches data into the input port. In the case of the 8703, N1 enables the data output. (5) During the "read" part of the INP instruction, the microprocessor reads the data into the data register and simultaneously into the RAM.

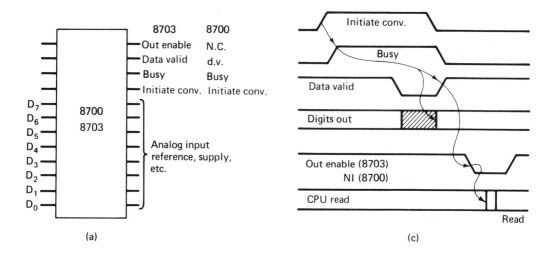

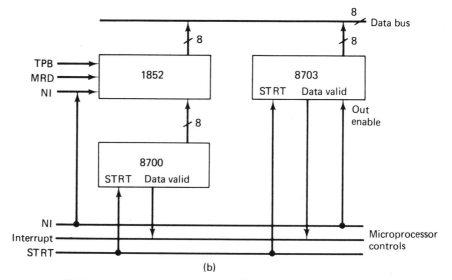

FIGURE 6.18 Analog-to-digital conversion. (a) Teledyne 8700 and 8703. (b) Interfaces to the COSMAC microprocessor. (c) A/D conversion timing diagram.

6.7 MICROCOMPUTER DEVELOPMENT*

We can divide the design of a microcomputer into two parts: (1) the CPU, I/O ports, and control components; and (2) the memory and its decoding circuit. Figure 6.19 shows the block diagram of the microcomputer system developed for our

---

*Section 6.7 written by Nitish V. Thakor.

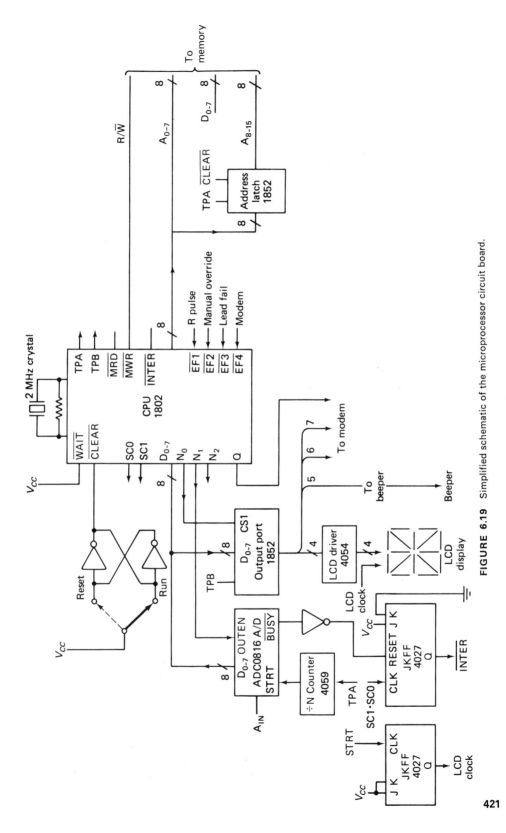

FIGURE 6.19 Simplified schematic of the microprocessor circuit board.

421

application. The COSMAC microprocessor communicates with the memory and the output port through a bidirectional 8-bit data bus and an 8-bit unidirectional address bus. The higher-order 8 bits of an address are latched into an address latch during the early part of the instruction cycle. Two of the CPU port control lines are set under program control. Port control line N0 activated by an OUT 1 instruction selects the output port, which in turn operates the liquid-crystal display and the audible beeper. Port control line N1, activated by an INP 2 command, enables the A/D converter digital output, which is read from the data bus by the COSMAC.

All four software-testable input flags of the COSMAC are utilized. At every occurrence of the R wave, the R-wave detector sets flag EF1 for 200 ms. Flag EF2 is set under manual control in case the patient wishes to override the automatic analysis and initiate the data collection. The lead-fail detector sets flag EF3 if there is a lead failure. Flag EF4 is used by the modem circuit for receiving serial communication by telephone or by hardwire link to the central computer.

Memory design

Figure 6.20 shows that the 4 kbytes of memory required in the design specification consist of four Intersil 6654 CMOS UV EPROM chips (Intersil, 1979) and 16 RCA CDP 1821 CMOS RAM chips. Each EPROM is organized as 512×8 bits and each RAM is 1024×1 bits.

Memory addressing. The COSMAC provides a time-multiplexed, 16-bit address. The higher 8 bits are put out first, as signaled by the TPA pulse and latched into an 8-bit latch. The lower 8 bits are put out during the remainder of the instruction cycle. Since the memory contains 4096 (2^{12}) bytes, the least-significant 12 address bits are routed to the memory.

Memory decoding. The EPROM chips (lower 2 kbytes) are selected by decoding bits 9 and 10 of the address bus. The decoding itself is done by dual 2-out-of-4 decoders. The EPROMs are edge-triggered devices (see the next section, on memory timing), and they are strobed by line STR at an appropriate time in the CPU instruction cycle. STR is derived by delaying the TPA pulse by two clock cycles, at which time the memory address lines are stable.

The CDP 1821 RAM chips (upper 2 kbytes) are level-triggered devices selected by decoding bits 10 and 11 of the address bus. Any memory chips not being accessed remain in a standby mode, thus conserving power. The following example illustrates the addressing scheme.

EXAMPLE

During the next phase in the development of the arrhythmia monitor, we anticipate that 8 kbytes of memory will be required. Can we easily expand the existing memory? Suggest a design. What is the maximum memory that can be addressed by the COSMAC?

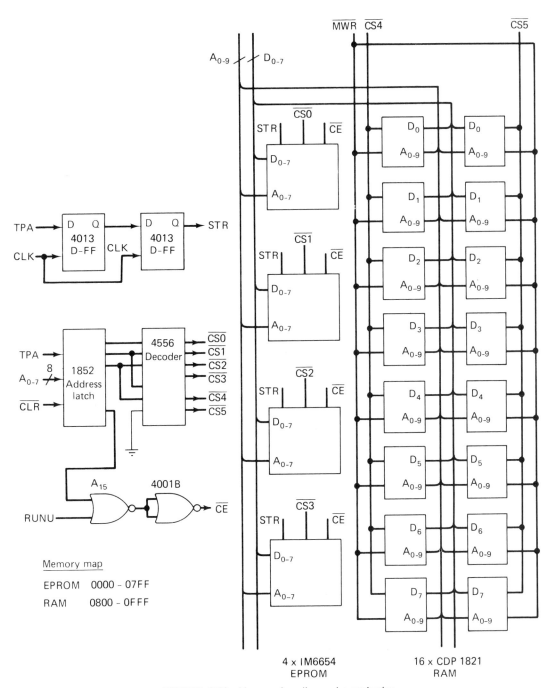

FIGURE 6.20 Memory decoding and organization.

Solution

Figure 6.21 shows the decoding to support an additional 4 kbytes of RAM. The new memory resides in locations 1000_{16} through $1FFF_{16}$. Note that bit $A_{12} = 1$ for this bank of memory. Hence

$$\overline{EN2} = \overline{A}_{12} \cdot (\overline{MRD} + \overline{MWR})$$

This can be interpreted as: memory is enabled ($\overline{CE} = 0$) only if $A_{12} = 0$ and $\overline{MRD}$ or $\overline{MWR}$ is zero.

Also, the other 4 kbytes are enabled when $A_{12} = 1$; therefore,

$$\overline{EN1} = A_{12} \cdot (\overline{MRD} + \overline{MWR})$$

Note that very little extra hardware was required to provide decoding for an additional 4 kbytes of RAM.

Memory timing.   Memory timing is a crucial part of the memory design. Memories from different manufacturers are specified differently, and hence the control signals such as read, write, and chip enable should be provided at the correct times during the instruction cycle, when the address and data buses have valid information.

We illustrate this important timing consideration via a timing comparison for two different CMOS memory chips used with the COSMAC. The first type shown in Fig. 6.22(a) is the RCA 1822, 256 × 4-bit RAM, and the other [Fig. 6.22(b)] is the Harris 6508, 1024 × 1-bit RAM.

Figure 6.22(c) and (d) gives the timing signals for the two RAM chips. Note that (1) a single R/$\overline{W}$ line is available with the 6508; consequently, it is normally held high for the read operation and pulled low for the write; and (2) the 1822 reads data out of the memory specified by the address on the address bus when all chip selects become active. On the other hand, the 6508 requires a falling edge on the $\overline{CE}$ line to strobe in the address. Hence for the 6508 a strobe pulse must be provided for $\overline{CE}$ that goes low only after the 8 least-significant address bits are stable (the upper 8 address bits are already stable since they are latched). Since no such strobe pulse is provided by the COSMAC at the proper time in the instruction cycle, it is necessary to derive $\overline{CE}$ from a delayed TPA pulse. Figure 6.22(e) shows these two memory-access schemes.

Display and alarms

An alarm is given upon detection of (1) an arrhythmia or (2) a lead failure. Each of these alarm conditions is indicated by lighting up a different segment of liquid-crystal display (LCD). Figure 6.16 shows the circuit for the LCD and its driver circuits. To provide feedback to the patient regarding the proper operation of the whole system, the display blinks for every R wave detected. This feature also provides a hardware and software condition check. The display driver is enabled via an output port. An audio beeper signals the patient to look at the LCD for the alarm condition.

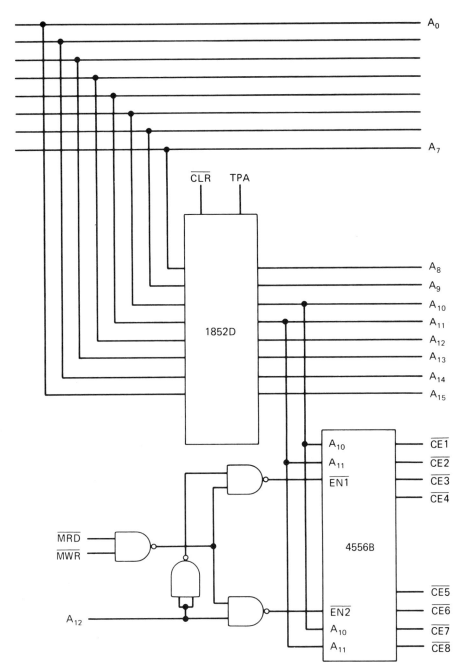

FIGURE 6.21 Memory decoding.

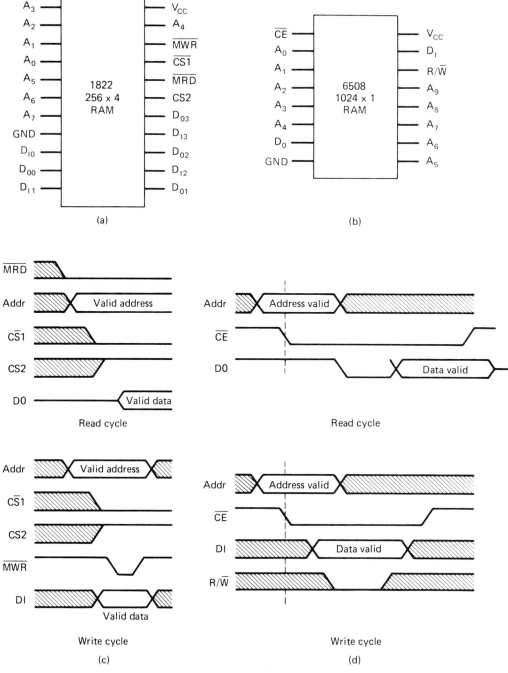

FIGURE 6.22 RAM memory timing. (a) RCA 1822 RAM. (b) Harris 6508 RAM. (c) RCA 1822 memory timing. (d) Harris 6508 memory timing. (e) Complete memory timing diagram for RCA COSMAC.

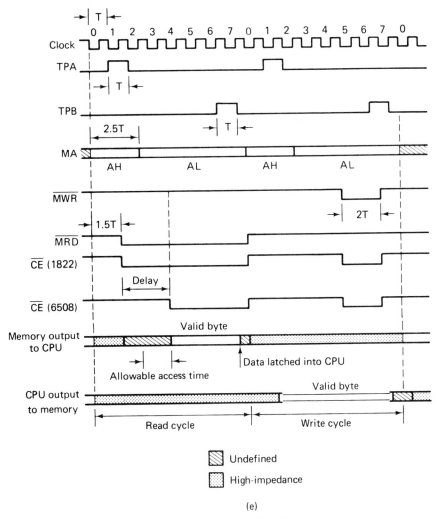

FIGURE 6.22 (continued)

A/D converter handling

The A/D converter of Fig. 6.17 is signaled to start conversion (STRT) by a timing signal derived from the system clock using a divide-by-N counter (Fig. 6.19). The A/D converter signals completion of conversion by pulling the $\overline{\text{BUSY}}$ line low. The $\overline{\text{BUSY}}$ line sets a flip-flop, the output of which interrupts the COSMAC. Once the COSMAC is interrupted, it enables the A/D converter data output lines, thereby putting the converter data on the data bus by turning on line N1 (INP 2 command). The A/D converter thus appears as an input port to the microprocessor. The INP 2 instruction is used to read the data into the microprocessor accumulator and into

RAM (as pointed to by register R(X)). When the COSMAC has been interrupted, its state-code lines SC0 and SC1 both go high. The AND combination of these processor outputs resets the JK flip-flop in preparation for the next interrupt.

Briefly, the sequence of operations is as follows:

$$\text{STRT} \longrightarrow \overline{\text{BUSY}} \longrightarrow \overline{\text{INTER}} \longrightarrow \text{N1}$$

where STRT means to start conversion, $\overline{\text{BUSY}}$ means that conversion is complete, $\overline{\text{INTER}}$ interrupts the COSMAC and causes an acknowledge signal, and N1 enables the A/D converter to read data onto the data bus.

Communication links

We use a telephone communication system to transmit data between the portable arrhythmia monitor and the central computer. Using inductive or acoustic coupling to a telephone handset, a modem circuit transmits and receives in a half-duplex mode over the voice-grade telephone system. The software-testable EF4 input flag and the software-settable Q output flag manage serial bit streams between the modem circuit and the COSMAC. The flag approach to serial communication could have been handled by a single large-scale-integrated (LSI) chip, a Universal Asynchronous Receiver Transmitter (UART). Although such an approach would require less software, the chip would consume significant space and power, so we decided on a software-oriented approach. Standard frequency-shift-keying (FSK) modem protocols result in a transmission rate of 300 baud. Since the transmitter and receiver circuits require significant current compared to the total requirements of the monitor, the COSMAC controls solid-state switches to turn their power off until they are needed.

Hardware design.   The Motorola MC14412 modem IC (Motorola, 1976) shown in Fig. 6.23(a) is used for telephone communication. Digital I/O signals from the microprocessor are converted to the standard FSK signals shown in Fig. 6.23(b). The modem IC synthesizes a transmission frequency of 1180 Hz for a 1, also called *mark*, and 980 Hz for a 0, or *space*. The chip also converts an incoming frequency of 2225 Hz to mark and 2025 Hz to space. For design simplicity and reliability, only half-duplex communication is used. Transmission and reception do not take place simultaneously. Under microprocessor control, the transmitter is shut off while receiving.

Two alternatives available to implement a portable modem for telephone communications are an inductive coil or a loudspeaker and a microphone [Fig. 6.23(e)]. An advantage of the inductive coil is that it is a compact, single unit which is easy to carry around and use. By placing the coil on the telephone earpiece, we can both transmit and receive, since the telephone has internal cross coupling. We found that a commercially available coil gave us a high error rate, so we designed our own coil with separate receiver and transmitter windings. By separating the

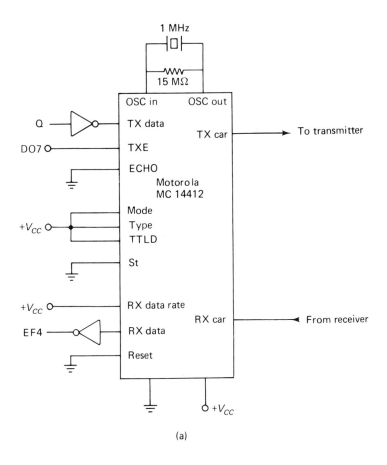

(a)

Mode		Tx data		Rx data
Originate	"1"	Mark	"1"	1180 Hz
Originate	"1"	Space	"0"	980 Hz
Answer	"0"	Mark	"1"	2225 Hz
Answer	"0"	Space	"0"	2025 Hz

(b)

FIGURE 6.23 Telephone communication. (a) Modem interface. (b) Modem specifications. (c) Receiver circuit. (d) Transmitter circuit. (e) Telephone inductive and acoustic couplers.

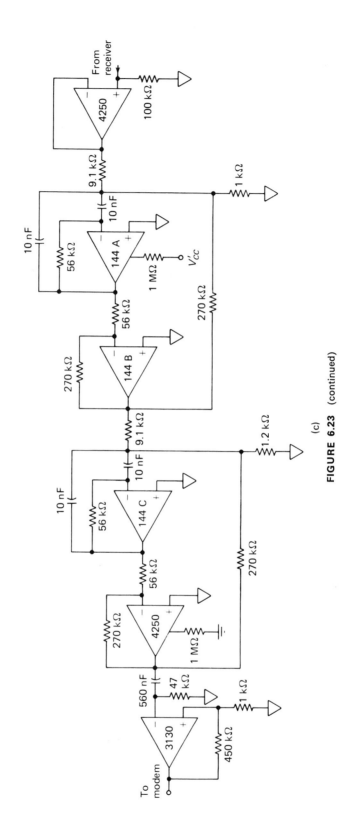

FIGURE 6.23 (continued)

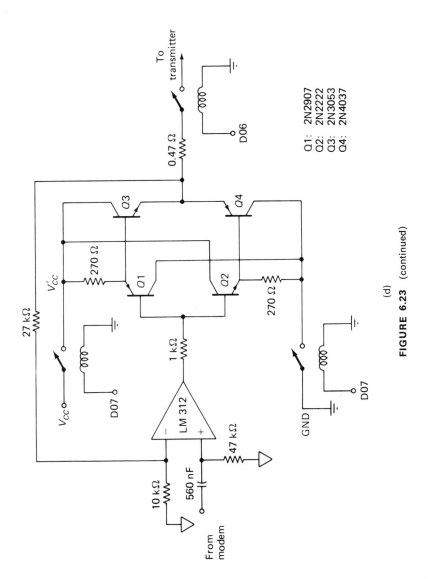

FIGURE 6.23 (continued)

(d)

Q1: 2N2907
Q2: 2N2222
Q3: 2N3053
Q4: 2N4037

431

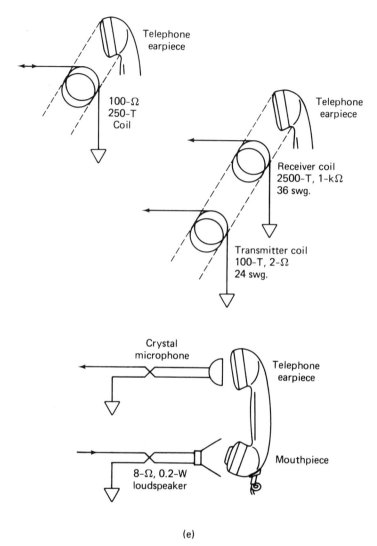

(e)

FIGURE 6.23 (continued)

receiver and transmitter coils, we were able to optimize each separately. By providing a large number of turns in the receiver coil, we achieve a high received-signal amplitude. By having a small number of turns in the transmitter coil, we reduce the resistive loss in the coil and boost the transmitter power. With the same transmitter and receiver circuits, we have explored using a loudspeaker and a microphone and have found the acoustic transmission to be more reliable than the inductive coil approach. The disadvantage here is that the loudspeaker and microphone are much larger than the coil.

The modem transmits over the telephone using either an inductive coil or a loudspeaker. To generate sufficient output for error-free transmission, the output power must be boosted. Figure 6.23(d) shows a complementary symmetry push-pull circuit to drive the transmitter. By cascading two such stages, we can obtain sufficient current to drive either an 8-Ω loudspeaker or a coil having a 20-Ω reactive impedance. Since this transmitter circuit consumes a significant amount of power, its power supply is turned off except when modem communication is required.

The receiver in Fig. 6.23(c) is a high-gain amplifier with bandpass character-istics that pass the incoming mark and space frequencies (2025 Hz and 2225 Hz). High gain is required because signals can be as low as 500 μV from the inductive coil. To reduce the group delay distortion, the amplifier's phase characteristic must be linear with frequency. The amplifier has a passband of 1900 to 2400 Hz and a gain of 900.

6.8 DATA REDUCTION ALGORITHMS*

The monitor samples the ECG at 200 samples/s. This produces a large number of data that are difficult to store and transmit. We need a process that reduces the amount of data without losing the clinical information content. This section intro-duces three different algorithms that are useful for biopotential data reduction.

Turning point

The turning-point data-reduction algorithm is the easiest to implement and fastest running of the algorithms discussed here (Mueller, 1978). It analyzes the trend of sampled points and stores only one of each pair of consecutive points. The term "turning point" derives from the fact that this algorithm retains turning points of the signal (points at which the sign of the signal slope changes or turns).

The algorithm developed from the following observations and assumptions:

1. According to sampling theory, sampling at 100 samples/s adequately represents the ECG recorded for this project with a 40-Hz bandwidth.
2. QRS complexes with large amplitudes and/or extremely high slopes often have diminished wave amplitudes at a 100-samples/s sampling rate because the key data points are missed. This can result in significant loss of ampli-tude or entire loss of small waves.
3. A sampling rate of 200 Hz gives excellent resolution.
4. The best visual time resolution of a standard ECG taken at 25 mm/s is about 10 ms.

A conclusion from the information given above is that except for clinically signif-icant high-frequency signals (making up a small fraction of the total ECG signal),

---

*Section 6.8 written by John P. Abenstein.

a sampling rate of 100 samples/s is adequate. Therefore, a signal sampled at 200 samples/s can be reduced to an effective sample rate of 100 samples/s while retaining key attributes (turning points) of the signal. The turning-point algorithm reduces every two data points in the original signal to one data point in the coded signal. An array of 1000 points becomes an array of 500, and we give the amount of data reduction as a ratio—500/1000.

The algorithm proceeds as follows. The first sampled point is stored and assigned as the reference point (X_0). The next two consecutive points become X_1 and X_2. Figure 6.24 shows all the possible configurations that three points could have. The circled point is then stored and becomes the new reference point (X_0) for the next iteration. The point not circled (either X_1 or X_2) is discarded. The next two points are sampled, their values are assigned to X_1 and X_2, and the process is repeated.

The retained point preserves the sense of the original three-point grouping.

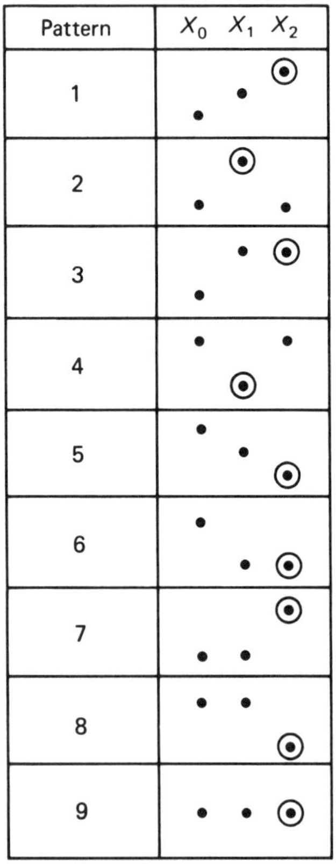

FIGURE 6.24 Turning-point algorithm. All possible 3-point configurations with the circle indicating the saved point. (From Mueller, W. C. 1978. Arrhythmia detection software for an ambulatory ECG monitor. Biomed. Sci. Instrum. 14 : 81–85. Used with permission of ISA.)

Note that in all cases except where there is a turning point, X_2 is the chosen point. X_1 is the chosen point only when there is a turning point in the three-sample configuration.

Since the computer cannot visually inspect the points to decide which point to save, it uses a mathematical criterion. $(X_2 - X_1)$ and $(X_1 - X_0)$ are the slopes of the two pairs of consecutive points. Figure 6.25 lists the signs of these two slopes for each possible configuration and the sign of the product of the two slopes. Examination shows that X_1 is saved only if the product is less than zero, while X_2 is retained when the product is greater than or equal to zero. Therefore, a very simple criterion emerges for implementation by the computer.

Figure 6.26 shows the flowchart of the turning-point algorithm, where

$$\text{if } (X_2 - X_1)(X_1 - X_0) < 0 \qquad X_0 = X_1$$
$$\text{if } (X_2 - X_1)(X_1 - X_0) \geq 0 \qquad X_0 = X_2$$

It is also possible to further reduce the data to an effective sample rate of 50 samples/s by a second application of the algorithm. Although the first application

Pattern	Sign of $X_1 - X_0$	Sign of $X_2 - X_1$	Sign of $(X_2 - X_1)(X_1 - X_0)$	Point choice
1	$+$	$+$	$+$	X_2
2	$+$	$-$	$-$	X_1
3	$+$	$\bigcirc$	$\bigcirc$	X_2
4	$-$	$+$	$-$	X_1
5	$-$	$-$	$+$	X_2
6	$-$	$\bigcirc$	$\bigcirc$	X_2
7	$\bigcirc$	$+$	$\bigcirc$	X_2
8	$\bigcirc$	$-$	$\bigcirc$	X_2
9	$\bigcirc$	$\bigcirc$	$\bigcirc$	X_2

FIGURE 6.25 Turning-point algorithm. Derivative signs and products. (From Mueller, W. C. 1978. Arrhythmia detection software for an ambulatory ECG monitor. Biomed. Sci. Instrum. 14: 81–85. Used with permission of ISA.)

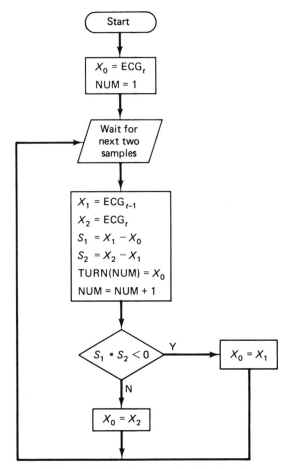

FIGURE 6.26 Turning-point algorithm flowchart.

of the algorithm produces little distortion of the signal, the second application can widen the QRS complex and produce sharp edges as shown in Fig. 6.27 for three different ECGs.

The turning-point algorithm has the advantage that it is easy to implement and is very fast, the latter being especially important for real-time computation. The algorithm yields an image that closely resembles that which a physician is accustomed to viewing.

To reduce the data so that a clinically significant sample of ECG data can be quickly transmitted, two applications of the algorithm must be applied to the original data. This is the primary disadvantage of the reduction method, for it introduces nontrivial distortion of the signal that can be unacceptable to the physician or coronary care nurse. A disadvantage of the turning-point algorithm is that saved points do not represent equally spaced time intervals. Although there is no long-term time distortion, there is short-term time distortion.

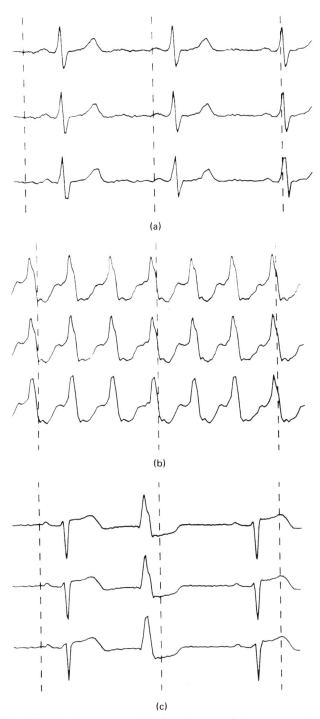

FIGURE 6.27 Turning-point algorithm. In each group of three traces, top is original ECG, center is ECG after one application of turning-point algorithm (data reduction of 500/1000), and bottom is ECG after two applications of turning-point algorithm (data reduction of 250/1000). (a) Normal sinus rhythm. (b) Tachycardia. (c) PVC.

AZTEC

The Amplitude Zone Time Epoch Coding (AZTEC) data-reduction algorithm has become an accepted form of data reduction for ECG monitors and data bases recently (Cox et al., 1968). AZTEC takes raw ECG data and produces short lines and slopes. Figure 6.28 shows a flowchart of the AZTEC algorithm. A description of this flowchart follows.

Horizontal lines. As the monitor samples the ECG, the first sample is set equal to the initial conditions, V_{mx} (for maximum value) and V_{mn} (for minimum value). The next sample is compared to V_{mx} and V_{mn}. If this sample is greater than V_{mx}, then V_{mx} is made equal to the value of the sample. Conversely, if the sample is less than V_{mn}, then V_{mn} is made equal to the value of the sample. This process is repeated until either the difference between V_{mx} and V_{mn} is greater than a predetermined threshold, V_{th}, or more than 50 samples have been gathered. Either event produces a line. To store the line, first the number of samples examined minus one is saved at T_1 (time or length of the line). Then the values of V_{mx} and V_{mn}, previous to the present sample, are averaged and set to V_1, which is saved [i.e., value of the line, $V_1 = (V_{mx} + V_{mn})/2$ at time $t - 1$]. V_{mx} and V_{mn} are then set equal to the present sample and the process is continued. This is the first part of the AZTEC algorithm and is called zero-order interpolation (ZOI). ZOI produces lines of zero slope. The first value saved is the length of the line, while the second value is the amplitude of the line. Figure 6.29 shows original data and the output.

Sloping lines. If the number of samples required to produce a line is less than three, a slope is produced (a constant rate of voltage change). If the length of a line is less than three, the line parameters are not saved. Instead, the algorithm begins to produce a slope. First, the value of the line is assigned to V_{s1} (value of the slope). Second, the length of the line is assigned to T_{s1} (time or length of the slope). The direction of the slope ($+$ or $-$) is also recorded. The algorithm then returns to line detection, beginning with resetting the values of V_{mx} and V_{mn} to equal the present sample. When the next line is produced, AZTEC determines whether or not the slope data should be updated or terminated. If the length of the new line is greater than 2 or if the direction of the slope is changed, the slope is terminated. Otherwise, the slope is updated. V_{s1} is made equal to the value of the new line and the length of the line is added to T_{s1}. AZTEC again returns to line detection.

When the slope is finally terminated, the slope parameters are determined and saved. First, T_{s1} is multiplied by -1 and stored. If the slope was terminated by a change in direction *and* the line length is less than 3 (i.e., a new slope), V_{s1} is saved, T_{s1} is made equal to the line length, V_{s1} is made equal to the terminating line amplitude, and AZTEC returns to sample for a new line but is producing a new slope.

If the slope was terminated by a change in direction and/or the terminating line length is greater than 2, the amplitude of that line is saved, then the length of that line, and finally the amplitude of the line is saved again (in other words, the updated T_{s1} times -1, V_1, T_1, and V_1 are saved in this order). After all four values are saved, AZTEC returns to reinitialize V_{mx} and V_{mn} and begins to produce a new line.

AZTEC's data reduction is not constant. The reduction is frequently as great as 100/1000 or more, depending upon the nature of the signal itself and the value of the empirically determined threshold. Figure 6.30 shows the same three ECGs as Fig. 6.27, encoded using the AZTEC algorithm.

Curve smoothing through parabolic fitting. When the arrhythmia monitor alarms, the patient goes to a telephone and transmits the recorded data for examination by a coronary care nurse. A central computer receives, processes, and displays the data on either a graphic terminal or a strip-chart recorder. Although AZTEC produces a recognizable ECG signal, the steplike quantization is unfamiliar to most nurses and physicians. Therefore, a curve-smoothing algorithm to process the AZTEC data produces a more acceptable output for the nurses and physicians.

The least-squares, polynomial-fitting technique described in Chapter 3 is an easy and fast method to smooth the signal. This method finds the best fit to each set of seven sample points in the original signal. The first step is to take the AZTEC straight-line data and expand it into a set of discrete data points. AZTEC describes lines and slopes; therefore, if a line 20 samples long at an amplitude of 35 is defined (i.e., AZTEC returns . . . , 20, 35, . . .), then 20 points equal to 35 are stored. The same process is done for a slope. After all the AZTEC data are translated into data points, curve smoothing can begin. Parabolic fitting provides a smooth-curve approximation to each set of seven points in the original waveform.
From Chapter 3,

$$P_0 = \tfrac{1}{21}(-2a_{k-3} + 3a_{k-2} + 6a_{k-1} + 7a_k + 6a_{k+1} + 3a_{k+2} - 2a_{k+3})$$

where P_0 is the new data point, $a_{k \pm n}$ the original data points (AZTEC), and $k \pm n$ defines the time relationship. This equation is a new waveform similar to AZTEC's, but with reduced noise and no discontinuities (i.e., low-pass filtered). Figure 6.30 shows waveforms produced by the parabolic fitting algorithm. Although this waveform smoothing does not produce a perfect reconstruction of the original ECG signal, it does make AZTEC's bizarre output more familiar for a nurse or physician. Therefore, we can take advantage of AZTEC's superior data compression while retaining the clinical information content of the ECG for diagnostic purposes.

Although the AZTEC flowchart appears to be much more complicated than that of the turning-point flowchart, in reality application of AZTEC is straightforward and not significantly slower. For the majority of samples, AZTEC only updates the minimum and maximum values of the window. When a line is produced only a few checks are made and either a slope is begun, updated, or terminated, or the line is stored. Therefore, the longest path through the flowchart is fairly short and is not executed that often.

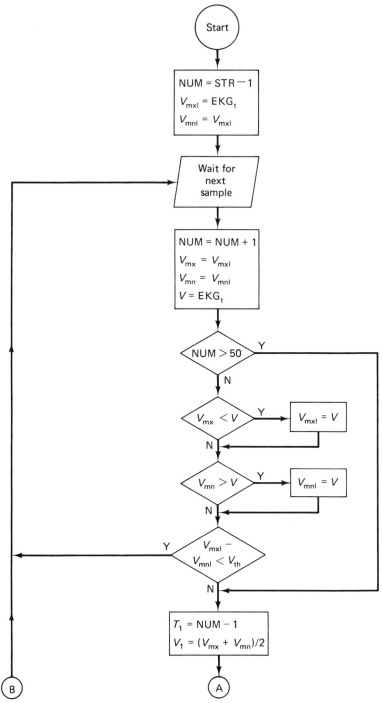

FIGURE 6.28 AZTEC algorithm flowchart. (From Abenstein, J. P. 1978. Algorithms for real-time ambulatory ECG monitoring. Biomed. Sci. Instrum. 14 : 73–79. Used with permission of ISA.)

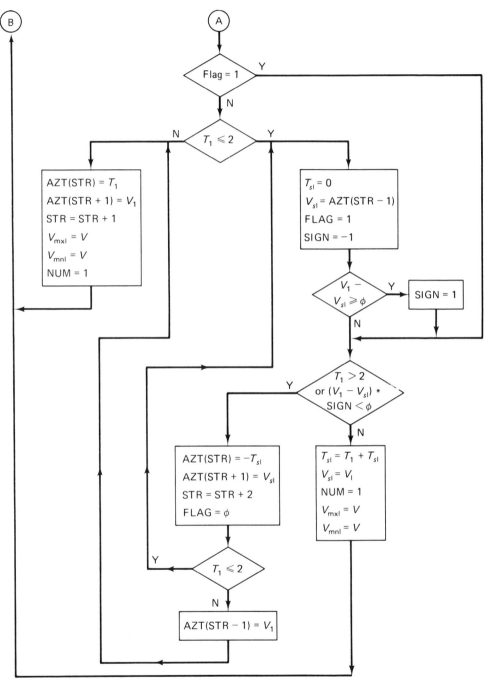

FIGURE 6.28 (continued)

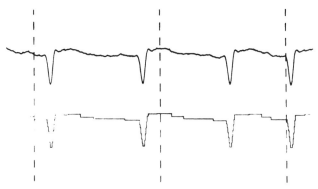

FIGURE 6.29 Atrial premature beat. (a) Amplifier output, sampled at 200 samples/s. (b) Zero-order interpolation (ZOI) output.

CORTES

Both the turning-point and AZTEC data-reduction algorithms have advantages and disadvantages. The turning-point algorithm keeps the resolution of the QRS complex after the first application, but after the second introduces a fair amount of distortion. The turning-point algorithm applies the same data reduction to low-information signal regions such as the isoelectric regions, the low-frequency P and T waves, and noise signals as it does to the high-information-content QRS complex. AZTEC has great data-reduction properties and adapts its coding mode to the nature of the signal region itself. AZTEC also eliminates baseline noise, but even after smoothing with a parabolic filter, an AZTEC signal is not visually acceptable to a cardiologist (even though it preserves the clinical content of the signal).

A new data-reduction algorithm, called the Coordinate Reduction Time Encoding System (CORTES), is a hybrid of the turning-point and AZTEC algorithms that attempts to take advantage of the strengths of each while sidestepping the weaknesses. We can make the following observations:

1. The turning-point algorithm produces great resolution at 100 Hz.
2. AZTEC discards clinically insignificant data in the isoelectric region of the ECG signal with greater than 10 : 1 data reduction in this region.

Therefore, CORTES applies AZTEC to the isoelectric region of the ECG signal and applies the turning-point algorithm to the clinically significant high(er) frequency parts of the ECG signal. To do this, AZTEC and the turning-point algorithm are applied in parallel to the incoming ECG data. When an AZTEC line is produced, a decision based on the length of the line is made whether to save the AZTEC data or the turning-point data. If the line is longer than an experimentally determined threshold, V_{1n}, the AZTEC line is saved. If the line is shorter or equal to V_{1n}, the turning-point data are saved. To speed up the process, the turning-point data are stored directly into the reduction array. By the use of two array pointers,

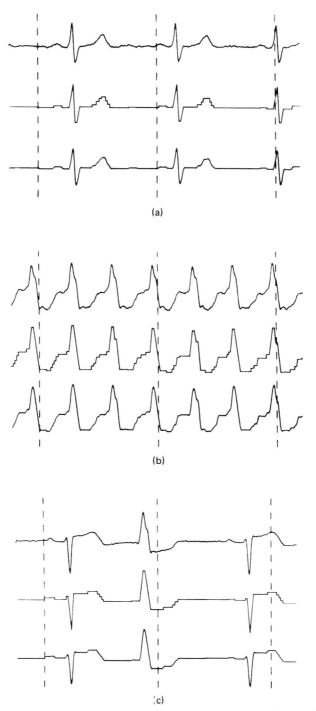

FIGURE 6.30 AZTEC algorithm. In each group of three traces, top is original ECG, center is AZTEC-coded ECG, and bottom is AZTEC-coded ECG after smoothing with a parabolic digital filter. (a) Normal sinus rhythm. Data reduction of 170/1000. (b) Tachycardia. Data reduction of 340/1000. (c) PVC. Data reduction of 138/1000.

P1 and P2, the difference between probationary and permanent data is determined. A marker is used to identify transitions between AZTEC and turning-point data. In the 8-bit COSMAC, any number will do as a marker (say zero), thus reducing the quantization of the ECG signal to 255 levels instead of 256.

CORTES flowchart. Figure 6.31 is a flowchart of the CORTES data-reduction algorithm. The first ECG sample is set equal to V_{mn}, V_{mx}, and X_0. The first CORTES array location is made equal to the marker, P1 is set equal to 1, and P2 is set equal to 2. Finally, the flags are zeroed. After this initialization, the algorithm can begin.

The next point is made equal to X_1 and compared to V_{mx} and V_{mn}, changing the values if need be. The third point is set equal to X_2 and compared to the AZTEC window limits. X_0 is then stored and P2 incremented. This continues until an AZTEC line is found. If the line is longer than V_{1n}, an AZTEC line is stored [Fig. 6.32(a)] and the pointers are moved. If the line is not long enough, the turning-point data are made permanent [Fig. 6.32(b)]. After the data are stored permanently (P1 is moved forward), the algorithm begins to produce another line while storing turning-point data on a probationary status at the same time.

Figure 6.32 shows the transitions from storing AZTEC data to storing either new AZTEC or new turning-point data, and vice versa. The most important change is the location of the marker that identifies what follows the marker.

If the produced AZTEC line is too short to be stored and the present data point was just set equal to X_1, then the next data sample must be captured before the turning-point data can be made permanent. This is done so that the new data point can be made equal to X_2 and a determination of the new value for X_0 can be made. This new value is needed, since V_{mn1} and V_{mx1} are made equal to the new X_0 and the new location of P1 points to X_0. Therefore, if the next line is long enough, it will write over the beginning of the turning-point data it is supposed to represent and will keep the correct time base.

Again the flowchart seems complicated, but the data flow is even shorter than AZTEC, since there is no slope coding. Termination of lines and decisions on what to store are very simple and therefore fast. Figure 6.33 shows the same three ECGs as Figs. 6.27 and 6.30 processed by CORTES.

Reconstruction of CORTES data. Unlike the turning-point and AZTEC algorithms, the reconstruction of the data in the CORTES array is not straightforward. Fortunately, this reconstruction is done on the central computer and does not have the constraints of real-time computations.

Since the lengths recorded in the AZTEC data section of CORTES represent single units of sampling rate, while the turning-point data points are two units apart, some manipulations are needed. Also, the transitions between lines and turning points follow other rules. If a line is followed by a marker as in Fig. 6.34(a) (i.e., next data is turning point), the length of the line is decremented, and the distance between this short, end line and the first turning point is 1 (versus 2 between turning points). If a turning point is followed by a marker (the next data set is an AZTEC line), the length between the turning point and the value of the line is 2 time units, as shown in Fig. 6.34(b) Therefore, to reconstruct CORTES, we must follow four rules:

1. Lengths of AZTEC lines are single time units.
2. Distance between turning-point values is 2 time units.
3. Transition from AZTEC line to turning point.
   a. Length of AZTEC line decremented.
   b. Distance between end of shortened AZTEC line and turning point equals 1.
4. Transition from turning point to AZTEC, distance from last turning point and beginning of line equals 2.

Parabolic fitting of CORTES data. Although the CORTES algorithm preserves the required QRS resolution, there are still discontinuities in the isoelectric region. Therefore, some smoothing is necessary. The first step, as with AZTEC, is to expand the data into a set of discrete data points. The same rules hold for this expansion as for reconstruction. In order to get consistent distances between points, the mean of each pair of turning points is found and stored. After the set of points is produced, parabolic smoothing can be applied to low-pass-filter the CORTES signal. Figure 6.33 shows examples of CORTES data after smoothing with parabolic fitting.

Other data-reduction algorithms

Within the world of ECG signal processing there are innumerable data-reduction methods. Many of these others use so-called Hoffman encoding or linear prediction theory. These have serious disadvantages. The first is that they require a great deal of bit manipulation, which is completely unsuited for the COSMAC in real time. Second, the nature of the encoding precludes any straightforward pattern recognition (QRS morphology analysis), to be included at a later date.

Conclusions

We have discussed these three data-reduction algorithms in depth. The purpose of this section was to introduce each algorithm and give enough detail so that the reader could implement any or all of the algorithms. Obviously, the best data are the raw data, but because we do not have that choice, we must make a decision. The turning-point algorithm is by far the fastest and easiest to implement. Unfortunately, significant data reduction (i.e., 250/1000) causes distortion of the signal.

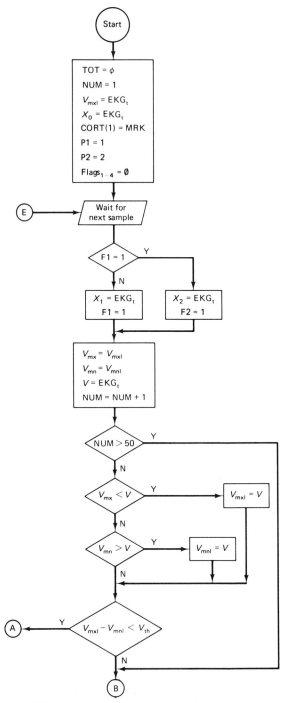

FIGURE 6.31 Flowchart of CORTES algorithm.

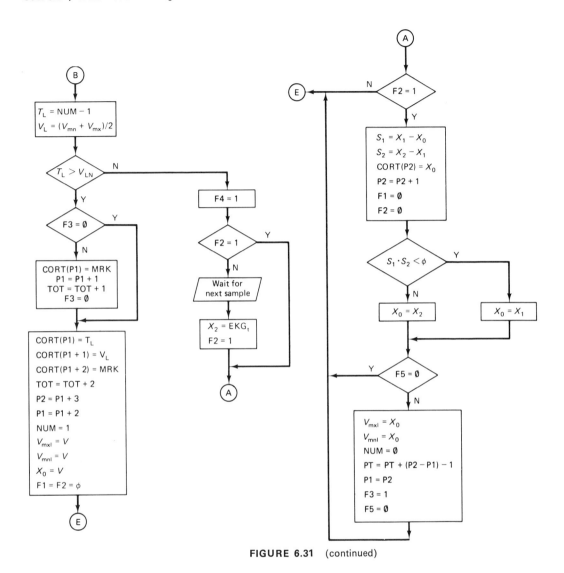

FIGURE 6.31 (continued)

AZTEC, on the other hand, produces fairly unacceptable output even with curve smoothing. CORTES seems to be a fair compromise, since the QRS, T, and P waves keep their basic morphologies while the major data reduction is done on the clinically insignificant isoelectric regions. However, CORTES is not the most straightforward algorithm. At the time of this writing no physician survey has been made of the acceptability of CORTES, but we plan it as part of the clinical testing of the device. The ability to change critical software modules while development is in progress is another example of the flexibility of the monitor.

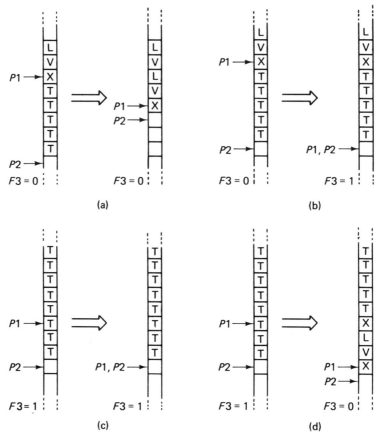

FIGURE 6.32 Pointer and data transition in CORTES array. (a) Last permanent data AZTEC, new data also AZTEC. (b) Last permanent data AZTEC, new data turning point. (c) Last permanent data turning point, new data turning point. (d) Last permanent data turning point, new data AZTEC. L, AZTEC line length; V, AZTEC line amplitude; X, mark—delimits AZTEC from turning-point data; T, turning-point data; F3, equals 1 when last permanently stored data was turning point; P1, pointer marking beginning of probationary data; P2, pointer marking next free space. [*Note:* (a) and (b) represent the top of the array.]

6.9 SOFTWARE DEVELOPMENT*

COSMAC software development package (CSDP)

When we received the COSMAC hardware evaluation kit from RCA, it became quickly evident that the software development was not going to progress at a very rapid pace without additional software development resources. The kit includes a

---

*Section 6.9 written by John P. Abenstein.

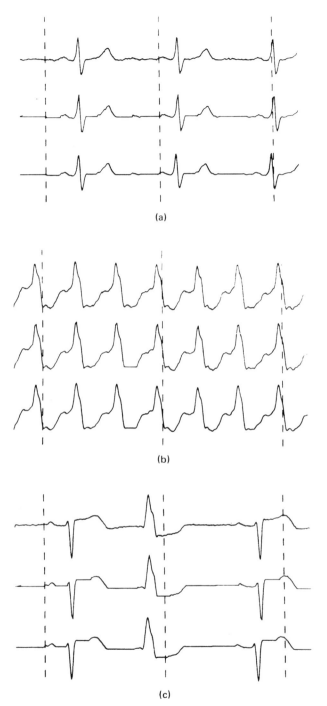

FIGURE 6.33 CORTES algorithm. In each group of three traces, top is original ECG, center is CORTES-coded ECG, and bottom is CORTES-coded ECG after smoothing with a parabolic digital filter. (a) Normal sinus rhythm. Data reduction of 202/1000. (b) Tachycardia. Data reduction of 266/1000. (c) PVC. Data reduction of 175/1000.

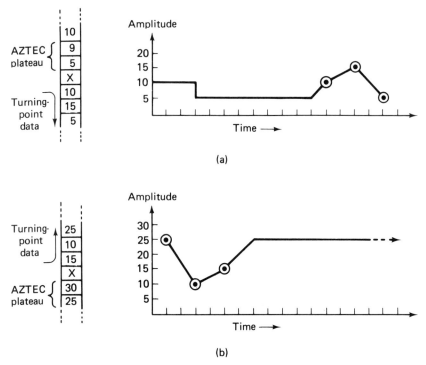

FIGURE 6.34 Reconstruction of CORTES data. (a) Transition from AZTEC to turning-point data. (b) Transition from turning-point to AZTEC data.

very simple monitor that allows the user with an interfaced terminal to load data one hexadecimal character at a time into memory. Therefore, the programmer is forced to write out a program and then hand-assemble the code into the equivalent hexadecimal codes. After assembly, the hexadecimal codes must be typed into the machine. Besides being tedious, this process is so error-prone that nontrivial program development is all but impossible.

Fortunately, RCA had contributed to the University of Wisconsin–Madison a copy of the COSMAC Software Development Package (CSDP) in four boxes of computer cards. Along with the cards was documentation explaining how to get it up on the computer. CSDP was not ready to be read into our minicomputer and run; there were a few nontrivial problems.

First, the cards could not be read correctly on any card reader available. The card reader made "+" into ">" and "=" into "<" and other such transpositions. Also, the minicomputer we bought had only dual-density floppy disks, which were not media-compatible with many computers on campus. We got the program into our PDP-11 by a rather roundabout method. We read the cards into a computer with a disk cartridge, then transferred the file to DECtape. From DECtape we copied the program to a single-density floppy disk and from this floppy to nine-track magtape. Finally, from nine-track tape we were able to transfer the program to a dual-density floppy disk that could be accessed by our PDP-11. The transposition problem was solved by manually correcting all the copying errors with the PDP-11 text editor.

Now we had a program that could be compiled and run. Unfortunately, there were still two small problems. CSDP was originally written to be run on an IBM VM/370 CMS system and required about 260 kbytes of memory. The version we received from RCA was made to run on a PDP-11 with 56 kbytes of memory under DEC's old DOS (disk-operating system) with substantial overlaying (overlaying is a method by which a program is swapped in and out of the computer from the disk in order to give a very large program the capability to run on a small system). Our PDP-11 has 56 kbytes of memory, and we use the RT-11 operating system. Therefore, we had to do some debugging. First, the DOS and RT-11 overlay structures are completely different. Second, DOS calls from FORTRAN are not functionally similar to the equivalent calls in RT-11.

Therefore, CSDP needed substantial work to get it operational. The unattractive alternative would have been to write our own cross assembler or do hand coding. We decided to get CSDP operational with particular emphasis on the cross assembler. The cross assembler took about 3 worker-months to implement with one person working on the project. The cross assembler then speeded up software development significantly. After another 4 months of part-time effort, the CSDP simulator was functional, making CSDP completely operational. CSDP is just a tool for software development. But like most useful tools, it is required for effective software development.

In a microprocessor project, software development is an important part of the project. Industrial evidence shows that the software part of a project can take up to 80% of the development time. Therefore, when choosing a microprocessor for a project, we should not examine only the power consumption and speed; the software support the manufacturer will (or can) supply is just as important as the hardware support.

Finally, a last word about CSDP. The documentation that RCA provides with CSDP is the best that we have seen for a computer program, especially for a product. The program itself is well written and fairly straightforward—it is easy to understand its function. The cross assembler has excellent error messages that facilitate debugging. The simulator is another tool that decreases development time significantly. Having the ability to run any number of instructions, stop the simulated execution, and examine any location or register is helpful. It is an excellent system well worth the time required to get it operating.

COSMAC software development

Figure 6.35 shows the software flowchart for both the portable monitor and the central computer. The COSMAC program was developed as a modular system so that modifications could easily be made in one module without having to modify the other modules.

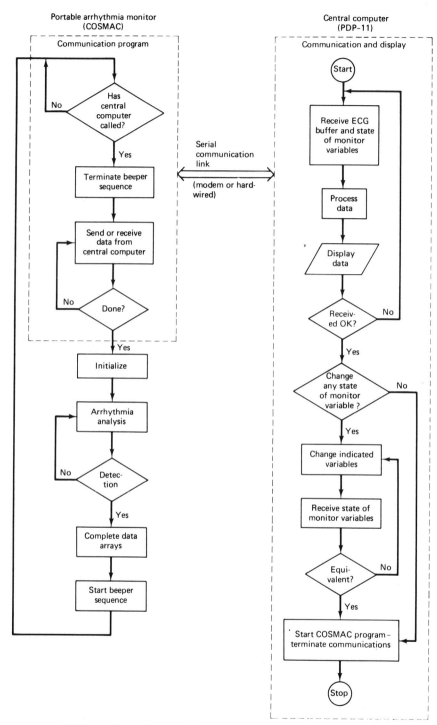

FIGURE 6.35 Ambulatory ECG monitoring system software flowchart.

Initialization. Initialization is the time required to fill all the buffers that are required for proper operation of the arrhythmia algorithm. These buffers include one to hold 16 s of ECG data, another to contain eight R-to-R intervals, and another to save the current and previous averages of the eight R-to-R intervals. Initialization begins by collecting 16 s of data, after which an R wave is required to establish a time base for interval computation. After the program detects the first R wave, it must locate eight more R waves to supply the eight R-to-R intervals required for the running-average calculation. This requires an additional 4-10 s of initialization time for heart rates between 120 and 50 beats/min. Therefore, it takes on the average 23 s for initialization to take place.

Arrhythmia detection. After initialization, the system becomes sensitive to single R-to-R interval changes and changes in the R-to-R interval averages, as outlined in Section 6.1. The program now stays in the arrhythmia-detection section until predefined limits are met for an alarm or manual override occurs.

Alarm. When an alarm condition is calculated, arrhythmia detection ceases, the program closes all buffers except the data buffer, and takes one of two paths. Depending upon the arrhythmia detected, either sampling continues for another 10 s before the 16-s buffer is closed or the buffer closes immediately upon alarm, as shown in Fig. 6.36.

If closure is immediate, the event causing the alarm is at the end of the 16-s buffer. If 10 s more data are to be gathered before the buffer is closed, the event that caused the alarm will be found 6 s into the buffer. After all the buffers are

Arrhythmia	Data buffer closure time after detected arrhythmia
Tachycardia ≥ 120 beats/min.	Immediate
Bradycardia ≤ 50 beats/min.	
Asystole	
Dropped beat	10 s
R on T	
15 premature beats/min.	

FIGURE 6.36 Arrhythmias currently detected and buffer closure times. (From Mueller, W. C. 1978. Arrhythmia detection software for an ambulatory ECG monitor. Biomed. Sci. Instrum. 14 : 81–85. Used with permission of ISA.)

closed, the program gives visual and audible alarms to signal the patient to make contact with the central computer for transmission of the calculated data and the ECG data buffer.

When the patient first contacts the central computer facility, the PDP-11 sends a carriage return to signal the monitor to leave the alarm mode and wait for a command. A command of the form

$$?AAAA \ NNNN \ \rangle$$

where AAAA is a hexadecimal address and NNNN a hexadecimal number, tells the COSMAC monitor to send NNNN bytes starting at address AAAA. A command of the form

$$!AAAA \ XXXX.\dots \ \rangle$$

where AAAA is a hexadecimal address and XXXX. . . . a string of hexadecimal characters, tells the COSMAC monitor to load bytes XXXX. . . . starting at address AAAA. A command of the form

$$\$ \ \rangle$$

tells the COSMAC to restart the arrhythmia program.

Manual override. Should symptoms arise that the patient thinks are cardiac-related, a manual override switch is available. Once this switch is pressed the program samples and stores 16 s of data for transmission and review. As with the alarm condition, activating this option stops all activity except the software clock after the 16-s buffer is closed.

PDP-11 software development

The responsibility of the central computer as a remote host is to receive the data the monitor has saved after an alarm, process and display the received data, and give the coronary care nurse or physician the ability to change the state of such monitor variables as the tachycardia limits, the bradycardia limits, and the time of day.

When a patient calls the central computer, the coronary care nurse puts the phone into the modem and runs the communication program. This program first sends over a carriage return to the monitor and then commands the monitor to send over the collected ECG data and the state of monitor variables. When all the data are received, the central computer reconstructs the ECG and displays the signal on the graphics terminal. The operator is then asked if the received data are correct (i.e., does it look like an ECG or did something get scrambled during transmission?). If the data are not correct, the monitor is asked to send the data again. When the data are received correctly, the operator has the option to store them on disk or output them via the D/A converter to a strip-chart recorder (ECG machine).

The operator can then change detection limits or the time of day. If these are changed, the monitor echoes the changes back to guarantee that the data were received correctly. If what was sent and received do not match, the program tries again. When the data sent and received are the same, the program restarts the monitor program and terminates communication.

6.10 SYSTEM TESTING*

Hardware testing

Development of microprocessor-based hardware is considerably facilitated by a hardware development system. We use an RCA COSMAC evaluation kit to aid in the rapid development of hardware (as well as software). The evaluation kit comes equipped with a monitor program (residing in a ROM) which enables reading from and writing into any specific memory location. We can start execution of a program at any specified location. The kit allows single stepping through the program. At any time we can monitor the contents of the address bus and data bus in LED registers. We can also observe the status of the program (run, load, pause, reset) in a LED register.

We can also use this evaluation kit to develop equipment prototypes. By coupling the address and data bus and the control lines via an "umbilicus," we can monitor the status of the prototype from the evaluation kit LEDs. For example, we can test the correct operation of the LCD and beeper by loading a small test program into the evaluation kit memory. We monitor the contents of the data bus for correct appearance of data bytes that should reach the LCD/beeper. Upon proper execution of the OUT 1 instruction, the LCD should light up according to data latched into the output port. Another example of the hardware support of such a configuration is the testing of memory boards. We use the monitor program in the evaluation kit ROM to test (read, write, and run) programs in the prototype memory.

We now describe the test devices used to develop microprocessor-based instruments. In addition to the oscilloscope and multimeter, debugging and testing of a microprocessor-based system is facilitated by a logic analyzer, such as the Tektronix Model 7D01. The logic analyzer has three modes:

1. In the time-domain mode, we simultaneously view many data channel signals in the manner of a normal multitrace oscilloscope.

2. In the map mode, we sequentially view the address of each program step on an x-y dot matrix.

3. In the state display mode we view lists of alphanumeric characters that represent the data and address of every instruction.

---

*Section 6.10 written by Nitish V. Thakor.

Analog system testing

To test various R-wave detector designs and subsequently to test the complete monitor for ambulatory ECGs, we have developed a test tape. We recorded 30 min of ECG data on an FM tape recorder in the format shown in Fig. 6.37.

Block	
1	Normal sinus rhythm
2	Tachycardia
3	Bradycardia
4	Couplets, triplets, bigeminy
5	Heart block
6	Atrial flutter/fibrillation
7	Ventricular fibrillation/asystole
8	Premature atrial beats
9	Premature ventricular beats
10	Paced rhythms
11–15	Not allocated
16	QRS morphologies
17	QRS morphologies
18	EMG noise
19	60–Hz interference
20	RF and other electrical interference
21	Skin-electrode motion artifact
22	Baseline drift
23	Amplifier saturation
24	Exercise ECG
25	Exercise ECG
26–30	Not allocated

FIGURE 6.37 Organization of ECG test tape (each block 1 min : six sections of 10 s each).

The tape is divided into 30 blocks of 1-min duration each. Each block is subdivided into six sections. Each section contains a different set of ECG data. Fifteen minutes of the tape contain various arrhythmias. The other 15 min contain noisy data typically encountered under ambulatory conditions.

To provide efficient compiling as well as future editing, we have used a PDP-11 computer to prepare the tape. Figure 6.38 shows the technique used. The computer converts analog data to digital data and stores them on a floppy disk. The program easily controls any revisions. After complete compilation the computer provides output data through a D/A converter and a low-pass filter for storage on the FM tape recorder.

Software testing

As with the analog system testing, the primary, preclinical testing method for the software is to make use of a test tape. This method discovers the most blatant errors in the software. This testing is not for just the monitor program. After an alarm

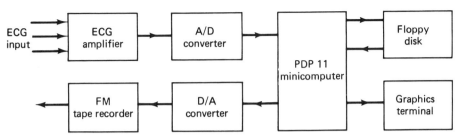

FIGURE 6.38 Test-tape development system. (From Thakor, N. V. 1978. Reliable R-wave detection from ambulatory subjects. Biomed. Sci. Instrum. 14 : 67–72. Used with permission of ISA.)

the central computer program must also be tested. The test tape is both a convenient and relatively rigorous criteria for software performance. Once the software passes the test tape, we must perform one more preclinical test. Normal subjects serve as "patients" for the device. With human subjects we can perform more rigorous tests for saturation and motion artifacts.

Clinical testing

Testing with "real" patients will consist of four phases:

1. Volunteers will determine the acceptability, function, and reliability of the monitor.
2. Volunteers will simultaneously wear this device and a Holter monitor.
3. Patients who are chosen for Holter monitoring will simultaneously wear this device.
4. Post-CCU patients will wear this device.

These phases are designed to test both the reliability of the device as a cardiac monitor and also to test the "human factors," which can only be guessed at until testing begins. For example, we have no idea how a heart patient will react to a device that beeps when something may be wrong with his or her heart.

The clinical testing will need a full-time programmer. As new bugs are found or adjustments of alarm criteria crop up, a programmer will need to make these adjustments. A goal of the clinical testing is to phase out the technical personnel. The monitor will only become clinically useful when highly trained individuals are no longer needed to keep the device(s) functional. Another goal of the clinical tests is to determine which alarm criteria must be adjustable and which can be fixed.

Finally, this device is designed to be used in the real world. An ultimate goal is to have this monitor at primary medical care sites in addition to academic hospitals, where the flexibility of the instrument is potentially supportive of research endeavors.

6.11 PROJECT EVALUATION*

It is instructive at this point to review the overall effort involved in developing the arrhythmia monitor. This section therefore reviews the project costs, labor effort, and development time. We estimate the cost of producing such a device on a commercial scale.

Project costs

The project costs are divided into three subgroups: (1) salaries, (2) equipment and hardware costs, and (3) miscellaneous and overhead. Figure 6.39 gives the estimates for each of these costs.

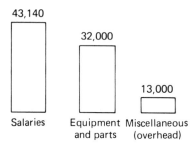

FIGURE 6.39 Project costs (in dollars).

Salaries. The salaries support six people (all part-time): two project leaders (in this case, professors at 30% time); one computer programmer (50% time); one hardware development engineer (graduate student at 50% time); one software development engineer (graduate student at 50% time); and one technician (student help at 10% time).

Equipment and hardware costs. Following a substantial initial capital equipment investment, the major costs in this group are for the prototype hardware. Note the hardware cost breakdown in terms of components and parts. Figure 6.40 shows the costs involved in major subgroups: (1) microprocessor and digital circuits, (2) memory, (3) analog circuit and components, and (4) miscellaneous (wires, batteries, case, boards, sockets, converters, switches). Figure 6.41 gives the detailed breakdown of the component costs involved in the development of the arrhythmia monitor.

Software development costs. Software development is a considerable fraction of the overall development costs. This aspect has become all the more evident with the advent of large-scale-integrated circuits (LSI), which limit the scope of hardware development and stabilize it fairly quickly. Software development and innovations

---

*Section 6.11 written by Nitish V. Thakor.

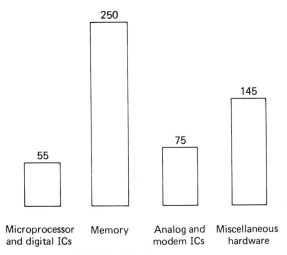

FIGURE 6.40   Hardware costs.

traditionally lag behind those in the hardware area. It has been generally accepted that one line of code requires one worker-hour of effort by an experienced programmer. A program that is about 2 kbytes long (as in our project) requires about 2000 worker-hours of effort, which itself forms a substantial fraction of the project costs.

Manpower effort and development time

Figure 6.42 shows the development time and the nature of the efforts involved. Note the long development time involved for the second prototype compared to the short development time of the first prototype, which used an evaluation kit. Note the short software development time for high-level language components of the project (PDP-11) compared to the time for developing COSMAC code.

We plan a considerable clinical testing period (6 months). Throughout this period, construction of new prototypes as well as software development will continue.

IC type	Description	Quantity	Unit cost	Total cost
Microprocessor board				
1802D	CPU	1	24.75	24.75
1852D	I/O port/latch	2	9.50	19.00
CD4069B	Rep inverter	1	0.45	0.45
CD4025A	Triple 3-input NOR	1	0.34	0.34
CD4027A	Dual JKFF	1	0.85	0.85
CD4054B	LCD driver	1	2.51	2.51
CD4059A	Prog. divide by N	1	6.00	6.00
CD4556B	Decoder	1	0.84	0.84
Memory board				
1821D	1024 x 1-bit RAM	16	18.50	296.00
6654	512 x 8-bit EPROM	4	24.00	96.00
Analog board				
LM4250C	Prog. op amp	3	1.75	5.25
L144	Prog. triple op amp	3	7.50	22.50
CD4098B	Dual monostable	1	1.50	1.50
MC14412	Modem	1	14.14	14.14
CD4016	Quad switch	1	0.69	0.69
CA3130	Op amp	1	1.00	1.00
2M2222A	Transistor	1	0.20	0.20
2M2907	Transistor	1	0.20	0.20
IN4148	Diodes	8	0.50	4.00
ADC0816	A/D converter	1	20.00	20.00
LM301	Zener regulator	1	9.00	9.00
	IC sockets	50		77.00
	Prototype boards	3		20.00
	Passive components			10.00
	Switches			3.00
	Connectors, cables			15.00
	Wire, solder			5.00
	Batteries (Ni–Cd)	4		16.00
			Total	667.22

FIGURE 6.41 Parts list.

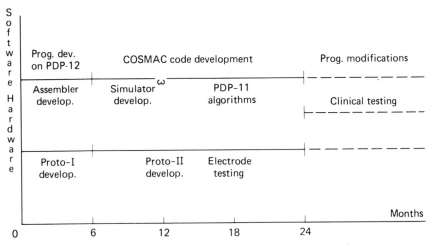

FIGURE 6.42 Labor effort and development time.

REFERENCES

ABENSTEIN, J. P. 1978. Algorithms for real-time ambulatory ECG monitoring. Biomed. Sci. Instrum. 14: 73–79.

ANALOG DEVICES. 1976. CMOS 10-bit monolithic A/D converter. Data sheet. Norwood, MA.

BRYDON, J. 1976. Automatic monitoring of cardiac arrhythmias. IEE Med. Electron. Monogr. 18–22. Peter Peregrinus, Stevenage, England, pp. 27–41.

COX, J. R., NOLLE, F. M., FOZZARD, H. A., AND OLIVER, G. C., JR. 1968. AZTEC: a preprocessing program for real-time ECG rhythm analysis. IEEE Trans. Biomed. Eng. BME-15: 128–129.

COX, J. R., NOLLE, F. M., AND ARTHUR, R. M. 1972. Digital analysis of the electroencephalogram, the blood pressure wave, and the ECG. Proc. IEEE. 60: 1137–1164.

HARRIS SEMICONDUCTOR. 1976. HM-6508/HM6518 1024 × 1 CMOS RAM. Data sheet. Melbourne, FL.

INTERSIL. 1979. IM6653/IM6654 4096 bit CMOS UV erasable PROM. Data sheet. Cupertino, CA.

MOTOROLA. 1976. Semiconductor data library, Vol. 5, Ser. B. Semiconductor Products, Austin, TX.

MUELLER, W. C. 1978. Arrhythmia detection software for an ambulatory ECG monitor. Biomed. Sci. Instrum. 14: 81–85.

NATIONAL SEMICONDUCTOR. 1976. LM4250/LM4250C programmable operational amplifier. Data sheet. Santa Clara, CA.

NATIONAL SEMICONDUCTOR. 1977. ADC0816/ADC0817 single chip data acquisition system. Data sheet. Santa Clara, CA.

POWER CONVERSION. 1976. The revolutionary lithium primary battery. Catalog 200. Mount Vernon, NY.

RCA. 1976a. RCA Integrated circuits. Solid State Div., Somerville, NJ.

RCA. 1976b. User manual for the CDP1802 COSMAC microprocessor. MPM-201A. Solid State Div., Somerville, NJ.

SILICONIX. 1973. L144: low-power triple operational amplifier integrated circuit. Data sheet. Santa Clara, CA.

STEINBERG, C. A., ABRAHAM, S., AND CACERES, C. A. 1962. Pattern recognition in the clinical electrocardiogram. IRE Trans. Biomed. Electron. BME-9: 35–42.

TAM, H. W., AND WEBSTER, J. G. 1977. Minimizing electrode motion artifact by skin abrasion. IEEE Trans. Biomed. Eng. BME-24: 134–139.

TELEDYNE SEMICONDUCTOR. 1976. CMOS 8700 series monolithic A/D converters. Mountain View, CA.

THAKOR, N. V. 1978. Reliable R-wave detection from ambulatory subjects. Biomed. Sci. Instrum. 14: 67–72.

THAKOR, N. V., AND WEBSTER, J. G. 1977. Two electrode ECG amplifier. Proc. Annu. Conf. Engr. Med. Biol. 18: 3.

TOMPKINS, W. J. 1978. A portable microcomputer-based system for biomedical applications. Biomed. Sci. Instrum. 14: 61–66.

UNGER, P. N. 1973. Cardiac warning device. U.S. patent 3,724,455.

VOGT, F. B., AND HALLEN, T. O. 1964. Cardiotachometer input processing unit, NASA Manned Spacecraft Center. Contract NAS-9-1461 Amd-1: 1–19.

WALTERS, J. B. 1976. A microprocessor-based arrhythmia monitor for ambulatory subjects. Rep. BMEC TR004. Biomedical Engineering Center for Clinical Instrumentation, MIT, Cambridge, MA.

WEBSTER, J. G., 1978. An intelligent monitor for ambulatory ECGs. Biomed. Sci. Instrum. 14: 55–60.

PROBLEMS

6.1   Redesign the ECG amplifier in the text to provide a bandwidth of 0.05 to 100 Hz (the diagnostic ECG bandwidth), with a 60-Hz notch filter and RF filtering. What other steps should be taken to reduce the electrical interference?

6.2   The arrhythmia monitor software is completely ready. We would now like to put the program in the 2758 (a 5-V version of 2708 described in Chapter 4). Two kbytes of program storage and 2 kbytes of data storage must be provided. Note that data storage is in a read/write memory such as the CDP1821. Design the memory system.

6.3   The arrhythmia monitor described in this chapter uses the BUSY signal from the A/D converter [which in turn is derived from the start conversion (STRT) signal] to interrupt the microprocessor. The R wave is detected via a flag. Design an alternative system with the R pulse as an interrupt. Make a flowchart for a program that times the interval between two consecutive R waves. What did you use as the timing generator?

6.4 Justify the use of low battery voltage to reduce the power consumption of the microprocessor. What other factors affect the microprocessor power consumption?

6.5 We would like to study the software versus hardware R-wave detector trade-offs. List the criteria for and against either scheme. Write a program in COSMAC assembly language for a software R-wave detector. This detector may be based on simple level detection of the ECG signals.

6.6 Note the considerable memory costs in the arrhythmia monitor system. Suppose that we decide to use instead a microcassette that can store 15 min of data. Devise a scheme for loading the ECG data serially from the COSMAC on an endless loop cassette. The recording should be stopped when an arrhythmia is detected.

6.7 Note that the arrhythmia monitor is a general-purpose, portable microcomputer. What are alternative applications for this device (as related to health care).

6.8 We would like to evaluate typical trade-offs involved in making a decision as to whether a given job should be done by software or dedicated hardware. A case in point is the QRS detector. A hardware implementation (see the text) needs four op amps (one 144 and one 4250 or four 4250) and one dual monostable. Hardware "overheads" include extra space, power consumption, and weight—let us say a "penalty" of 50% of the overall hardware costs. Calculate the total hardware costs, assuming that each 4250 op amp costs $1.50, monostable 14S28 $1.50, and miscellaneous components $1.50. On the other hand, a software QRS detector will need 100 bytes of memory (memory costs 1 cent/bit) and program execution time of 5 ms, a "penalty" of 50%, for time in a real-time system is at a premium, too. Calculate the costs for a software QRS detector. (Note that we have ignored the development costs; presumably they are the same for both approaches.)

6.9 Give a block diagram of a "physician's computer" which is to be used in conjunction with the arrhythmia monitor described in the text. That is, the patient should be able to get in touch with the physician via a telephone line and dump all the data collected into a memory. The physician, via a keyboard, should be able to play the data out into a chart recorder (after D/A conversion).

6.10 Design an R-wave detector with the following features: (1) A differentiator that differentiates the ECG signal up to 21 Hz; beyond that, the signal is low-pass-filtered (to limit noise). Draw the Bode plot of this filter. (2) A peak-and-valley detector to detect the peak of the ECG signal for either polarity. Compare this approach with a fixed threshold for R-wave detection. (3) An output pulse width of 200 ms. How is this R-wave detector different from the one described in the text?

6.11 We have selected an 8-bit A/D converter for digitizing the ECG signal. What is the analog signal resolution possible as seen at the amplifier input? Suppose that we feel it necessary to use a 12-bit A/D converter to obtain greater resolution. Suggest various schemes of interfacing it with an 8-bit microprocessor such as the COSMAC.

6.12 Using the ECG data below sampled at 200 samples/s for 0.5 s, implement the following data-reduction algorithms: (a) turning-point; (b) AZTEC (assume that $V_{th} = 27$); (c) CORTES (assume that $V_{th} = 27$ and $V_{in} = 20$). Use ***** as the mark.

51, 74, 82, 82, 78, 86, 92, 96, 95, 96, 91, 85, 84, 83, 82, 75, 68, 70, 68, 62, 62, 56, 63, 58, 54, 60, 72, 82, 95, 110, 136, 178, 244, 298, 295, 219, 83, −36, −86, −85,

−71, −50, −20, 11, 37, 56, 64, 72, 66, 68, 68, 71, 72, 70, 76, 76, 75, 83, 78, 80, 82, 83, 88, 88, 88, 91, 89, 93, 91, 90, 96, 102, 106, 113, 118, 126, 130, 138, 146, 158, 163, 171, 179, 182, 186, 192, 189, 188, 178, 162, 147, 137, 126, 108, 106, 98, 92, 86, 76, 72

6.13 Given the AZTEC data below, reconstruct the ECG signal.

−2, 83, 22, 83, 18, 77, 4, 101, −5, −232, −4, 141, 24, 141, 21, 164

6.14 Given the CORTES data below, reconstruct the ECG signal. Use ***** as the mark.

*****, 42, *****, 22, 83, *****, 66, 71, 68, 72, 64, 68, 75, 70, 79, 100, 115, 16, −189, −238, −71, 83, *****, 25, 144, *****, 160, 168, 166, 171, 174, 171, 172, 168, 162, 155

6.15 When the ECG is being sampled and reduced, a continuous stream of data must be stored. Unfortunately, storing the data and incrementing a pointer will not work, since the memory will be filled quickly (remember that the system only has 2 kbytes for data storage). Develop a method that can store a finite amount of data, say 1600 bytes, into a data array that is continuously being updated.

6.16 Several of the arrhythmias that are detected only alarm when their rate exceeds a limit. Develop a method that can determine when arrhythmia XYZ occurs more often than five times per minute.

6.17 After initial clinical testing, the QRS shape will be analyzed for arrhythmia detection. In the detection of PVCs the width of the QRS can be an important criterion of whether a QRS complex is indeed a PVC. Develop a method to determine the width of a QRS complex.

6.18 Because of real-time computing constraints, it may not be practical to implement CORTES as discussed in Section 6.8. Instead, it may be more practical to store the output of the turning point algorithm (one pass) and after an alarm pass these data through zero-order interpolation (ZOI). Redraw the flowchart, Fig. 6.31, to implement this system.

6.19 When CORTES is implemented, we must choose a value for the mark. Since the COSMAC is an 8-bit machine with an 8-bit A/D converter, one of the quantization levels must be sacrificed. Suggest a solution or method around this, if one can be found. Explain the compromises of your solution.

6.20 Discuss the social and clinical implications of (1) an audio beeper, (2) a manual override that suppresses the arrhythmia alarm, (3) the impact of the alarm on the patient's psychological state, and (4) the effect of false positives and negatives on device acceptance. However sophisticated the device might be, such considerations may limit its acceptance. An engineer should be well aware of this.

Appendices

1 GLOSSARY

access time. The time required to move data between the microprocessor and memory.

accumulator. A register that holds an operand used in logical or arithmetic operations.

address. The binary number that defines a location in memory.

ALGOL. ALGOrithmic Language. A high-level scientific language.

algorithm. The procedure for performing a specific task.

ALU. *See* arithmetic logic unit.

analog-to-digital (A/D) converter (or ADC). An interface device that converts an analog signal into a digital signal.

APL. A Programming Language. A high-level language with special instructions for operating on groups of data.

architecture. The internal construction of a processor; includes registers, arithmetic logic unit, and instruction set.

arithmetic logic unit (ALU). A section of the microprocessor that performs the arithmetic and logical operations.

ASCII (American Standard Code for Information Interchange). A 7-bit code for a 128-character set which includes upper- and lowercase letters, numerals, special symbols, and control codes. Usually, a parity bit is attached, which makes a total of 8 bits per character. One character is stored in 1 byte of memory.

assembler. A specialized program that converts assembly-language mnemonics into machine-language code.

assembly language. A set of letters grouped to form mnemonics that represent machine-language instructions which are easier to remember than machine-language codes.

asynchronous operation. Circuit operation without a common clock such that each operation ends when the destination signals completion.

BASIC. Beginner's All-purpose Symbolic Instruction Code. Currently, the most popular high-level language for microcomputers.

baud. A unit of serial data transmission rate that is equal to bits per second.

BCD. *See* binary-coded decimal.

benchmarking. Generally, a method of comparing the relative performance of different microprocessors by writing a program for each that does a specific task. The amount of memory required and speed of execution for each processor serve as figures of merit to compare them.

binary. The number system consisting of only the digits 0 and 1.

binary-coded decimal (BCD). A number system that represents the decimal digits (0 through 9) with 4-bit binary codes.

bit. Binary digit equal to 0 or 1.

bootstrap. A technique of loading a few instructions of a program into the memory which are used to bring in the rest of the program.

breakpoint. A prespecified location in a program at which execution stops to aid in debugging.

buffer. A segment of memory used for temporary storage of information until the processor is ready to use it. Buffers permit microprocessors to process data in one segment of memory at the same time data are arriving at another segment. In hardware, a buffer is a device such as a tristate buffer that separates one part of a circuit from another. It may provide a higher current output than the device driving its input is able to provide.

bus. A set of wires that carry data to any number of devices. Three buses are typically present in a microcomputer: address bus, data bus, and control bus.

byte. An 8-bit binary number.

central processing unit (CPU). The computational unit of a computer. It usually contains the ALU, program counter, stack pointer, general-purpose registers, timing and control units, instruction register, and bus interface drivers. The CPU is typically completely implemented on a single microprocessor chip.

clock. A signal used for timing and synchronization of system operations.

COBOL. COmmon Business-Oriented Language. A high-level language for business applications.

compiler. A specialized program that converts a high-level language such as FORTRAN into machine code.

CPU.   *See* central processing unit.

crash.   A computer system shutdown caused by a hardware or software problem.

cross assembler.   An assembly-language translation program that runs on one computer (usually a minicomputer or large-scale computer) to produce the machine code for a microprocessor.

cycle time.   The time needed to perform a fundamental sequence of operations.

daisy chain.   A simple hardware method for assigning relative priority to a number of devices linked together in a chain.

digital-to-analog (D/A) converter (or DAC).   An interface device that converts digital (binary) numbers into analog voltages.

direct memory access (DMA).   A hardware technique that permits transfer of data between RAM and an input/output device without software control.

DMA.   *See* direct memory access.

DOS.   Disk Operating System.

EAROM.   *See* read-only memory.

editor.   A specialized program that manipulates text data in a source program to provide a means of changing mistakes or inserting new material.

emulator.   Hardware and software that replaces a microprocessor in a circuit and operates as if it were the microprocessor. The designer can monitor the performance of his or her design by inspecting register contents, executing subroutines, and the like through the emulator processor resources, such as a display terminal.

EPROM.   *See* read-only memory.

execute.   The process of interpreting an instruction and performing the indicated operation.

fetch.   The process of addressing memory and transferring the contents of that location into the microprocessor's instruction register.

FIFO.   First-In, First-Out stack. The first piece of data put in is the first to come out.

firmware.   Software stored in ROM.

floating.   Term used to describe the output of a tristate device that is in the high-impedance state.

floating point.   A type of arithmetic where the decimal point may occupy any position.

FORTRAN.   FORmula TRANslator. The most popular high-level scientific language. It was the first high-level language.

glitch.   Any error or malfunction that occurs in hardware or software.

handshaking.   The exchange of a certain sequence of control signals by two devices to synchronize an operation, typically input/output.

hardware.   The electronic circuits that make up a device.

hexadecimal.   The number system that uses 16 digits (0 through F) to represent 4-bit binary words.

higher-level language.   A language such as FORTRAN, BASIC, or COBOL that is derived from user-oriented functions.

input/output (I/O).   The peripheral equipment that communicates with the microprocessor, usually through special circuits called ports.

instruction. A machine code or group of bits that defines a specific microcomputer task such as an arithmetic or logical operation.

instruction set. The complete collection of individual instructions in a microprocessor.

interpreter. A specialized program that provides for interactive operation of a high-level language such as BASIC.

interrupt. A signal that causes the microprocessor to jump to another routine at the completion of the current instruction. The microprocessor saves the location of the next instruction in sequence, performs the interrupt service routine, and returns to the main program at the saved location.

interrupt service routine. A set of instructions that processes data for an interrupting device.

large-scale integration (LSI). High-density monolithic integrated circuits that contain more than 100 gates on a single chip.

latch. A flip-flop capable of storing 1 bit that is the basic building block for registers.

LIFO. Last-In, First-Out stack. The last piece of data pushed in is the first popped out.

LSI. *See* large-scale integration.

machine cycle. The shortest sequence of machine operations that repeats itself. There are usually four steps in each cycle:

1. Fetch an instruction.
2. Increment the program counter.
3. Set up the internal gates to execute the instruction.
4. Execute the instruction.

machine language. The set of binary codes that specify the operation of the microprocessor by controlling the logic gating of the internal circuits.

medium-scale integration (MSI). A monolithic integrated circuit that contains between 20 and 100 gates on a single chip.

memory. The section of the computer that stores data and instructions. Each memory word has a unique location or address.

microprocessor. A computer that contains the CPU, on one chip or small set of chips.

mnemonic code. A unique alphabetic assignment given to each binary machine code to facilitate remembering the machine codes.

modem (modulator-demodulator). A device used to convert the voltage levels for binary 0 and 1 to tones for transmission over the telephone network, and vice versa.

MROM. *See* read-only memory.

MSI. *See* medium-scale integration.

nibble. A 4-bit unit that is operated on as a unit by machine codes.

object program. A binary machine-language program that is in a form ready for execution. An assembler produces an object program.

octal. The numbering system that uses 8 digits (0 through 7) to code all combinations of 3 bits.

operation code. Synonym of instruction.

page. A segment of memory. In an 8-bit processor with 16-bit addressing, a page is 256 bytes long and there are a total of 256 pages or 65,536 bytes.

parse. The technique of analyzing a string of characters and breaking it down into more easily processed components, such as commands and their arguments.

PASCAL. A high-level language which is becoming popular in part because it produces an intermediate code, called the p code, which is not specific to any microprocessor. A relatively simple interpreter program can be implemented for any processor to convert the p code to a runnable program.

PL/M. Programming Language/Meta. A subset of PL/1.

PL/1. Programming Language/One. A high-level language with attributes of several languages, particularly ALGOL.

program. A set of instructions that direct the operation of the computer to perform a sequence of data manipulations.

PROM. A programmable ROM. *See* ROM.

queue. A waiting line, such as data waiting to be processed.

RAM. *See* random-access memory.

random-access memory (RAM). Also referred to as read/write memory, because its contents can be both accessed and changed during execution of a program. The contents of any address can be accessed in any sequence.

read-only memory (ROM). A memory used to store programs or data. The contents of a ROM are preset and are not alterable during execution of a microprocessor program. The following definitions describe some of the types of ROM available.

Electrically Alterable ROM (EAROM) is similar to EPROM except that electric current rather than ultraviolet light erases the contents. The electric current initializes the memory bits to all ones or all zeros and the bits are selectively reversed to program the device. EAROM requires complex logic for read/write control. It is the most expensive and least-used type of ROM. It has been used for special applications, such as machine controllers, where programs need to be changed from time to time.

Erasable PROM (EPROM) can be erased with ultraviolet light and reprogrammed. An EPROM consists of an array of MOS field-effect transistors having electrically isolated gates. Charge is selectively injected into these gates during the programming process to represent ones (or zeros). Exposing an EPROM to UV light for several minutes causes the stored charge to leak away from the gates to erase its contents and return all addresses to an all zeros (or all ones) condition. The cost per bit for EPROM is slightly higher than for fuse PROM, but EPROM is reusable, making it the most popular ROM for program development.

Fusible-link Programmable Read-Only Memory (PROM) consists of an array of fuses that represent zeros. The user programs the PROM by selectively injecting a high-enough current to blow the fuses at locations where ones are to be stored. Fuse PROM is permanently altered during programming and hence is not reusable like EPROM.

Mask-programmed Read-Only Memory (MROM) is programmed during chip fabrication with a pattern of ones and zeros provided by the user. MROM is most economical in production applications where 1000 or more units will be produced. MROM is highly reliable and permanently saves its contents, but it is not reprogrammable.

register. A circuit that temporarily stores 1 or more bits of data.

ROM. *See* read-only memory.

RS232. A standard interface for serial data communication.

S100 bus. A 100-pin microcomputer-system bus.

scratchpad memory. A temporary-storage, random-access memory which is used to store intermediate results or data.

simulator. A program that simulates the execution of a machine-language program on another computer. This approach is useful in debugging, since the simulator computer usually has peripherals, such as mass-storage devices, which the microprocessor-based device under development does not have.

small-scale integration (SSI). A monolithic integrated circuit that contains only several gates per chip.

SNOBOL. A high-level, string-oriented language.

software. A set of instructions that control the operation of a computer.

source program. A program written using mnemonic codes (assembly language) ready for the assembler to convert to machine codes.

SSI. *See* small-scale integration.

stack. A set of registers or memory locations that are used to hold data temporarily.

stack pointer (SP). A register or counter that points to the last entry in the stack.

synchronous operation. Circuit operation with a common clock timing all events, such as data transfers.

Universal Asynchronous Receiver/Transmitter (UART). A single-chip device that converts two-wire serial data to parallel (receiving) and converts parallel data to serial for transmission over a two-wire line (transmitting).

UV EPROM. *See* read-only memory.

volatile memory. Memory such as RAM which loses its contents when power is removed.

word. The number of bits that represents the primary data length manipulated by the computer, usually 8 bits in a microprocessor.

2 ASCII/HEXADECIMAL CONVERSION

Figure A.1 provides a method for converting between the hexadecimal code and the American Standard Code for Information Interchange (ASCII). Any character can be coded in hexadecimal by matching the column and row hexadecimal digits corresponding to the location of the character. For instance, the hexadecimal code for the letter H is found to be 48. Alternatively, the character represented by any two-digit hexadecimal number can be found. For example, the hexadecimal number 5A represents the character Z. Although the most significant binary bit is set to 0 for the table, it is sometimes set to 1 or used as a parity bit. In these cases the first hexadecimal digit for all the characters will be different.

Each of the control characters in the two left columns is generated on a computer terminal by holding down the special CTRL key and simultaneously depressing the character indicated in Fig. A.1. For example, depressing key C simultaneously with CTRL creates the ASCII code for ETX, which is hex 03. Alternatively, if a microprocessor sends a control character to a terminal, the terminal interprets it as a nonprinting control character. For example, the terminal rings its bell (modern terminals usually beep) if it receives hex 07 (i.e., the ASCII code for BEL).

		0	1	2	3	4	5	6	7
				First hex digit					
	0	NUL	DLE	SP	0	@	P	--	p
	1	SOH	DC1	!	1	A	Q	a	q
	2	STX	DC2	''	2	B	R	b	r
	3	ETX	DC3	#	3	C	S	c	s
	4	EOT	DC4	$	4	D	T	d	t
Second hex digit	5	ENQ	NAK	%	5	E	U	e	u
	6	ACK	SYN	&	6	F	V	f	v
	7	BEL	ETB	'	7	G	W	g	w
	8	BS	CAN	(	8	H	X	h	x
	9	HT	EM	)	9	I	Y	i	y
	A	LF	SUB	*	:	J	Z	j	z
	B	VT	ESC	+	;	K	[	k	{
	C	FF	FS	,	<	L	\	l	--
	D	CR	GS	-	=	M	]	m	}
	E	SO	RS	.	>	N	^	n	≈
	F	SI	US	/	?	O	—	o	DEL

Control character abbreviations:

NUL	null, or all zeros (CTRL/@)	DC1	device control 1 (CTRL/Q)
SOH	start of heading (CTRL/A)	DC2	device control 2 (CTRL/R)
STX	start of text (CTRL/B)	DC3	device control 3 (CTRL/S)
ETX	end of text (CTRL/C)	DC4	device control 4 (CTRL/T)
EOT	end of transmission (CTRL/D)	NAK	negative acknowledge (CTRL/U)
ENQ	enquiry (CTRL/E)	SYN	synchronous idle (CTRL/V)
ACK	acknowledge (CTRL/F)	ETB	end of transmission block (CTRL/W)
BEL	bell (CTRL/G)	CAN	cancel (CTRL/X)
BS	backspace (CTRL/H)	EM	end of medium (CTRL/Y)
HT	horizontal tabulation (CTRL/I)	SUB	substitute (CTRL/Z)
LF	line feed (CTRL/J)	ESC	escape (CTRL/[)
VT	vertical tabulation (CTRL/K)	FS	file separator (CTRL/\)
FF	form feed (CTRL/L)	GS	group separator (CTRL/])
CR	carriage return (CTRL/M)	RS	record separator (CTRL/^)
SO	shift out (CTRL/N)	US	unit separator (CTRL/_)
SI	shift in (CTRL/O)	SP	space (SPACE BAR)
DLE	data link escape (CTRL/P)	DEL	delete (RUBOUT OR DEL)

FIGURE A.1   ASCII/hexadecimal code conversion table.

3 HEXADECIMAL-TO-DECIMAL CONVERSION

A four-digit hexadecimal number can represent any of 64 k addresses. The memory space is divided into 256 pages, numbered from page 00 to FF hex. Each page has 256 byte addresses, numbered from 00 to FF hex. Figure A.2 gives conversion values to find the decimal equivalent of any four-digit hexadecimal number.

Page number				Byte address			
HEX	DEC	HEX	DEC	HEX	DEC	HEX	DEC
0	0	0	0	0	0	0	0
1	4,096	1	256	1	16	1	1
2	8,192	2	512	2	32	2	2
3	12,288	3	768	3	48	3	3
4	16,384	4	1,024	4	64	4	4
5	20,480	5	1,280	5	80	5	5
6	24,576	6	1,536	6	96	6	6
7	28,672	7	1,792	7	112	7	7
8	32,768	8	2,048	8	128	8	8
9	36,864	9	2,304	9	144	9	9
A	40,960	A	2,560	A	160	A	10
B	45,056	B	2,816	B	176	B	11
C	49,152	C	3,072	C	192	C	12
D	53,248	D	3,328	D	208	D	13
E	57,344	E	3,584	E	224	E	14
F	61,440	F	3,840	F	240	F	15

FIGURE A.2 Hexadecimal-to-decimal conversion table. Any address in 64 kbytes can be represented by four hexadecimal digits—the two most significant digits are the page number and the two least significant are the address on the page.

Examples of the use of this chart are:

1. Address $1FFF_{16}$ (8191_{10}) is the last address in an 8-kbyte system ($1 k = 1024$), since it has 8192 bytes, numbered from 0 to 8191. Address 2000_{16} (8192_{10}) is the starting address of the second 8 kbytes of a larger system.

2. Address 8000_{16} is midway through a 64-kbyte memory.

3. The first addresses on pages A0 and C0 are separated by 8 kbytes.

4. The number $2345_{16} = 8192_{10} + 768_{10} + 64_{10} + 5_{10} = 9029_{10}$.

4 INSTRUCTION SETS FOR THE COSMAC AND THE Z80

The COSMAC has more than 90 instructions, which are summarized in Fig. A.3. Most are 1-byte instructions.

The Z80 instruction set summarized in Fig. A.4 includes more than 150 instructions. The Z80 can execute the 78 instructions of the 8080A, so most 8080A programs run without modification on the Z80.

Memory and logic instructions**

Instruction	Mnemonic	Op Code
Increment reg N	INC	1N
Decrement reg N	DEC	2N
Increment reg X	IRX	60
Get low reg N	GLO	8N
Put low reg N	PLO	AN
Get high reg N	GHI	9N
Put high reg N	PHI	BN
Load via N	LDN	0N
Load advance	LDA	4N
Load via X	LDX	F0
Load via X and advance	LDXA	72
Load immediate	LDI	F8
Store via N	STR	5N
Store via X and decrement	STXD	73
OR	OR	F1
OR immediate	ORI	F9
Exclusive OR	XOR	F3
Exclusive OR immediate	XR	FB
AND	AND	F2
AND immediate	ANI	FA
Shift right	SHR	F6
Shift right with carry	SHRC } RSHR	76*
Ring shift right		
Shift left	SHL	FE
Shift left with carry	SHLC } RSHL	7E*
Ring shift left		

Arithmetic instructions**

Instruction	Mnemonic	Op Code
Add	ADD	F4
Add immediate	ADI	FC
Add with carry	ADC	74
Add with carry immediate	ADCI	7C
Subtract D	SD	F5
Subtract D immediate	SDI	FD
Subtract D with borrow	SDB	75
Subtract D with borrow immediate	SDBI	7D
Subtract memory	SM	F7
Subtract memory immediate	SMI	FF
Subtract memory with borrow	SMB	77
Subtract memory with borrow immediate	SMBI	7F

Branch instructions

Instruction	Mnemonic	Op Code
Short branch	BR	30
No short branch (see SKP)	NBR	38*
Short branch if D = 0	BZ	32
Short branch if D not 0	BNZ	3A
Short branch if DF = 1	BDF	33*
Short branch if pos or zero	BPZ	
Short branch if equal or greater	BGE	
Short branch if DF = 0	BNF	3B*
Short branch if minus	BM	
Short branch if less	BL	
Short branch if Q = 1	BQ	31
Short branch if Q = 0	BNQ	39
Short branch if EF1 = 1	B1	34
Short branch if EF1 = 0	BN1	3C
Short branch if EF2 = 1	B2	35
Short branch if EF2 = 0	BN2	3D
Short branch if EF3 = 1	B3	36
Short branch if EF3 = 0	BN3	3E
Short branch if EF4 = 1	B4	37
Short branch if EF4 = 0	BN4	3F
Long branch	LBR	C0
No long branch (see LSKP)	NLBR	C8*
Long branch if D = 0	LBZ	C2
Long branch if D not 0	LBNZ	CA
Long branch if DF = 1	LBDF	C3
Long branch if DF = 0	LBNF	CB
Long branch if Q = 1	LBQ	C1
Long branch if Q = 0	LBNQ	C9

*Note: This instruction is associated with more than one mnemonic. Each mnemonic is individually listed.

**Note: The arithmetic and logic instructions are the only instructions that can alter the DF.

Skip and control instructions

Instruction	Mnemonic	Op Code
Short skip (see NBR)	SKP	38*
Long skip (see NLBR)	LSKP	C8*
Long skip if D = 0	LSZ	CE
Long skip if D not 0	LSNZ	C6
Long skip if DF = 1	LSDF	CF
Long skip if DF = 0	LSNF	C7
Long skip if Q = 1	LSQ	CD
Long skip if Q = 0	LSNQ	C5
Long skip if IE = 1	LSIE	CC
Idle	IDL	00
No operation	NOP	C4
Set P	SEP	DN
Set X	SEX	EN
Set Q	SEQ	7B
Reset Q	REQ	7A
Save	SAV	78
Push X,P to stack	MARK	79
Return	RET	70
Disable	DIS	71

Input/output byte transfer instructions

Instruction	Mnemonic	Op Code
Output 1	OUT 1	61
Output 2	OUT 2	62
Output 3	OUT 3	63
Output 4	OUT 4	64
Output 5	OUT 5	65
Output 6	OUT 6	66
Output 7	OUT 7	67
Input 1	INP *1	69
Input 2	INP 2	6A
Input 3	INP 3	6B
Input 4	INP 4	6C
Input 5	INP 5	6D
Input 6	INP 6	6E
Input 7	INP 7	6F

FIGURE A.3 COSMAC instructions. (Reprinted with permission from Electronic Design, Vol. 24, No. 22, October 25, 1976, © Hayden Publishing Co., Inc. 1976.)

Mnemonic	Description
8-bit load instructions	
LD r, r	Load register r with r
LD r, n	Load register r with n
LD r, (HL)	Load r with location (HL)
LD r, (IX + d)	Load r with location (IX + d)
LD r, (IY + d)	Load r with location (IY + d)
LD (HL), r	Load location HL with r
LD (IX + d), r	Load location IX + d from register r
LD (IY + d), r	Load location IY + d from register r
LD (HL), n	Load location HL with value n
LD (IX + d), n	Load location IX + d with n
LD (IY + d), n	Load location IY + d with n
LD A, (BC)	Load AC with location BC
LD A, (DE)	Load AC with location DE
LD A, (nn)	Load AC with location nn
LD (BC), A	Load location BC with AC
LD (DE), A	Load location DE with AC
LD (nn), A	Load location nn with AC
LD A, I	Load register A from I
LD A, R	Load AC with register R
LD I, A	Load register I with AC
LD R, A	Load register R with AC
16-bit load instructions	
LD dd, nn	Load registers dd with nn
LD IX, nn	Load register IX with nn
LD IY, nn	Load register IY with nn
LD HL, (nn)	Load L with contents of location nn and H with (nn + 1)
LD dd, (nn)	Load registers dd with location nn
LD IX, (nn)	Load IX with location nn
LD IY, (nn)	Same but for IY
LD (nn), HL	Load location nn with HL
LD (nn), dd	Load location (nn) with register pair dd
LD (nn), IX	Same but for IX
LD (nn), IY	Same but for IY
LD SP, HL	Load stack pointer from HL
LD SP, IX	Load stack pointer from IX
LD SP, IY	Load stack pointer from IY
PUSH qq	Load register pair qq onto stack
PUSH IX	Load IX onto stack
PUSH IY	Load IY onto stack
POP qq	Load register pair qq with top of stack
POP IX	Load IX with top of stack
POP IY	Load IY with top of stack
Exchange, transfer and search instructions	
EX DE, HL	Exchange contents of DE and HL
EX AF, A'F'	Exchange contents of AF and A'F'
EXX	Exchange all six general purpose registers with alternates
EX (SP), HL	Exchange stack pointer contents with HL contents
EX (SP), IX	Same but use IX register
EX (SP), IY	Same but use IY register
LDI	Load (HL) into DE, increment DE and HL, decrement BC
LDIR	Same but loop until (BC) = 0
LDD	Load location (PE) into register (HL) and decrement DE, HL and BC
LDDR	Same but loop until (BC) = 0
CPI	Compare contents of AC with (HL), set Z flag if =, increment HL and decrement BC,
CPIR	Same but repeat until BC = 0
CP s	Compare operand s with AC
CPD	Same as CPI but decrement HL
CPDR	Same as CPIR but decrement HL
8-bit arithmetic and logic instructions	
ADD A, r	Add contents of r to AC
ADD A, n	Add byte n to AC
ADD A, (HL)	Add contents of HL to AC

ADD A, (IX + d)	Add location (IX + d) to AC
ADD A, (IY + d)	Same but (IY + d)
ADC A, s	Add with carry operand s to AC
SUB s	Subtract contents of r, n, HL, IX + d or IY + d from AC
SBC s	Same but also subtract carry flag
AND s	Logic AND of operand s and AC
OR s	Same but OR with AC
XOR s	Same but EX-OR with AC
INC r	Increment register r
INC (HL)	Increment location (HL)
INC (IX + d)	Same but use (IX + d)
INC (IY + d)	Same but use (IY + d)
DEC m	Decrement operand m
16-bit arithmetic instructions	
ADD HL, ss	Add register pair ss to HL
ADC HL, ss	Same but include carry flag
SBC HL, ss	From HL subtract contents of ss and carry flag
ADD IX, pp	Add register pair pp to IX
ADD IY, rr	Same but use rr and IY
INC ss	Increment register pair ss
INC IX	Increment IX register
INC IY	Same but IY register
DEC ss	Decrement register pair ss
DEC IX	Same but IX register
DEC IY	Same but IY register
General purpose arithmetic and control instructions	
DAA	Decimal adjust accumulator
CPL	Complement (AC)
NEG	Complement (AC) and add 1
CCF	Complement carry flag
SCF	Set carry flag = 1
NOP	No operation
HALT	Halt, wait for interrupt or reset
DI	Disable interrupts
EI	Enable interrupts
IMØ	Set μP to interrupt mode Ø
IM1	Set μP to interrupt mode 1
IM2	Set μP to interrupt mode 2
Rotate and shift instructions	
RLCA	Rotate AC left
RLA	Same but include carry flag
RRCA	Rotate AC right
RRA	Same but include carry flag
RLC r	Rotate register r left
RLC (HL)	Rotate location (HL) left
RLC (IX + d)	Same but location (IX + d)
RLC (IY + d)	Same but location (IY + d)
RL m	Same as any RLC but include carry flag
RRC m	Same as RLC but shift right
RR m	Same as RL m but shift right
SLA s	Shift left (any RLC register)
SRA s	Same but shift right and keep MSB
SRL s	Same as SLA but shift right
RLD	Simultaneous 4-bit rotate from AC_L to L, L to H and H to AC_L
RRD	Simultaneous 4-bit rotate from AC_L to H, H to L and L to AC_L
Bit set, reset and test instructions	
BIT b, r	Test bit b of register r
BIT b, (HL)	Test bit b of location (HL)
BIT b, (IX + d)	Test bit b of location (IX + d)
BIT b, (IY + d)	Test bit b of location (IY + d)
SET b, r	Set bit b in register r to 1
SET b, (HL)	Same but use contents of location HL
SET b, (IX + d)	Same but use contents of location IX + d
SET b, (IY + d)	Same but use contents of location IY + d
RES b, s	Reset bit b of operand m

Jump, call and return instructions	
JP nn	Unconditional jump to location nn
JP cc, nn	If condition cc True, do a JP nn otherwise continue
JR e	Unconditional jump to PC + e
JR C, e	If C = 0 continue. If C = 1 do JR e
JR NC, e	Reverse of JR c, e
JR Z, e	If Z = 0 continue. If Z = 1 do JR e
JR NZ, e	Reverse of JR Z, e
JP (HL)	Load PC from (HL)
JP (IX)	Load PC from (IX)
JP (IY)	Load PC from (IY)
DJNZ, e	Decrement register B and jump relative if B = 0
CALL nn	Unconditional call subroutine at location nn
CALL cc, nn	Call subroutine at location nn if condition cc is True
RET	Return from subroutine
RET cc	If cc false continue, otherwise do RET
RETI	Return from interrupt
RETN	Return from nonmaskable interrupt
RST p	Store PC in stack, load 0 in PC_H and restart vector in PC_L
Input/output instructions	
IN A, n	Load AC with input from device n
IN r, (C)	Load r with input from device C
INI	Store contents of location specified by C in address specified by HL, decrement B and increment HL
INIR	Same but repeat until B = 0
IND	Same as INI but decrement HL too
INDR	Same as INIR but decrement HL too
OUT n, A	Load output port (n) with AC
OUT (C), r	Load output port (C) with register r
OUTI	Load output port (C) with location and increment HL and decrement B
OTIR	Same but repeat until B = 0
OUTD	Same as OUTI but decrement HL
OTDR	Same as OTIR but decrement HL

Notes

b represents a 3-bit code that indicates position of the bit to be modified

cc represents a 3-bit code that indicates which of eight condition codes are to be used

d is an 8-bit offset value

dd refers to register pairs BC, DC, HL or the stack pointer

e represents a signed two's complement number between −126 and +129

m is an 8-bit number

n is an 8-bit number

nn refers to two 8-bit bytes

p represents one of eight restart vector locations on page 0

pp refers to register pairs BC, DE, the IX register or the stack pointer

qq refers to register pairs AF, BC, DE or HL

r or r refers to registers A, B, C, D, E, H or L or their alternates

rr refers to register pairs BC, DE, the IY register of the stack pointer

s refers to either the r registers, the n data word or the contents of locations specified by the contents of the HL, IX + d or IY + d registers

ss refers to register pairs BC, DE, HL or the stack pointer

FIGURE A.4 Z80 instructions. (Reprinted with permission from Electronic Design, Vol. 25, No. 14, July 5, 1977, © Hayden Publishing Co., Inc. 1977.)

5 COMPARISONS OF MICROCOMPUTER-BASED MEDICAL INSTRUMENTS

Figure A.5 gives comparisons of instruments discussed in Chapter 5. We obtained this information from questionnaires which we sent to the developers of the instruments.

Device Name	Section	Processor	ROM (bytes)	RAM (bytes)	Development time (worker-months)		Programming technique				Evaluation kit used
					Hardware	Software	Hand code	Cross-assembler	Emulation	High-level language	
Norland NI2001A	5.1	8080	24 k								
Nicolet 2090	5.1	AMD 2900		4 k							
Histogram–averager	5.1	6800	1 k	1 k							
Flight recorder	5.1	8080	11 k								
Biomedical computer module	5.1	8080A	8 k	256							
Augmented cardiograph	5.2	6800	2 k								
Cardiac monitoring	5.3	Z80									
Intensive care unit	5.3	8080	4 k	1 k							
Space Labs Alpha system	5.3	PPS8			20	14	Yes		Yes		
Arrhythmia analyzer	5.3	8085									
Fetal monitor	5.3	8080	512	4 k							
Fetal monitor	5.3	6502	2 k	1 k				Yes			
Apnea monitor	5.3	6502					Yes	Yes			KIM-1
Apnea monitor	5.3	8080	512	32 k							
Animal motion monitor	5.3	6800	128	512							
Uterine pressure	5.3	Z80		24 k							
Animal data recorder	5.3	8080	32 k								
Impedance pneumograph	5.4	8080A	512	128		2	Yes				
Honeywell MEDDARS	5.4	CP–1600									
Lung function	5.4	8080	8 k	8 k							
Spirometry	5.4	6502									KIM-1
Flow-volume loops	5.4	8080	12 k	12 k							
Pulmonary compliance	5.4	6502		4 k							
Whole Body plethysmograph	5.4	8080									
Pulmonary edema	5.4	6502									KIM-1
Ventilator monitor	5.4	4004	512	80							
Animal respiratory monitor	5.4	8008									
Boston anesthesia	5.5	8080			$150,000					PL/M	
Anesthesia monitoring	5.6	LSI-11	1	18 k							
Trend monitoring	5.6	Z80		34 k							
Compressed spectral array	5.7	TI990/4									
Zero-crossing analysis	5.7	8080A	2 k	1 k							
Biofeedback training	5.7	8748									
SMR activity	5.7	6100									
Blood-pressure monitor	5.8	4040	1256	80	18	18	Yes	Yes			
Arterial tonometer	5.8	Z80	5 k	12 k							
Net charge transport	5.9	TI990/4									
Blood gases	5.9	8080	3 k	256							
Blood-gas monitor	5.9	Z80	6 k	16 k							
Chemical analyzer controller	5.9	8080									
Clinical chemical analyser	5.9	6501	2 k	10 k							

FIGURE A.5 Comparison of microcomputer-based medical instruments.

Device Name	Section	Processor	ROM (bytes)	RAM (bytes)	Development time (worker-months) Hardware	Software	Hand code	Cross-assembler	Emulation	High-level language	Evaluation kit used
Visual-field analyzer	5.10	6800			4-5	12					
Visual-field analyzer	5.10	8080									
Nystagmus analyzer	5.10	8080			36 (total)					STOIC	
Nystagmus overshoot	5.10	8080		32 k							
Vestibular testing	5.10	8080									
Visual contrast	5.10	M6800	1 k	256							
Glaucoma diagnosis	5.10	6502									KIM-1
Eyeglass prescription	5.10	TI9900									
Training Aid	5.11	6502		1 k					Yes		KIM-1
Auto-Com	5.11	RCA 1802	>2 k	256				Yes			
Speech communication	5.11	8080									
Communication for disabled	5.11	M6800	3 k	4 k							
Vocal communicator	5.11	6800			2-3	4			Yes		
Treatment of aphasics	5.11	4040					4	Yes			
Ophthalmic ultrasound	5.12	Z80									
Pacemaker tracking	5.13	8080A	4 k	16 k							
Bone scanner	5.14		4 k	1280							
Optic disk blood flow	5.14	6502									KIM-1
Microdensitometer	5.14	6800		8 k						BASIC	
Programmable stimulator	5.15	8080			12	18			MDS 800		Intel 8020
Wisconsin programmable stimulator	5.15	6800			$1\frac{1}{2}$	4		Yes			EPA MICR068
Wisconsin lower limb	5.15	F8									
Colorado prosthesis	5.16	8080		4 k							
UCLA prosthesis	5.16	RCA 1802		1 k							
Spinal-curve monitor	5.17	6800	512	128							
Penile tumescence	5.17	8080	8 k	5 k	$\frac{1}{2}$	1	MDS 800				SBC 80/10
Esophageal manometry	5.17	8080	4 k	32 k							
Intra aortic timer	5.17	6800									
Intra aortic timer	5.17	8008	4 k								
Programmed exerciser	5.17	PPS-4/2	4 k	128							
X-ray control	5.17	8080A									
Psychometric testing	5.17	8080									
Independent living	5.17	6502		4 k							
Physician's office	5.17	SOL-20				$\frac{1}{5}$					

FIGURE A.5 (continued)

6 LABORATORY MICROCOMPUTER SYSTEMS

We are frequently asked what microcomputer system is best for biomedical laboratory applications. Although each laboratory has different computing needs, typical laboratory problems are acquisition and analysis of analog signals such as electrocardiograms or parallel digital data such as the output of a clinical laboratory instrument. In this appendix, we discuss a diversity of available microcomputers, examples of possible laboratory microcomputer configurations, and a set of questions to answer before choosing a system.

Basic microcomputer systems

Many of the inexpensive (less than $1000) microcomputer systems in the consumer marketplace include the basic resources to do general purpose computing. They each have a keyboard/display, a small amount of RAM (usually between 4 and 16 kbytes), and a mass storage device (usually an audio cassette) to store programs and data. Examples of such computers are the Apple II, Radio Shack TRS-80, and Commodore PET. Although they are general-purpose microcomputers with significant computing power, these systems are designed for the consumer market and consequently do not have the versatility necessary for most laboratory environments. They each provide a high-level programming language called BASIC as the primary system software. BASIC is adequate for equation solving but awkward for control or data acquisition tasks. Also, on these computers it is implemented as an interpretive language which runs programs inherently much slower (20 to 100 times) than a compiled language like FORTRAN. Peripheral devices, such as floppy disk drives which we feel are necessities in a laboratory environment, are usually add-on hardware to a system which was not originally designed to use them. They are normally available from only a small number of sources and mostly from just the primary manufacturer. The user is at the mercy of one manufacturer for both hardware and software support. Therefore we do not recommend these personal computers for most laboratory applications.

Altair developed the first home computer around the 8080 microprocessor in 1975. They called their address/data/control bus the S100 bus because it is a system bus that uses 100-pin edge-card connectors. This is the only microcomputer bus that has a proposed IEEE standard. The S100 bus has been adopted by a number of mainframe manufacturers including Imsai, Cromemco, North Star, and Exidy. About 100 manufacturers produce a diversity of S100-compatible boards including memories, floppy disk controllers, video graphics display generators, speech and music synthesizers, and many other specialized boards. The availability of a diversity of compatible hardware makes a S100-bus mainframe a good choice for a laboratory system.

Examples of laboratory microcomputer systems

We have configured and use two microcomputer systems for general laboratory applications. The Cromemco model Z2 is based on the 8-bit Z80 microprocessor. The General Robotics Corporation (GRC) model GRC 11/X3 is based on the 16-bit LSI 11 microprocessor and is similar to the DEC PDP 11/03.

We use the Digital Research CPM (Control Program for Microprocessors) disk operating system on the Cromemco and the DEC RT11 disk operating system on the GRC. CPM and RT11 appear very similar to the user since the designers of CPM modelled it after RT11. The format of the command string is identical for both, and many system programs such as the editor (ED) and the peripheral interchange program (PIP) have the same name and similar function in both systems.

Our overall investment for the Cromemco system is about $8000 for hardware and $400 for software. For the LSI 11 system we have invested about $25,000 for hardware and $1500 for software. We find that initial costs for a 16-bit microcomputer system are approximately double for both hardware and software compared to an 8-bit system with similar features. A reasonable maintenance budget is 10 to 15% of the initial hardware cost annually.

Z80-based system. Our Z80-based Cromemco computer is an S100-bus system that permits us to purchase from a diversity of different boards provided by many different manufacturers. Our system currently includes

1. High-speed version of the Z80 processor (Cromemco ZPU with 4-MHz clock),
2. 48 kbytes RAM (3 16-kbyte boards from different manufacturers),
3. 8 kbytes EPROM (Cromemco Bytesaver board),
4. 7 A/D and 7 D/A 8-bit converter channels (Cromemco D+7A),
5. Twin UART board with 2 RS232 serial I/O interfaces, 32 parallel I/O lines, and 10 software-programmable timers (Cromemco TUART),
6. Point-plot, raster-scan video graphics board with 256 × 256-point resolution (Matrox),
7. Dual double-density microfloppy disk drives (Micropolis),
8. Console terminal (Lear-Siegler ADM-3A), and
9. Printer (Centronics 761).

We routinely interface to analog devices such as ECG amplifiers and strip-chart recorders and to digital devices such as digital voltmeters and seven-segment LED displays.

The CPM operating system is available from several sources including Digital Research, Microsoft, and Lifeboat Associates for about $150. In addition to the basic operating system, this price includes

1. Editor (ED) for creating and modifying programs,

2. 8080 assembler (ASM) for converting assembly language programs to Intel-standard hexadecimal format files,

3. Loader for formatting the hexadecimal files to run under CPM,

4. Peripheral interchange program (PIP) for transferring programs and data from one I/O device to another,

5. Dynamic debugging tool (DDT) for getting the bugs out of user programs, and

6. A number of additional utility programs.

Additional CPM-compatible system software that can be purchased for prices ranging from $100 to $400 includes a powerful macro-assembler (MAC), BASIC, FORTRAN IV, PASCAL, and a diversity of word-processing and data base management packages.

The CPM operating system is to software compatibility what the S100 bus is to hardware compatibility. This disk-operating system is available for a multitude of different manufacturers' 8080 and Z80 systems and is likely to propogate to different microprocessors as well. By masking the personalities of different computers, CPM makes the user-to-machine software interface the same for every computer. Once learning CPM, a user employs the same operating protocols and command strings for writing and executing programs on computers from several different manufacturers. Programs developed on one type of computer under CPM are directly transferrable to other CPM-based computers regardless of hardware differences such as terminal type or disk-drive manufacturer. Thus CPM is promoting the development of compatible, transportable 8080 software.

LSI 11-based system. Our LSI 11-based laboratory computer has a system bus called the Q bus designed by DEC. Although several manufacturers sell Q-bus-compatible boards, there is far less competition for this market than for the S100-bus market. This is undoubtedly in part because there are more 8-bit than 16-bit microprocessors in the field. Also DEC exerts some control on the market as the sole manufacturer of the LSI 11 processor board. Our system currently includes

1. LSI 11 CPU board (DEC),

2. 56 kilobytes RAM (Mostek),

3. 16 A/D and 2 D/A converter channels plus a software-controllable real-time clock (Adac Corporation model 600-LSI 11),

4. 2 RS232 serial I/O boards,

5. Dual double-density, full-size floppy disk drives (AED 6200),

6. Graphics console terminal (Tektronix 4006), and

7. Hard copy unit (Tektronix 4631).

The LSI 11 is a microprocessor that completely emulates the instruction set of the DEC PDP 11/40 minicomputer. Although its hardware and bus structure are completely different from the PDP 11/40, the LSI 11 is completely software compatible. However, it executes programs at only about 20% of the speed of the PDP 11/40. A more recent DEC microprocessor, the LSI 11/23, is not only software compatible with the newer DEC PDP 11/34 minicomputer but also its execution speed is about the same.

The RT11 operating system has features similar to CPM. A wide diversity of system software is available, primarily developed and supported by DEC. There is also available a large amount of inexpensive, user-developed software available through a user's group called DECUS.

A primary advantage of the LSI 11 and a major reason that we purchased it is that its operating system and user-developed software are upward compatible with larger, more powerful DEC computers. Programs are transportable to the larger systems with minimal difficulty. This compatibility is important for only a select few applications, however. The 8-bit processors should be given serious consideration when choosing a laboratory computer.

Selection of a laboratory microcomputer system

Before purchasing a laboratory system, consider the following questions. The answers will provide direction to help in selecting the proper system for a given application.

Definition of the task. For what tasks should a microcomputer be used? One-of-a-kind research instruments? Controllers? Data processing? Volume production that requires servicing in the field? Laboratory computing?

Hardware requirements. What hardware should be purchased? Chips? Kits? Larger computers for development? Emulators? Logic analyzers? Turn-key microcomputer system?

Software requirements. What software must be purchased? Monitors? Assemblers? Cross assemblers? Compilers? Interpreters? Simulators?

Hardware skills. What hardware skills are required? Logic design? Board construction? Interfacing? Debugging? Is a circuit designer required?

Software skills. What software skills are required? Machine code programming? Assembly language programming? Higher level language programming? Knowledge of compilers? Knowledge of interpreters? Is a programmer necessary?

Development costs. What are the total system development costs? For system hardware purchase? For test equipment? For system software purchase? Worker-hours for hardware design, development, and debugging? Worker-hours for software development and debugging?

Usage costs. What are documentation and user training costs? What are the costs for supplying maintenance and repair? Is a service contract desirable?

Index